Breast
Surgery

2nd Edition

Take a look at the other great titles in the *Companion Series*...

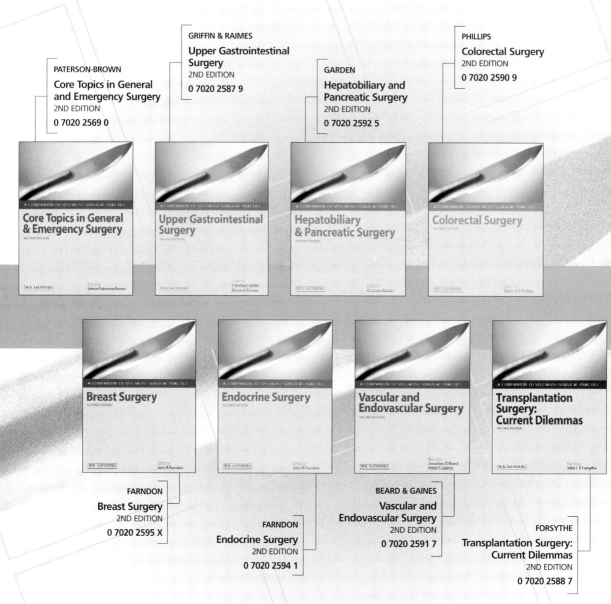
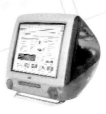
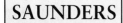

A Companion to Specialist Surgical Practice

Series editors
O. James Garden
Simon Paterson-Brown

Breast Surgery

2nd Edition

Edited by

John R. Farndon

Professor and Head of Department
University Department of Surgery
Bristol Royal Infirmary
Bristol

SAUNDERS
Edinburgh London New York Oxford Philadelphia St Louis Sydney Toronto 2001

First edition published in 1997
Second edition published in 2001
    Reprinted 2002 (twice)

ISBN 0 7020 2595 X

British Library Cataloguing in Publication Data
A catalogue record for this book is available from the British Library

Library of Congress Cataloging in Publication Data
A catalog record for this book is available from the Library of Congress

Note
Medical knowledge is constantly changing. As new information becomes available, changes in treatment, procedures, equipment and the use of drugs become necessary. The editors and the publishers have taken care to ensure that the information given in this text is accurate and up to date. However, readers are strongly advised to confirm that the information, especially with regard to drug usage, complies with the latest legislation and standards of practice.

Existing UK nomenclature is changing to the system of Recommended International Non-proprietary Names (rINNs). Until the UK names are no longer in use, these more familiar names are used in this book in preference to rINNs, details of which may be obtained from the British National Formulary

Printed in China by RDC Group Limited
P/03

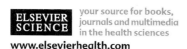

your source for books,
journals and multimedia
in the health sciences
www.elsevierhealth.com

Commissioning Editor:	Miranda Bromage
Associate Editor:	Paul Fam
Project Development Manager:	Sheila Black
Project Manager:	Cheryl Brant
Production Manager:	Mark Sanderson

The
publisher's
policy is to use
**paper manufactured
from sustainable forests**

Contents

Contributors

Tom Bates FRCS
Consultant Surgeon, The Breast Unit, The
William Harvey Hospital, Ashford, Kent, UK

J. Michael Dixon BSc(Hons) MBChB MB
FRCS(Edinburgh) FRCS(England)
Senior Lecturer in Surgery, University of
Edinburgh; Consultant Surgeon, Edinburgh
Breast Unit, Western General Hospital,
Edinburgh, UK

Julie C. Doughty FRCS (Gen)
Consultant Surgeon, University Department
of Surgery, Glasgow, UK

Janet Hardy MBChB FRACP MD
Consultant Physician, Department of Palliative
Medicine, Royal Marsden Hospital, Surrey,
UK

Anthony R. Hyett FRACS
Consultant Surgeon, Department of Academic
Surgery, Royal Marsden Hospital, London,
UK

Mark W. Kissin MChir FRCS
Consultant Breast Surgeon and Quality
Assurance Co-ordinator for Breast Screening
in South Thames, Royal Surrey and St Lukes
Hospitals Trust, Jarvis Breast Screening
Centre, Guildford, Surrey, UK

Robert C.F. Leonard BSc MBBS MD
FRCP FRCPE
Consultant Medical Oncologist, Edinburgh
Breast Unit, Western General Hospital,
Edinburgh, UK

Peter Malycha FRCS FRACS
Breast, Endocrine Unit, Department of
Surgery, University of Adelaide, Royal
Adelaide Hospital, Adelaide, Australia

Robert E. Mansel MS FRCS
Professor of Surgery, University of Wales
College of Medicine, Cardiff, UK

Michelle H. Mullan MRCS
Research Fellow, Breast Unit, Royal Surrey
County Hospital, Guildford, Surrey, UK

Robert F. Parkyn MBBS FRACS
Senior Visiting Surgeon and Head of Breast
and Endocrine Surgery Unit, Queen Elizabeth
Hospital, Adelaide, Australia

Nigel P.M. Sacks MS FRACS FRCS
Consultant Surgeon, Department of Academic
Surgery, Royal Marsden Hospital, London,
UK

Richard Sainsbury MD FRCS
Consultant Surgeon, Department of Surgery,
Royal Free and University College of London
Hospitals NHS Trust, London, UK

Hemant Singhal MBBS FRCS
Northwick Park NHS Trust
Northwick Park, UK

Christopher Wilson MD
University Department of Surgery, Glasgow,
UK

Foreword

In their Preface to the first edition, the series editors expressed the hope that the series would meet the needs of the higher surgical trainee and busy practising surgeon, providing up-to-date information on recent developments and succinct coverage of key topics within each specialty area. The outstanding success of the first edition suggests that these ambitions have been fulfilled and that the product is indeed meeting demand and expectations. Throughout the initiative there has been great emphasis on rapid publication, with all of its attendant stresses and strains, so that the reader could be provided with the very latest information. The fact that the second edition is now emerging within three years of the first indicates that O. James Garden and Simon Paterson-Brown and their now established team of volume editors are determined to follow through and maintain the momentum of this excellent series.

Contributors have been hand-picked with great care. They are a widely respected and authoritative group of surgeons and supporting specialists who are at the very forefront of their respective fields. The second edition retains the attractively format of the first, is well illustrated and eminently readable. The needs of the general surgeon are balanced nicely with those of the true surgical sub-specialist, and there are significant additions to the range of topics covered. The series has been expanded from seven to eight volumes due to the separation of breast and endocrine surgery. There will be a widespread welcome for the emphasis on evidence-based practice and the highlighting of key references both within the text and the supporting bibliography. I am pleased to see that the authors have endeavoured to use references that are as up-to-date as possible, and readers will welcome their consistent emphasis on recent developments.

A Companion to Specialist Surgical Practice series has filled an important niche in surgical publishing and with the quality and industry of the team now established, it seems destined to continue to do so. I am proud to have been associated with the first edition of the series and feel privileged to have been asked to provide this introduction to its successor. I congratulate all those who have worked so hard to ensure the continued success of the series and wish it well over the years to come. I have no doubt that the second edition will be very well received and recommend it unreservedly.

Sir David Carter MD, Hon DSc, Hon LID, FRCS (Ed), FRCS (Eng), FRCS (Glas), Hon FRCS (Ire), Hon FACS, Hon FRACS, FAMedSci, FRSE.

Vice Principal, University of Edinburgh, Formerly Chief Medical Officer in Scotland and Regius Professor of Clinical Surgery, Royal Infirmary, Edinburgh, UK

Preface

A Companion to Specialist Surgical Practice series has been designed to meet the needs of the higher surgeon in training and busy practising surgeon who require access to up-to-date information on recent developments in relation to their sub-specialty surgical practice. Many major surgery texts cover the whole of 'general surgery' and may contain information which is not of specific interest to the specialist surgeon. Similarly, specialist texts may be outwith the reach of the trainee's finances and, though comprehensive, may fall out-of-date during production or as a consequence of rapid new developments in practice. As with the successful first edition, this edition has also been written and produced in a very short time frame, so that the contents are as up-to-date as possible.

Each volume in the *Companion to Specialist Surgical Practice* series provides succinct summaries of all key topics within a specialty and concentrates on the most recent developments and current data. A specialist surgeon, whether in training or in practice, need only refer to the volume relevant to his or her chosen specialist field in addition to the *Core Topics in General and Emergency Surgery*.

We are grateful to our series editors for their perseverance and for their out-standing response to our repeated promptings over the last year. We would like to thank Rachel Stock and Linda Clark from WB Saunders for their help in getting this project safely launched in the past, and would give special thanks to Sue Hodgson, Sheila Black, Paul Fam and Miranda Bromage for piloting this series to its second edition. We appreciate very much the guidance and assist-ance of Sir David Carter as a series editor in the first series and for writing the foreword to this second series.

We hope that our aim of providing affordable up-to-date specialist surgical texts has been met, and that all surgeons, whether in training or in practice, will find the second edition of this series to be a valuable resource.

Addition of new chapters has led to the separation of the breast and endocrine volumes. Although the two specialist subjects are often spoken of in tandem, practitioners do not always have specialist expertise in both of these two areas. A recent survey of members of the British Association of Endocrine Surgeons, for example, showed that only about half of endocrine practitioners also specialised in breast disease.

Some of the most exciting developments are the chapters on clinical govern-ance and medicolegal aspects of surgical practice. These chapters complement each other and even if you do not buy both volumes you would be well advised to read the corresponding chapters in the sister book.

The endocrine volume includes a new chapter on the surgery of salivary glands, and the breast volume contains new chapters covering breast cancer in men and infective and inflammatory diseases.

We hope that you are not daunted by the lack of evidence which is beyond reasonable doubt in breast and endocrine disease. We do not think that evidence is present in any greater proportions in any of the other specialist areas. It is interesting to ponder on exactly what types of evidence actually influence innovation and inclusion of new techniques and treatments.

We hope that you enjoy these new volumes. We are grateful to previous contributors for bringing their chapters up-to-date, and to the new authors for their valuable chapters.

O. James Garden BSc, MB, ChB, MD, FRCS(Glas), FRCS(Ed)
Regius Professor of Clinical Surgery, Department of Clinical and Surgical Sciences (Surgery), Royal Infirmary, Edinburgh

Simon Paterson-Brown MB, BS, MS, MPhil, FRCS(Ed), FRCS(Eng), FCS(HK)
Consultant General and Upper Gastrointestinal Surgeon, Department of Clinical and Surgical Sciences (Surgery), Royal Infirmary, Edinburgh

John F. Farndon BSc, MD, FRCS
Professor and Head of Department, University Department of Surgery, Bristol Royal Infirmary, Bristol

Evidence-based Practice in Surgery

The second edition of the Companion to Specialist Surgical Practice series has attempted to incorporate, where appropriate, **evidence-based practice in surgery**, which has been highlighted in the text and relevant references. A detailed chapter on evidence-based practice in surgery written by Jonathan Michaels and Kathryn Rigby has been included in the volume on 'Core Topics in General and Emergency Surgery' to which the reader is referred for further information on assessing levels of evidence. We are grateful to them for providing this summary for each volume.

Critical appraisal for developing evidence-based practice can be obtained from a number of sources; the most reliable being randomised controlled clinical trials, systematic literature reviews, meta-analysis and observational studies. For practical purposes three grades of evidence can be used, analogous to the levels of 'proof' required in a court of law:

1) **Beyond reasonable doubt** – such evidence is likely to have arisen from high quality randomised controlled trials, systematic reviews, or high quality synthesised evidence such as decision analysis, cost effectiveness analysis or large observational data sets. The studies need to be directly applicable to the population of concern and have clear results. The grade is analogous to burden of proof within a criminal court and may be thought of as corresponding to the usual standard of 'proof' within the medical literature (i.e. $p < 0.05$).

2) **On the balance of probabilities** – in many cases a high quality review of literature may fail to reach firm conclusions due to conflicting or inconclusive results, trials of poor methodological quality, or the lack of evidence in the population to which the guidelines apply. In such cases it may still be possible to make a statement as to the best treatment on the "balance of probabilities". This is analogous to the decision in a civil court where all the available evidence will be weighed up and the verdict will depend upon the balance of probabilities.

3) **Not proven** – insufficient evidence upon which to base a decision or contradictory evidence.

Depending on the information available three grades of recommendation can be used:

a) strong recommendation, which should be followed unless there are compelling reasons to act otherwise.

b) a recommendation based on evidence of effectiveness, but where there may be other factors to take into account in decision-making, for example the user of the guidelines may be expected to take into account patient preferences, local facilities, local audit results or available resources.

c) a recommendation made where there is no adequate evidence as to the most effective practice, although there may be reasons for making a recommendation in order to minimise cost or reduce the chance of error through a locally agreed protocol.

Having highlighted the text and references which are considered to be associated with reasonable evidence in this volume with a "scalpel code", the reader can then reach his or her own conclusion.

1 Developmental abnormalities and benign breast disease

Robert E. Mansel
Hemant Singhal

Benign breast disease

Symptoms of benign breast disease are very common, with an estimate that over half the female population will, at some time, seek medical attention for a breast problem, and approximately 1 in 4 women will undergo a surgical breast biopsy. These figures are being modified by modern methods of triple assessment, which allow evaluation of breast lesions without the need for surgical biopsy. Benign conditions of the breast have been neglected in research efforts and literature output compared with cancer, despite the fact that only 6–10% of patients presenting to a breast clinic will have cancer.[1] The initial step in any patient presenting with breast symptoms is the exclusion of cancer by appropriate triple assessment.

The multiplicity and diversity of the terminology for benign breast disease in the past has resulted in some confusion. The situation can be clarified by abandoning morphological terminology that implies disease and substituting terms that describe a functional range of normality and change. The breast is under constant systemic hormonal influence, and it might be expected that the breast would show a uniform morphology and function throughout its parenchyma. This is not usually the case, and great variation exists in one part from another. Both the epithelial and stromal elements in the lobule are hormonally responsive, and normality depends on a balanced relationship between the two elements. The normal cyclical changes of heaviness and fullness are not associated with major histological change but have been shown to be correlated to changes in breast volume. The more radical hormonal changes occurring in pregnancy and during lactation are associated with the morphological changes of lobular growth and differentiation. After the conclusion of childbearing the onset of the menopause produces a decline in hormonal concentrations leading to lobular involution, ductal ectasia and fat replacement of the breast parenchyma. These changes occur over a reproductive life of nearly 40 years and give ample opportunity for minor aberrations to occur.[2]

Aberrations of normal development and involution: the concept

The management of benign breast conditions depends on the understanding of the normal processes within the breast and the aberrations that lead to clinical presentation. Most benign breast complaints are due to aberrations of the normal processes of development, cyclical change and involution. Most benign conditions, therefore, show a predominance in a particular period of reproductive life. It has increasingly become obvious that the concept of fibrocystic disease is quite inadequate in describing benign breast disease as it implies a clinical and histological equivalence that is fallacious.[3] For each disorder there is a spectrum from normal through mild abnormality (aberration) to disease. The common occurrence of these benign changes on histology with no clinical correlations has led to the suggestion that they be called aberrations rather than disease.[4] The 'aberrations of normal development and involution' (ANDI) concept has been proposed as a framework for benign breast disorders that is

Reproductive period	Normal process	Benign breast disease	
		Common	Uncommon
Development	Ductal	Nipple inversion Single duct obstruction	Mammary duct fistula
	Lobular	Fibroadenoma	Giant fibroadenoma
	Stromal	Adolescent hypertrophy	(severest form)
Cyclical change	Hormonal activity	Mastalgia Nodularity Focal Diffuse	(Severest form)
	Epithelial activity	Benign papilloma	
Pregnancy and lactation	Epithelial hyperplasia	Blood-stained nipple discharge	
	Lactation	Galactocoele and inappropriate lactation	
Involution	Lobular involution	Cysts and sclerosing adenosis	
	Ductal involution	Nipple retraction	Periductal mastitis
	Fibrosis	Duct ectasia	with suppuration
	Dilation		
	Micropapillomatosis	Simple hyperplasias	Lobular hyperplasias with atypia Duct hyperplasias with atypia Intracystic papilloma

Table 1.1 A framework of pathogenesis for the classification of benign breast disorders[4]

comprehensive, accurate in terminology and based on pathogenesis.[4] This concept encompasses pathogenesis, clinical and histological importance and general principles of management. The concept of ANDI has now been extended to include duct ectasia cystic change and duct sclerosis (**Table 1.1**).

Aetiology

Few epidemiological studies clarify the aetiology of benign breast disease. The literature comprises badly designed studies in selected populations with poorly defined diagnostic groups, based principally on historic biopsy proven disease. Several important factors can be found consistently through case–control epidemiological studies, notably that biopsy for benign breast disorders is more common in thin nulliparous women with a family history of breast cancer, suggesting considerable surgical selection.[5] Necropsy studies in asymptomatic women who died from accidental trauma consistently showed the presence of histological changes that would have been labelled as benign breast disease in the past. This casts considerable doubt on the importance of these lesions as disease entities in most women.

Role of dietary factors

Much interest has been shown in the role of dietary factors in the aetiology and progression of benign breast disease. Owing to its wide consumption and diverse biochemical and physiological effects, caffeine has been extensively examined in clinical and experimental studies. Early reports linking caffeine to breast pain have not been confirmed by later studies. Deficiency of essential fatty acids in the diet can lead to a deficient production of prostaglandin E_1, which may potentiate the effects of prolactin on the breast. Higher tissue concentration ratios of saturated to unsaturated fatty acids may lead to similar potentiation of the endocrine response. A high red meat intake with low consumption of fresh vegetables and vitamin A increases the risk of proliferative benign breast disease. Conversely, a reduction in fat intake reduces breast pain. Endocrine factors such as increased oestrogen, decreased progesterone and increased prolactin concentrations have been considered, but serum concentrations of these hormones during the menstrual cycle have not shown any difference between those with mastalgia and those without. Breast pain and cyst formation, however, are found in the menopausal age group but are rarely seen in the absence of oestrogen. Oestrogen is necessary for the development of these conditions. Although measurement of hormonal profiles for groups of patients may show little variation, it is possible that minor individual variations in hormonal concentrations and end-organ responsiveness may play a part in the aetiology.

The widespread use of the contraceptive pill has prompted numerous detailed studies of its effect on breast disease. Results from large studies have shown a decrease in benign breast disease in long-term users of oral contraceptives. Fewer biopsies for benign breast disease were performed in this group in the large prospective Oxford FPA study. The protective effects seem to be related to the progesterone component of oral contraceptives. Controversy still exists on the effects of oral contraceptives on epithelial hyperplasia.

Periductal mastitis is linked to cigarette smoking. Women who smoke and have periductal mastitis develop more inflammation and recurrence of the disease after corrective surgery. This effect may be due to altered oral bacterial flora in smokers leading to breast duct colonisation or direct ischaemic effects of nicotine on breast ducts.

Factors altering hepatic metabolism of oestrogen, with an alteration in the ratio of C2 hydroxylation products (inactive metabolites) to C16 hydroxylation (active metabolites) may play a part. Exercise and intake of vegetables containing indole-3-carbinol both increase C2 hydroxylation whereas smoking increases the active C16 metabolites. These studies emphasise a potentially important pathway for chemoprevention studies.

Studies are currently underway to examine the role of phyto-oestrogens in breast cancer and breast physiology.

Cancer risk

There have been many studies linking histological changes in benign breast biopsies and subsequent risk of breast cancer, but there was no attempt to standardise criteria, and patient populations were often small. Three groups did agree to use the same definition of benign changes and a unified set of criteria for the diagnosis of these lesions. The definitions combine cytological detail with the general architectural structure of the tissue associated with a measure of the degree of cellular proliferation. The resulting categories of mild proliferation, severe proliferation and marked atypia were predictive of concurrent cancer and/or future cancer development. In proliferative breast disease, the markers of cancer risk may be classified into histological categories of increased risk above the general population: slightly (1–2 times), moderately (4–5 times) and markedly (9–10 times).[6] The results from the three groups (Nashville, Nurses Health Study (NHS) and the Breast Cancer Detection Demonstration Project (BCDDP)) were similar and showed that if the biopsy revealed proliferative disease without atypia, the subsequent risk was approximately 1.5 times. If the biopsy revealed atypical hyperplasia, the risk was approximately 4.5 times (level III evidence). If the patients with atypical hyperplasia had a family history of breast cancer, the subsequent risk approached that of patients with *in situ* carcinoma (approximately 8–10 times). In patients with atypical hyperplasia, the breast cancer risk was much higher in premenopausal than postmenopausal patients. Although the classification scheme proposed by Page *et al.* is useful in assigning different levels of risk to women with benign breast disease, it has not been universally accepted. A major short-term goal should be to encourage pathologists to apply these criteria in a reproducible manner in daily practice.[6,7]

Diagnosis

Major progress in the assessment of breast complaints and early detection of malignancy has been achieved by improvement of mammographic technique and application of ultrasonography, cytology and stereotactic techniques. Problems in diagnosis are still encountered in patients where tissue distortion occurs after surgery or radiation therapy or in the presence of silicone implants. Ultrasonography has a major role as a primary and an ancillary modality in the modern diagnosis of breast abnormalities.[8] It differentiates cystic from solid abnormalities and thereby guides further interventions. Doppler ultrasonography has certain indications,[9] and newer techniques such as digital luminescence radiography and contrast-enhanced magnetic resonance imaging (MRI) are being developed and are likely to be clinically important. Magnetic resonance spectroscopy, positron emission tomography transillumination, ductoscopy and biomagnetism offer interesting new aspects for research, but the value of computed tomography (CT) and thermography is not established.[10–12]

Breast symptoms are assessed by a careful history and by the diagnostic triad ('triple assessment') of clinical breast examination, breast imaging (mammography or ultrasonography) and fine needle aspiration cytology (FNAC).[13,14] More recently wide-bore needle core biopsy guided by ultrasonography has become much more popular as it allows a histological diagnosis with the potential of immunohistochemical examination (e.g. for oestrogen receptors).

 When there is a palpable dominant mass, the diagnostic triad yields a reliable pathological diagnosis with a sensitivity approaching 100% (level III evidence).[15]

If there is a lack of concordance between the individual elements of triple assessment or if there is any doubt about the diagnosis either on the part of the physician or the patient, a wide-bore needle biopsy may obviate the need for open surgical biopsy and allows a definitive histological diagnosis. Indeed the widespread introduction of core biopsy and the increasing acceptance of the ANDI concept has led to a greatly reduced rate of open surgical biopsies and the virtual disappearance of the need to excise fibroadenomas.

In contrast, FNAC is a quick, accurate, cost-effective procedure and is best suited in a one-stop diagnosis setting, although it requires an experienced cytologist. Its sensitivity ranges from 90 to 97% in large series.[16,17] A positive result on FNAC is sufficiently accurate to justify one-stage diagnosis and treatment, if the other elements of the triple assessment are concordant.

All patients over the age of 35 presenting with breast symptoms should have mammography. Patients under 35 can be imaged using ultrasonography. Only the diagnosis of a simple cyst will obviate the need for further evaluation or therapy. Doppler ultrasonography of breast lesions may give further information, but this is currently not in routine clinical practice.

Congenital anomalies

Embryonic development

The breast is a distinguishing feature of the class mammalia and is a modified sudoriferous gland developing in the fifth and sixth week of fetal life as two ventral bands of thickened ectoderm ('milk lines'). The bands extend bilaterally from the axilla to the inguinal region, and normally only a single pair of glands develop in the pectoral area. Each mammary gland develops as an ingrowth of ectodermal tissue into the underlying mesenchyme. During 13 to 20 weeks of intrauterine life each primary bud initiates the outgrowth of 15–20 secondary buds. Epithelial cords develop from these secondary buds and extend into the surrounding mesenchyme. Canalisation of the outgrowths forms lactiferous ducts and their branches. The lactiferous ducts open into epithelial depressions, forming the mammary pit. Proliferation of the surrounding mesenchyme causes the mammary pit to elevate, forming the nipple.

Absence of breast or nipple

Amastia or absence of the breast is a rare condition and is presumably due to failure of the milk line to develop. The condition is usually unilateral. An association with the absence of pectoral muscles and syndactly has been described. Unilateral hypoplasia of the breast is found more commonly than complete absence. Some degree of asymmetry between the breasts is normal, with the left usually being slightly larger than the right. True asymmetry between the breasts can be treated by enlarging the smaller breast with implants or reducing or elevating the larger breast with plastic surgical procedures. Absence of the nipple, or athelia, is extremely rare and is usually associated with amastia. Absent nipples and areolas can be reconstructed with skin from the inner thigh, labial skin or by nipple sharing.

Supernumerary nipples and accessory nipples

Supernumerary or accessory nipples occur in 1–5% of people and result from the persistence of one or more nests of ectodermal cells in the milk line. Supernumerary nipples or breasts may occur in any size or configuration and are often mistaken for skin papillomas. Axillary breast tissue is usually bilateral and becomes more obvious with pregnancy and lactation. Supernumerary breasts have been reported at other sites, including the groin, labia majora, inner sides of thighs and buttocks. Accessory nipples rarely require treatment for other than cosmetic reasons. However, breast tissue in abnormal sites can develop breast cancer.

Disorders of development

Hypertrophic abnormalities of the breast

Prepubertal breast enlargement in girls in the absence of other signs of sexual maturation is a common occurrence. It is not a reason for investigation unless accompanied by other signs of early sexual maturation, when it may be due to hormone-secreting ovarian or adrenal tumours. The breasts do not develop synchronously, and reassurance should be given. A watch-and-wait policy should be adopted and biopsy or excision avoided at all costs as the whole developing breast could be removed accidentally.

Juvenile hypertrophy of the breast is a relatively rare condition, rapidly leading to gigantomastia in peripubertal females. The pathology is limited to the breast, with otherwise normal growth and development.

In adolescent girls the normal development of the breast can occasionally continue, with overgrowth of periductal tissue. Proliferation and increased branching of the ducts without lobule formation can lead to juvenile or virginal hypertrophy. Endocrine abnormalities have not been detected as an underlying cause, although a higher rate of infertility has been reported. The nipple and areola may be difficult to recognise as they are stretched over the pendulous breasts. The weight of the huge breasts results in neck and back pain with indentation of the shoulder skin by the bra straps. The patient may develop a stooping posture due to a combination of weight redistribution and embarrassment. Medical treatment with danazol and bromocriptine has been tried, but reduction mammoplasty is the treatment of choice. Occasionally the condition recurs, when a further resection may be needed. Histology of the resected breast tissue is remarkably normal, with a relative increase in the stromal component.

Several techniques are available for reduction mammoplasty, each aiming to reduce the breast size and correct the associated ptosis. The nipple and areola are preserved on a de-epithelialised pedicle, which may be inferior, superior or centrally based, depending on the technique chosen. Alternatively, a free graft of the nipple and areola may be used if the desired degree of nipple elevation is difficult to achieve with a pedicle technique. Immediate postoperative complications include haematoma, infection and fat necrosis. Scarring of the breast may make subsequent examination and imaging of the breast difficult. Studies have shown objective improvement in back pain and respiratory function after reduction mammoplasty for large breasts.

Gynaecomastia

Gynaecomastia is the commonest condition affecting the male breast and is an enlargement of ductal and stromal tissues that is structurally different from the surrounding subcutaneous fat. The condition is entirely benign and usually

Decreased androgens		
	Reduced production	Congenital anorchia
		Chromosomal abnormalities e.g. Klinefelter's syndrome
		Bilateral cryptorchidism
		Viral orchitis
		Bilateral torsion
		Granulomatous disease
		Renal failure
	Androgen resistance	Testicular feminisation
Increased oestrogens		
	Increased secretion	Testicular tumours
		Carcinoma lung
	Increased peripheral aromatisation	Adrenal disease
		Liver disease
		Starvation re-feeding
		Thyrotoxicosis
Drug induced		
	Antiandrogens	Spironolactone
		Cyproterone
	Oestrogenic activity or bound to oestrogen receptors	Digitalis
		Griseofulvin
		Cannabis
	Disturbance in gonadotrophin control	Phenothiazines
		Reserpine
		Cimetidine
		Methyldopa
		Isoniazid
		Metoclopramide
		Tricyclic antidepressants
		Anabolic steroids

Table 1.2 Causes of secondary gynaecomastia

reversible. It is usually physiological as in neonatal, pubertal and senescent hypertrophy, which are due to an excess of oestrogens relative to testosterone. Specific causes of gynaecomastia need to be considered in all patients, but many will be idiopathic in apparently healthy men. These include hypogonadism, neoplasms, drugs and systemic diseases (**Table 1.2**). The increasing use of anabolic steroids is increasing the incidence of gynaecomastia in weightlifters and body builders.

The presentation is usually with a tender enlargement of the breast, often unilateral. In non-obese patients, nearly 2 cm of subareolar breast tissue is required before the presence of gynaecomastia can be confirmed. Patients may be concerned about the cosmetic appearance, tenderness or pain or the possibility of underlying malignancy. Malignancy should be suspected when gynaecomastia presents with an eccentric, hard lump or ulcerating lesions. Investigation by mammography and FNAC or core biopsy are appropriate.

Treatment

Because most patients have hormonal imbalance or drug-induced disease, firm reassurance that gynaecomastia is a benign and self-limiting condition will suffice. Medical therapy is seldom of value except when a specific diagnosis has been established. Discontinuation of causative drugs or improvement in the medical condition leading to gynaecomastia often results in breast regression. Testosterone has been of variable value, but some dramatic results have been reported. Tamoxifen, clomiphene and danazol have been tried in small numbers of patients with a heterogeneous case-mix, with variable results. In general the evidence for specific drug interventions is based on small non-randomised studies, and there does not seem to be a drug of choice. Surgical removal of the breast tissue is indicated when medical treatment has failed or where the degree of breast enlargement is a cosmetic or psychological problem. Subcutaneous mastectomy is performed through a periareolar or inframammary incision, depending on the extent of tissue to be excised. With the increasing emphasis on cosmesis, even in men, the short periareolar incision is preferred. The nipple is elevated, leaving a small amount of adherent breast tissue and subcutaneous fat. Flaps are dissected only a small distance superiorly and interiorly in a deep subcutaneous plane, so that a good proportion of subcutaneous fat is retained with the flap. This ensures that the initial deformity of a swelling is not replaced by a hollow. Division of the cone of breast tissue into two or four pieces eases the dissection and subsequent haemostasis when a short periareolar incision is used.

Fibroadenoma

Fibroadenoma appears usually in young women as a rubbery, firm, smooth and mobile mass. These characteristic features make clinical diagnosis easy in most young women, but the situation is not so obvious in older women where fibrotic changes of involution decrease the mobility of the lump. Calcified fibroadenomas are sometimes found in elderly patients as a hard discrete but mobile mass, and they are readily demonstrated by the typical coarse calcification seen on mammography. Fibroadenomas arise from lobules and are therefore seen predominantly at the ages of development, i.e. 15–25 years. Hyperplastic lobules, which are histologically identical to fibroadenomas, are found so frequently as to be regarded as normal.[18] The full spectrum from hyperplastic lobules to fibroadenoma is seen, but without the continued growth characteristic of neoplasms and can, therefore, be regarded as aberrations of normal development. Fibroadenomas show hormonal dependence similar to the lobules from which they are derived. Lactational changes can be seen in the lobules during pregnancy, and changes of involution are evident in the perimenopausal period. Most fibroadenomas are 1–2 cm in size, and growth beyond 5 cm is unusual. They may be multiple, especially in Oriental and Negroid races.

The clinical diagnosis of fibroadenoma may be incorrect in up to 50% of patients, and definite proof of the diagnosis should be obtained in all patients using ultrasonography and FNAC/core biopsy. Excision of all fibroadenomas is not essential as only a small number increase in size, the majority get smaller and some disappear.[19,20] If clinical and diagnostic investigations confirm the lesion to be a fibroadenoma, the patient can be given the choice of observation or excision after reassurance.[21] In current practice, excision of a fibroadenoma is a rare operation but if necessary excision is performed through an incision along Langer's lines. The histological appearance is characteristically a combination of pale stroma and duct-like structures lined by regular epithelial cells. The risk of cancer within a fibroadenoma is small (1 in 1000 lesions). It is usually lobular carcinoma *in situ*, as would be expected from the lobular origin of fibroadenomas, and it carries an excellent prognosis. Ductal carcinoma is significantly less common and is usually direct infiltration by an adjacent cancer or cancer extending along the duct into the lobules. Treatment is directed to the primary cancer, and the presence of the fibroadenoma is irrelevant. Follow-up studies of fibroadenomas treated by observation show that around 30% reduce in size over 1 year.

Mastalgia and cyclical change

Mastalgia is one of the commonest breast symptoms, affecting up to 70% of women at some time in their lives. It accounts for approximately 50% of referrals to a specialised breast clinic and is also the most common reason for breast-related consultation in general practice. These figures are an underestimate of the real prevalence of the condition. A recent randomised study of primary care referrals (the Bridge study) has shown that general practitioners only refer 26% of symptomatic women to hospital clinics (**Fig. 1.1**).[22] Referrals for a discrete lump were much higher than for breast pain (78% vs. 26%). In hospital practice, mastalgia is cyclical in two thirds of patients, non-cyclical in the rest or due to pain arising from the chest wall.[23] Surprisingly, the Bridge study showed that the presentation of mastalgia is different in primary care as the ratio of cyclical/non-cyclical is 20%:65% compared with 75%:25% in hospital practice. A

Figure 1.1
Prevalence of mastalgia.

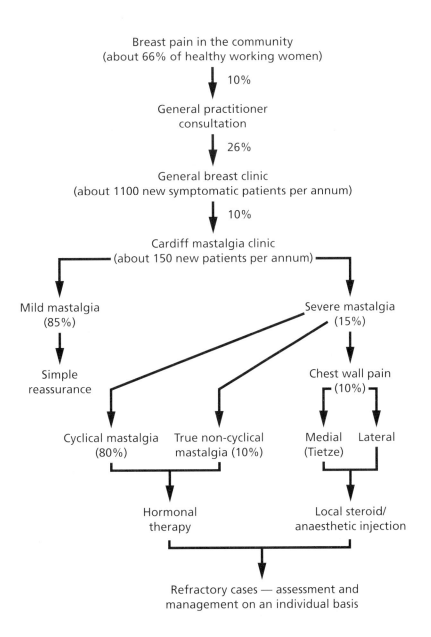

Breast pain in the community
(about 66% of healthy working women)

↓ 10%

General practitioner consultation

↓ 26%

General breast clinic
(about 1100 new symptomatic patients per annum)

↓ 10%

Cardiff mastalgia clinic
(about 150 new patients per annum)

Mild mastalgia (85%)

↓

Simple reassurance

Severe mastalgia (15%)

↓

Chest wall pain (10%)

Cyclical mastalgia (80%)   True non-cyclical mastalgia (10%)   Medial (Tietze)   Lateral

Hormonal therapy

Local steroid/anaesthetic injection

↓

Refractory cases — assessment and management on an individual basis

further difference is that the proportion of pain judged to be severe by the general practitioner is twice as high as assessed in hospital practice. These differences were unsuspected prior to this prospective randomised study (level IV evidence). Premenstrual discomfort and nodularity are so common that they should be considered to be normal. The aetiology of mastalgia remains obscure. Water retention has been suggested as a cause of mastalgia and premenstrual tension. Diuretics are often used to treat these conditions, but a study comparing total body water on day 5 and day 25 of the menstrual cycle using tritiated water, failed to show any differences between symptomatic patients and normal controls.[23] Some have suggested that psychological factors play a major part in the causation of mastalgia, but there is no scientific basis for this. Increased oestrogen, decreased progesterone and increased prolactin concentrations were thought to be likely factors, but measurement of serum concentrations of these hormones through the menstrual cycle have not shown any difference between those with mastalgia and controls.[24] Overstimulation of the breast cells due to interference with ATP degradation by methylxanthine consequent to high caffeine intake may have a role. Deficiency of essential fatty acids in the diet can lead to impaired production of prostaglandin E that may potentiate the effects of prolactin on the breast.

The most important factors in the evaluation and treatment of breast pain consist of a thorough history taking and physical and radiological evaluation. These can be used to reassure the patient that she does not have breast cancer. After exclusion of breast cancer, 85% of patients can be discharged from the clinic without specific treatment.[25] In 15% of patients, however, the pain is severe enough to affect lifestyle and thus warrants therapy and a systematic approach to achieve relief of pain (**Fig. 1.2**).[26,27] Therapy may consist of a well fitting bra, a decrease in dietary fat intake, manipulation to reduce saturated fat or to supplement essential fatty acid intake and discontinuance of oral contraceptives or hormone replacement therapy. Those women resistant to these simple measures may experience relief from γ-linolenic acid as first-line therapy. Treatment with γ-linolenic acid should be continued for about 3 months, and about 70% of patients with cyclical mastalgia will have a moderate to good response. Danazol or bromocriptine are usually used as second-line agents, both of which are effective treatments but have a much higher incidence of side effects. Danazol is started at a dose of 200 mg daily and continued for at least two menstrual cycles. Those obtaining a response can then be maintained on a dose of 100 mg on alternate days or 100 mg on days 14 to 28 of the menstrual cycle. About 25% of patients taking danazol experience side effects of weight gain, nausea or oily skin.

Bromocriptine, a prolactin-lowering drug, is used at a dose of 2.5 mg twice daily but is introduced at 1.25 mg daily for 3–4 days then increased by similar

Figure 1.2
Principles of mastalgia treatment. From Peplinski & Norton. Gastrointestinal endocrine cancers and nodal metastasis: biological significance and therapeutic implications. Surg Oncol Clin North Am 1996; 5: 159–71.

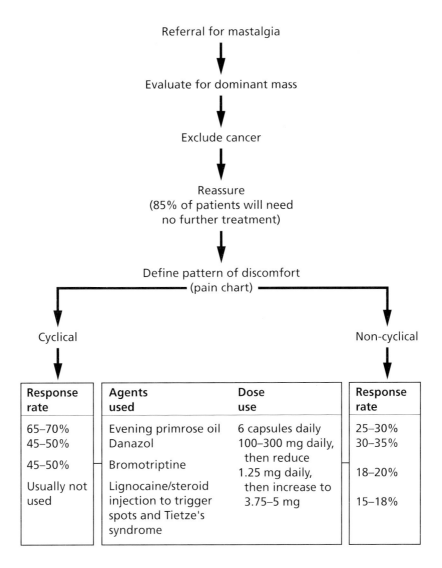

Referral for mastalgia

Evaluate for dominant mass

Exclude cancer

Reassure
(85% of patients will need
no further treatment)

Define pattern of discomfort
(pain chart)

Cyclical   Non-cyclical

Response rate	Agents used	Dose use	Response rate
65–70%	Evening primrose oil	6 capsules daily	25–30%
45–50%	Danazol	100–300 mg daily, then reduce	30–35%
45–50%	Bromotriptine	1.25 mg daily, then increase to	18–20%
Usually not used	Lignocaine/steroid injection to trigger spots and Tietze's syndrome	3.75–5 mg	15–18%

amounts at 3-day intervals to achieve the desired dose. Side effects have resulted in limited use of this drug in recent years. By using γ-linolenic acid as first-line therapy and danazol or bromocriptine as second-line agents, a clinically useful improvement in pain can be anticipated in 92% of patients with cyclical mastalgia and 74% with non-cyclical mastalgia. Patients with severe recurrent or refractory mastalgia may require treatment with tamoxifen, goserelin or testosterone, but the short-term and long-term adverse effects of these drugs preclude their use as first-line agents.

The efficacy of bromocriptine, γ-linolenic acid, danazol and tamoxifen have been proven in double blind randomised trials (level IV evidence).[28–31]

Predicting which treatment will be most efficacious for any particular woman is not easy because presenting features, personal or family history of breast disease or reproductive history are not predictive of success rates.[32] The aetiology of cyclical mastalgia is poorly understood, but lack of previous breast feeding and low levels of physical exercise are contributing factors. The consistent finding of an increased prolactin secretion in response to thyrotrophin-releasing hormone in patients with mastalgia, probably due to oestrogen dominance, has led to the use of treatment with prolactin-lowering drugs and antioestrogens. The efficacy and safety in mastalgia of gestrinone (which has androgenic, antioestrogenic and antiprogestogenic properties) and vaginal micronised progesterone have been investigated in recent studies, with gestrinone showing encouraging results. Progestogens may be an effective therapy although earlier studies were negative.[33] Chest wall pain (or Tietze's disease) is localised to the costochondral junctions and is usually self-limiting, but symptomatic relief can often be obtained with steroidal and local anaesthetic injections or non-steroidal anti-inflammatory drugs.

Disorders of involution

These changes become progressive from the age of 35 years. The involution of stroma and epithelium do not occur at the same rate or in an integrated fashion over the 20-year period of this process. When the stroma involutes faster than the epithelial acini, these remain and form microcysts, which are so common as to be regarded as a normal part of an involuting breast. Obstruction of the efferent duct leads to macrocyst formation. This concept fits well with the common occurrence of macrocysts and the fact that they are often multiple. Many are not clinically detectable. In sclerosing adenosis, the complex interrelationship between involution and stromal fibrosis superimposed on the cyclical changes leads to a complex picture of epithelial acini surrounded by fibrous tissue.

Cysts

Cysts are the commonest single abnormality found in patients attending a breast clinic, and most are a manifestation of ANDI. Less common cystic lesions include galactocoele, oil cysts of fat necrosis, papillary cystadenomas and those associated with necrosis in a phyllodes tumour or carcinoma. Hydatid cysts are very rare. Microcysts may be present in most women at some time during the process of involution, and some develop clinically detectable macrocysts. Cysts are most common between the ages of 38 and 53 years.

If a breast lump is suspected to be a cyst it should be aspirated directly or by using ultrasonographic guidance. The cyst fluid has a variable colour from pale yellow to brown or dark green. The routine cytological examination of cyst fluid is not rewarding and can be potentially misleading. It is essential to confirm that the cyst has disappeared after aspiration and that the fluid is not blood stained. If ultrasonography shows a solid component to the cyst, the cyst should be investigated as for a solid lesion with FNAC or wide-bore needle biopsy.

The fluid filling the cysts contains unusual amounts of biologically active substances, including hormones and metabolites. Measuring cations (K^+, Na^+) permits classification of cysts into two major subsets (type I and type II), conceivably associated with a difference in the apocrine cells in the lining epithelia. Type I cysts (high K^+:Na^+ ratio) accumulate huge amounts of dehydroepiandrosterone sulphate, oestrone sulphate, androstane-3a, 1 7-diol glucuronide and androsterone glucuronide and contain more testosterone and dihydrotestosterone than type III cysts. Conversely, type II cysts (low K^+:Na^+ ratio) contain more progesterone and pregnenolone than type I cysts.[34] The risk of cyst relapse is significantly higher in women with type I cysts or with multiple cysts at presentation.

Various proteins and several polypeptide growth factors, including EGF and IGF-I, are often found in cyst fluid. Biochemical analysis of these components may shed further light on the role of gross cysts in relation to cyst recurrence and the risk of breast cancer. Several reports indicate that patients with macrocysts have a two- to four-fold higher risk of developing cancer but long-term cohort studies have failed to show any relationship between cyst fluid type and cancer development.[35,36]

Epithelial hyperplasia

Epithelial hyperplasia is an increase in the number of layers of epithelial cells lining the terminal duct lobular unit. The degree of hyperplasia is graded as mild, moderate or severe. During the premenopausal period, mild and moderate changes are common and are known to regress spontaneously. They should be regarded as part of ANDI as they are common and are associated with a minimal or non-significant increased risk of breast cancer in the absence of other factors. Dupont and Page have classified epithelial hyperplasia into ductal and lobular on the basis of histological criteria. Atypia within the hyperplasia is important as this leads to an increased risk of subsequent cancer. There is no clinical counterpart to this pathology finding within the concept of ANDI. Most patients with epithelial hyperplasia are asymptomatic and this is a coincidental finding in a biopsy done for other reasons. Atypical epithelial hyperplasia may be found incidentally in up to 3% of such biopsies.

Residual breast tissue

Not all breast tissue involutes at the same rate, and this may lead to clinical and mammographic asymmetry, which may be difficult to differentiate from a carcinoma. Studies have shown that hormone replacement therapy increases the density of breast tissue on mammography, and this may reduce the sensitivity of screening mammography.

Nipple discharge

A small amount of fluid can be expressed in up to two thirds of all non-lactating women by application of suction to the nipple. This should be regarded as physiological. This fluid is not blood stained and varies in colour from clear off-white through yellow to dark green. The fluid may come from a single duct or multiple ducts. Nipple discharge is significant when it occurs spontaneously and is a dominant symptom, but is an uncommon presentation to the breast clinic, constituting fewer than 3% of patients.

Serous discharge is characterised by its yellow colour and is often sticky. A coloured opalescent discharge is seen most often in duct ectasia but can rarely occur with cysts. Milky discharge is on most occasions physiological and can be seen in the neonatal period (witch's milk) owing to hormonal stimulation of the neonatal breast. It is also seen in pregnancy, lactation and the postlactational period. Mechanical stimulation can lead to a milky discharge. Hyper-prolactinaemia produces galactorrhoea, and this may be caused by a pituitary tumour and drugs that block or deplete dopamine (e.g. phenothiazines, meta-clopramide, domperidone, methyldopa). Blood staining can vary from small amounts that produce a serosanguineous discharge to frank blood. Bloody discharge is often due to epithelial hyperplasia in the form of a duct papilloma. The condition is most often benign, but the risk of malignancy increases with age. Duct ectasia may lead to blood-stained nipple discharge with ulceration within the ducts. The discharge associated with breast cancer is usually blood stained and associated with a palpable lump. In a minority of patients no cause of the discharge is established even after operations such as major duct excision.

Investigation of the discharge should include Haemostix® testing for blood, cytological examination and assessment of the breast with examination and mammography. An algorithm for management is outlined in **Figure 1.3**. Surgical excision of the involved duct as a microdochectomy is preferred for a single discharging duct. Total duct excision is the favoured approach for a patient with multiple duct discharge and in patients over the age of 50 with a single duct discharge as the risk of malignancy is higher.

Duct ectasia/periductal mastitis

Periductal mastitis is characterised by mastalgia of a non-cyclical nature, nipple discharge and periareolar inflammation that may be associated with nipple

Figure 1.3
Management of nipple discharge. From Peplinski & Norton. Gastrointestinal endocrine cancers and nodal metastasis: biological significance and therapeutic implications. Surg Oncol Clin North Am 1996; 5: 159–71.

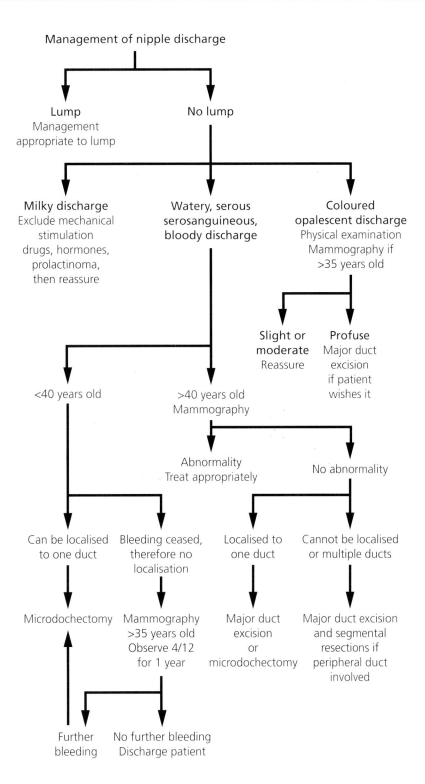

retraction. The formation of mammary fistulae and non-lactating breast abscess is often seen. In periductal mastitis the major ducts are not dilated but are surrounded by an inflammatory response that consists of polymorphs, plasma cells, lymphocytes and granulomas with giant cells and epithelioid cells. The aetiology of the inflammation is unknown.

Duct ectasia typically occurs in the perimenopausal or late premenopausal groups. Periductal mastitis and duct ectasia affect the major breast ducts. The dilation usually affects 3–4 of the ducts within 2–3 cm of the nipple. The reason why these particular segments and only some ducts are affected is unclear. The dilated ducts allow secretions to collect, leading to a discharge from the nipple. The leakage or secretion into the periductal tissue causes an inflammatory response, with infiltration by neutrophils, macrophages and plasma cells. This inflammation leads to periductal fibrosis and nipple retraction. This explanation of pathogenesis, however, does not explain the presence of periductal mastitis in the younger patient with no associated duct ectasia. An alternative theory suggests an autoimmune basis leading to destruction and weakening of the muscle layer with secondary dilatation of the ducts. It is possible that both processes contribute to the clinical picture. The role of bacterial infection in the pathogenesis is controversial, but the presence of anaerobic bacteria in the ducts has been confirmed in several studies. Infection is more common after biopsy of breasts showing duct ectasia on histology. *Bacteroides* species, together with coliforms and streptococci have been isolated. The presence of bacteria is more usual in the recurrent lesion. The absence of bacteria in many patients and the rapidity of resolution without antibacterial treatment would suggest that the inflammation may be a chemical response to leaked ductal secretion.[37]

Management of duct ectasia and periductal mastitis includes antibiotic therapy for the acute inflammatory episode. Ongoing symptoms are best resolved with the operation of total major duct excision. Special care is needed to excise all ducts to prevent recurrence of the condition. Free eversion of the nipple is indicative that all ducts have been sectioned.

Mammary fistula

Mammary fistula is a rare recurrent condition characterised by persistent draining abscesses at the areolar margin in one or both breasts. Because little is known about the disease, it is often misdiagnosed and inappropriately treated. The clinical and pathological findings are similar to duct ectasia or periductal mastitis, with a swelling or mass at the areola, draining fistula from the subareolar tissue, a chronic thick, pasty discharge from the nipple and pain. Histological examination reveals keratinising squamous epithelium replacing the lining of one or more lactiferous ducts for a variable distance into the subareolar tissue. Core excision of the fistula and all of the retroareolar fibroglandular tissue and the ductal tissue within the nipple is the usual definitive therapy. Where sepsis is present at the time of excision, perioperative antibiotics are mandatory, and the wound may be managed by packing if primary closure is difficult.

Benign tumours

Duct papilloma

Benign papillomas of the ducts are common and should be regarded as aberrations of cyclical change rather than true benign tumours. These lesions may be single or multiple. Symptoms are present usually when major ducts are affected. The most common finding is a discharge from the nipple that may be blood stained. Treatment consists of microdochectomy, excising the involved duct.

Lipoma

These soft, lobulated and radiolucent lesions are quite common in the breast. A similar soft mass, 'pseudolipoma,' can often be found around a carcinoma, caused by indrawing of the adjacent fat by the spiculated tumour. All patients over the age of 35 with a clinical diagnosis of a lipoma should be investigated by triple assessment as for a breast lump.

Mammary hamartomas

Mammary hamartomas are breast disorders currently underestimated and not well recognised. Hamartomas account for 1.2% of benign breast lesions and 4.8% of benign breast tumours. Clinically they present with a palpable lump, which is usually painless. Typically, but inconsistently, mammography shows a clearly circumscribed density, separated from adjacent normal breast by a thin radiolucent zone. Macroscopically, hamartomas are slightly larger and softer than fibroadenomas. They are well defined, white/pink and fleshy, with yellow islands of fat tissue. Histologically, hamartomas exhibit 'pushing' borders with pseudoencapsulation and consist of a combination of variable amounts of stromal and epithelial components. Stromal components mainly consist of a prominent fibrohyalin background with small islands of adipose tissue and oedematous changes. Epithelial structures show variable features of benign breast disease. The overall architecture is lobulated. Hamartomas result more from breast dysgenesis than from any tumorous process.

References

1. Hughes LE, Mansel RE, Webster DJT. Benign disorders and diseases of the breast. Concepts and clinical management. London: WB Saunders, 2nd edn, 1999.

2. Mansel RE. Benign breast disease. [Review.] Practitioner 1992; 236: 830–4.

3. Love SM, Gelman RS, Silen W. Fibrocystic disease of the breast—a non disease. N Engl J Med 1982; 307: 1010–4.

 4. Hughes LE, Mansel RE, Webster DIT. Aberrations of normal development and involution (ANDI): a new perspective on pathogenesis and nomenclature of human breast disorders. Lancet 1987; ii: 1316–9.

5. Bundred NJ. Aetiological factors in benign breast disease. Br J Surg 1994; 1: 788–9.

6. Page DL, Dupont WD. Risk factors for breast cancer in women with proliferative breast disease. N Engl J Med 1985; 312: 146–51.

7. Dupont WD, Parl FF, Hartmann WH et al. Breast cancer risk associated with proliferative breast disease and atypical hyperplasia. [Review.] Cancer 1993; 71: 1258–65.

8. Jokich PM, Monticciolo DL, Adler YT. Breast ultrasonography. Radiol Clin North Am 1992; 30: 993–1009.

9. Cosgrove DO, Kedar RP, Bamber JC et al. Breast diseases: color Doppler US in differential diagnosis. Radiology 1993; 189: 99–104.

 10. Donegan WL. Evaluation of a palpable breast mass. N Engl J Med 1992; 327: 937–42.

11. Jackson VP. The status of mammographically guided fine needle aspiration biopsy of nonpalpable breast lesions. Radiol Clin North Am 1992; 30: 155–66.

12. Sickles EA. Management of probably benign breast lesions. Radiol Clin North Am 1995; 33: 1123–30.

 13. Kaufman Z, Shpitz B, Shapiro M et al. Triple approach in the diagnosis of dominant breast masses: combined physical examination, mammography, and fine-needle aspiration. J Surg Oncol 1994; 56: 254–7.

14. Bland Kl, Love N. Evaluation of common breast masses. Postgrad Med 1992; 92: 95–7.

 15. Vetto J, Pommier R, Schmidt W et al. Use of the 'triple test' for palpable breast lesions yields high diagnostic accuracy and cost savings. Am J Surg 1995; 169: 519–22.

16. De Freitas R Jr, Hamed H, Fentiman I. Fine needle aspiration cytology of palpable breast lesions. Br J Clin Pract 1992; 46: 187–90.

17. Ciatto S, Bonardi R, Cariaggi MP. Performance of fine-needle aspiration cytology of the breast—multicenter study of 23 063 aspirates in ten Italian laboratories. Tumori 1995; 81: 13–7.

18. Parks AG. The microanatomy of the breast. Ann R Coll Surg Engl 1959; 25: 295–311.

19. Wilkinson S, Forrest AP, Rifkind E et al. Natural history of fibroadenoma of the breast. Br J Clin Pract 1988; 67–8.

20. Wilkinson S, Anderson TJ, Rifkind E et al. Fibroadenoma of the breast: a follow up of conservative management. Br J Surg 1989; 76: 390–1.

 21. Cant PJ, Madden MV, Close PM et al. Case for conservative management of selected fibroadenomas of the breast. Br J Surg 1987; 74: 857–9.

 22. The Bridge Study Group. The presentation and management of breast symptoms in general practice in South Wales. Br J Gen Pract 1999, 49: 811–2.

23. Preece PE, Hughes LE, Mansel RE et al. Clinical syndromes of mastalgia. Lancet 1976; ii: 670–3.

24. Preece PE, Richards AR, Owen GM, Hughes LE. Mastalgia and total body water. Br Med J 1975; 4:498–500.

25. Fentiman IS. Mastalgia mostly merits masterly inactivity [Editorial.] Br J Clin Pract 1992; 46: 158.

 26. Holland PA, Gateley CA. Drug therapy of mastalgia: what are the options? Drugs 1994; 48: 709–16.

27. Gateley CA, Miers M, Mansel RE et al. Drug treatments for mastalgia: 17 years' experience in the Cardiff mastalgia clinic. J R Soc Med 1992; 85: 12–15.

 28. Mansel RE, Dogliotti L. European multicentre trial of bromocriptine in cyclical mastalgia. Lancet 1990; 335: 190–3.

 29. Mansel RE, Wisbey JR, Hughes LE. Controlled trial of the antigonadotrophin danazol in painful nodular benign breast disease. Lancet 1982; i: 928–31.

 30. Pashby NL, Mansel RE, Hughes LE et al. A clinical trial of evening primrose oil in mastalgia. Br J Surg 1981; 68: 801.

 31. Fentiman I, Caleffi M, Brame K et al. Double blind controlled trial of tamoxifen therapy for mastalgia. Lancet 1986; i: 287–8.

32. Mansel RE. Reproductive factors associated with mastalgia. Cancer Detect Prev 1992; 16: 39–41.

33. Euhus DM, Uyehara C. Influence of parenteral progesterones on the prevalence and severity of mastalgia in premenopausal women: a multi-institutional cross-sectional study. J Am Coll Surg 1997; 184: 596–604.

34. Miller WR, Dixon JM, Scott WN *et al.* Classification of human cysts according to electrolyte and androgen conjugate composition. Clin Oncol 1983; 9: 227–32.

35. Bruzzi P, Dogliotti L, Naldoni C *et al.* Cohort study of association of risk of breast cancer with cyst type in women with gross cystic disease of the breast. BMJ 1997; 314: 925–8.

36. Dixon JM, McDonald C, Elton RA *et al.* Risk of breast cancer in women with palpable breast cysts: a prospective study. Edinburgh Breast Group. Lancet 1999, 353: 1742–5.

37. Webb AJ. Mammary duct ectasia—periductal mastitis complex. Br J Surg 1995; 82: 1300–2.

2 Breast screening and screen-detected disease

Michelle H. Mullan
Mark W. Kissin

In July 1985 a committee was set up in the UK under the chairmanship of Professor Sir Patrick Forrest to consider information available on breast cancer screening by mammography. The committee was to examine the provision of mammographic facilities in the UK, and the screening of symptomless women and to evaluate the means to implement a screening policy. The Forrest report was published in 1986 and the principal conclusion was that the introduction of mass screening by mammography would lead to a reduction in breast cancer mortality by 25%.[1] On the basis of these findings, UK population breast screening was introduced in 1988 and it is now universally available.

The breast screening programme in the UK was modelled on the randomised controlled trial carried out in the Swedish two counties, which screened women aged 40–74, with a screening interval of 24 months for those under 50 and 33 months for the older group, using a single 45 degree oblique mammographic view alone.[2] As the UK screening experience and audit of performance has been accumulating over 10 years, the results have been compared step by step with the outcomes of the Swedish two counties study. Modifications have been made to the UK programme to improve on the Swedish experience where possible, and current results suggest outcomes that will be superior to the original Swedish trials.

At the time the Forrest report was being prepared there was no evidence that clinical examination, breast ultrasonography or breast self-examination were effective tools for screening. Evidence did exist in the form of several randomised controlled trials and case-control studies showing that mortality from breast cancer could be reduced in women attending for mammographic screening. This evidence is summarised in **Table 2.1**. Using meta-analysis, Kertilowske *et al.* showed that for women in the age group 50–74 years, screening mammography reduced the death rate by 26% regardless of the number of mammographic views, the screening interval or the duration of follow-up.[3] For

Study	Date	Age	Study type	Interval (months)	No of views	Clinical examination	Screening Rounds of mammography	Follow-up year	Outcome (RR)	Last reported
Edinburgh	1979	45–64	RCT	24	2	✓	4	14	−21%	1999
Malmo	1976	45–69	RCT	18–24	2	✗	6	12	−9% to −14%	1995
Two counties	1977	70–74	RCT	24–33	1	✗	5–6	12	−26% to −36%	1995
Canada, 1	1980	40–49	RCT	12	2	✓	5	7	36%*	1992
Canada, 2	1980	50–59	RCT	12	2	✓	5	7	−3%*	1992
Health Insurance Plan	1963	40–64	RCT	12	2	✓	4	16	−29%	1995
Stockholm	1981	40–64	RCT	28	1	✗	3	11	−20%	1997
Gothenburg	1982	40–59	RCT	18	2	✗	3	7	−14%	1997
DOM	1974	50–64	C-C	26	2	✓	5	7–12	−70%	1997
Florence	1977	40–70	C-C	30	2	✗	3–7	7–10	−43%	1997
Nijmegen	1975	35–65	C-C	24	1	✗	4	7–8	−49%	1997
UK	1979	45–64	C-C	24	1	✓	4	16	−27%	1999

RR, relative risk of death; RCT, randomised controlled trial; C-C, case-control study. Negative score confers benefit. *Only two trials not showing significant benefit.

Table 2.1 Evidence for benefit of breast screening

younger women aged between 40 and 49 years the most reliable information at that time came from the Swedish randomised trials, showing a 13% reduction in mortality from cancer. This reduction in mortality only appeared after 8 years of follow-up, at which time survival curves seemed to diverge at a time coinciding with the women going through the menopause.

Despite strong evidence that screening saves lives (evidence 1A), it has recently been called into question.[4] Gotzsche and Olsen judged there was no reliable evidence that screening decreased deaths from breast cancer by excluding six of the eight large randomised trials. The basis for such action was minor statistical irregularities of the randomisation process. De Koning, commenting on this public health announcement, believed that the evidence for screening/ saving lives was still evidence grade 1A.[5] Furthermore, the directors of the NHS Breast Screening Programme (NHSBSP) firmly repudiated the finding of Gotzsche and Olsen and called their interpretation into question. The UK programme remains confident of its clear and significant achievements to date and for reduction in mortality in the future.[6]

In this chapter the screening process, changes in the surgical process mandated by screen-detected disease and the success of the programme are examined and new directions for the 21st century are considered.

The screening process

Organisation of service

The process of screening in the UK is undertaken under the supervision of 90 screening centres. The size and location of these vary from region to region and are a mixture of fixed and mobile units. A standard so-called 'Forrest' unit was designed to screen a population of 41 000 women in the target age group of 50–64 years. Sophisticated computer networks have been developed, in conjunction with general practitioner lists, to ensure women in the target group are identified and receive an invitation for screening. For screening to be successful, over 70% of the target population must accept their invitation, bearing in mind that the Swedish uptake was 86%. The number of women attending for first screening mammograms (prevalence screen) is usually lower than those attending subsequent screening rounds (incidence screen). The values for acceptance for invitation to screening in the UK in 1997/98 was 73% for the prevalent screen and 86.6% for the incident screen. Where individual general practices or screening centres start to fall below this level of acceptance, extra publicity campaigns are mounted to improve uptake. The levels of uptake are lower in inner city conurbations for a variety of reasons. In more remote areas of the country so-called 'clients' may not attend because of transport problems. Thus for 1998/99 uptake in south west London was 71% compared with 78% in mid-Surrey. In 1997/98 the lowest uptake was in the North Thames region (62%) and the highest in the Trent region (80%). The screening centres are staffed by healthcare professionals who are trained and well motivated in the screening process. This team works together with clear screening protocols, agreed patterns of referral, built-in quality assurance programmes and continuing audit and education. The first phase of the breast screening project was concerned mainly with development of the screening centres, recruitment of trained staff and setting standards to assess the whole process. The second phase was one of consolidation and learning as the first round of screening became complete. The third and current phase involves the development of end points, resetting new standards and defining treatment outcomes. The last involves true mortality statistics from patients screened in the early years and surrogate end points using prognostic variables for the more recent patients. Six training units were established to educate members of screening teams (Edinburgh, Guildford, King's College Hospital, Manchester, Nottingham and Cardiff). The organisation of the screening process is summarised in **Figure 2.1**, and the current standards for radiological and surgical quality assurance are listed in **Table 2.2**.

The basic screen

The basic screen is carried out on a series of mobile of static mammographic units sited on an assessment centre. The mobile units are parked for several weeks in a high profile location for the target community, e.g. supermarket car parks or large general practitioner health centres. At prevalence screening women have two-view mammography on each breast. After the publication of the UKCCCR trial results in 1995, a mandatory policy was introduced to use

Figure 2.1
The screening process. QA, quality assurance.

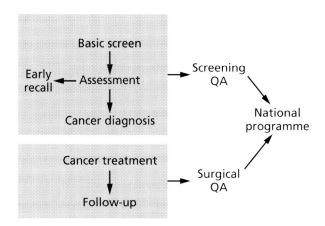

Objective	Criteria	Minimum standard	Target
To maximise the number of eligible women who attend for screening	The percentage of eligible women who attend for screening	≥70% of invited women to attend for screening	
To maximise the number of cancers detected[1]	a) The rate of invasive cancers detected in eligible women invited and screened b) The rate of cancers detected which are *in situ* carcinoma c) Standardised detection ratio	Prevalent screen ≥2.7 per 1000 Incident screen ≥3.0 per 1000 Prevalent screen ≥0.4 to ≥0.9 per 1000 Incident screen ≥0.5 to ≤1.0 per 1000 ≥0.75	Prevalent screen ≥3.6 per 1000 Incident screen ≥4.0 per 1000 ≥1.0
To maximise the number of small invasive cancers	The rate of invasive cancers less than 15 mm in diameter detected in eligible women invited and screened	Prevalent screen ≥1.5 per 1000 Incident screen ≥1.65 per 1000	Prevalent screen ≥2.0 per 1000 Incident screen ≥2.2 per 1000

To achieve optimum image quality	a) High contrast spatial resolution
	b) Minimal detectable contrast (approximately)
	  5–6 mm detail
	  0.5 mm detail
	c) Standard film density
		≥101 p mm^{-1}
		
		≤1%
		≤5%
		1.4–1.8	

To limit radiation dose	Mean glandular dose per film to standard breast using a grid	≤2 mGy	
To minimise the number of women undergoing repeat examinations	The number of repeat examinations	<3% of total examinations	<2% of total examinations
To minimise the number of women screened who are referred for further tests[1]	a) The percentage of women who are referred for assessment b) The percentage of women screened who are placed on early recall	Prevalent screen <10% Incident screen <7%
<1%	Prevalent screen <7% Incident screen <5%
≤0.25%
To ensure that most cancers, both palpable and impalpable, receive a non-operative tissue diagnosis of cancer	The percentage of women who have a non-operative diagnosis of cancer by cytology or needle histology	≥70%	
To minimise the number of unnecessary operative procedures	The rate of benign biopsies	Prevalent round <3.6 per 1000 Incident round <2.0 per 1000	Prevalent round <1.8 per 1000 Incident round <1.0 per 1000

Table 2.2 Standards for the NHS breast screening programme (updated August 1998)

To minimise the number of cancers in the women screened presenting between screening episodes[1]	The rate of invasive cancers presenting in screened women a) In the years after a normal screening episode b) In the third year after a normal screening episode	**Expected standard** 1.2 per 1000 women screened in the first 2 years 1.3 women per 1000 women screened in the third year	
To ensure that women are recalled for screening at appropriate intervals	The percentage of eligible women whose first offered appointment is within 36 months of their screen	≥90%	100%
To minimise anxiety for women who are awaiting the results of screening	The percentage of women who are sent their result within 2 weeks	≥90%	100%
To minimise the interval from the screening mammogram to assessment	The percentage of women who attend an assessment centre within 1 week of the decision that further investigation is necessary and within 3 weeks of attendance for the screening mammogram	≥90%	100%
To minimise the delay before examination screened who are referred for further tests[1]	Time interval between the first assessment appointment and surgical assessment	≤5 working days	Same day (surgeon present at an assessment clinic)
To minimise the interval between a surgical decision to operate for diagnostic purposes and the first offered admission date[2]	The percentage of women who are offered an admission date within 2 weeks of the surgical decision to operate for diagnostic purposes.	≥90%	100%
To minimise the interval between a surgical decision to operate for therapeutic purposes (i.e. where there is a preoperative definitive diagnosis of cancer) and the first offered date[2]	The percentage of women who are admitted within 3 weeks of informing the patient that she needs surgical treatment	≥90%	100%

Table 2.2 *continued*

two views for all prevalent screens.[8] This is significantly different from the Swedish study where only one oblique view was taken. Physical examination is not carried out. A questionnaire is filled in by the women, and details of any symptoms are noted by the radiographer for the benefit of the radiology team reading the mammograms; this may be enough to trigger recall for assessment. Screens are repeated every 3 years up to the age of 64, with a minimum of a single oblique view. Many centres now use two views. Women are invited practice by practice, and some are brought into the screening programme aged 50 or just under, 51 or 52 years. After the age of 64 women no longer receive invitations but are eligible for screening on demand. Relatively few women over the age of 65 routinely use this service, with only 86 000 doing so in 1997/98.[7] At the end of any screening day the mobile units return the films to the central base where they are processed and read by a radiologist with a specialist interest in breast imaging. Quality assurance standards ensure expertise in mammographic interpretation. In many units double reading is now carried out, with arbitration by a third opinion if the two film readers cannot agree. The results of the screening are communicated to the patient within two weeks.

Assessment

Women are recalled for assessment for two reasons. Firstly, a technical recall may occur when the mammographic films fail to reach standard quality features owing to errors in exposure, developing or positioning (**Fig. 2.2**). Secondly, women with a true radiological abnormality are recalled for clinical assessment. This process may include further standard or specialised views of the breast, including magnification and paddle compression views. Clinical examination and ultrasonography are performed and, where necessary, five needle aspiration cytology (FNAC) for palpable lumps and image-guided cytology and/or core biopsy for impalpable lesions. A small number of women are reviewed in early recall when the degree of abnormality is not sufficient to warrant an intervention but not so minor as to go back to triennial screening. In women found to have a definitive abnormality a positive diagnosis should be achieved. In 1998/99 1 668 476 women were invited for screening and 75.1% attended. Overall, 71 255 (5.3%) were recalled for assessment. In the same year 80% of women with cancers received a preoperative diagnosis either by cytology or by core biopsy, with a range for impalpable cancers of 47% (North Western region) to 85% (Northern Ireland) and for palpable cancer a range of 51% (East Anglia) to 89% (Trent).[7]

Cost

The cost of a basic screen for an individual client was £12 in 1986. The cost of the whole project is expensive in healthcare terms. In 1986 the capital cost at the outset of the screening project was estimated at £31 000 000 and an £18 000 000 annual running cost. The cost of a quality of life adjusted year

Figure 2.2
Technical problems, two view versus one view, interval cancer. Mammograms from 58-year-old woman with a left-sided cancer. (a) 45 degree oblique view 1995 showed no specific abnormality. At that stage a single view was taken. The star indicates the pectoralis major muscle and for technical reasons this muscle should come down further towards the back of the plate. The lower inner quadrant is not adequately imaged. (b) 45 degree view 1996 when presenting with interval lump in lower inner quadrant. Arrow shows an edge of a lesion again not well visualised. (c) Craniocaudal view with obvious tumour (arrowed) in most medial aspect of breast.

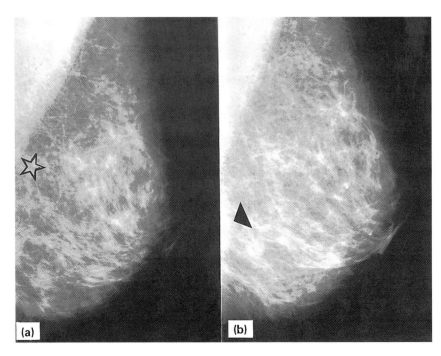

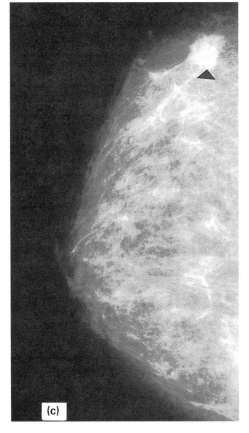

gained by screening was estimated at £3310. This translates to similar cost of the benefits of kidney transplantation. In 1992 the Humberside screening service found that the cost of each cancer detected was £5533, with an average cost of £32 per woman screened.[9] In 1996 the national running costs had increased to £25 000 000.

Trials

Number of views

The original Forrest report concluded that one 45 degree oblique mammogram was the screening gold standard.[1] A randomised controlled trial in nine breast screening centres in England involved 40 163 women who were randomised to have one view, two views or two views in which one view was read by one reader and both views were read by another. In addition to detecting 24% more cancers, two-view mammography was associated with a 15% lower recall rate. The cost of the two-view screening was higher but the average cost of each cancer detected was similar. The trial concluded that two-view mammography was medically more effective,[8] and in 1995/96 the basic screen consisted of two views (Fig. 2.2). Further studies went on to examine the potential for improved performance by introducing two views for the incident rounds. Blanks *et al.* found an increase in sensitivity of 9% and specificity of 5.4% with two views, with the second view being most beneficial when the tumour was off the oblique plate owing to a lower medial position or when an asymmetrical or round mass had a vague non-specific appearance, often clarified by the extra view as a spiculate density.[10] The double-view technique seems particularly important for small cancers of 10 mm or less, when sensitivity is increased from 71 to 85%.[11] These studies also indicated that the cancer detection rate would be increased by films being double read with arbitration, but this would unfortunately increase the cost of manpower. Computerised film reading has, therefore, been suggested.

Frequency of screening

Some European screening programmes have adopted a screening interval much shorter than the 3 years of the UK programme. A trial was therefore set up to compare 1- versus 3-year screening intervals, recruiting 100 000 women, but no hard data have yet emerged. There are some data, using surrogate end points, which have predicted mortality on the basis of the Nottingham Prognostic Index (NPI).[12] The predicted 10-year mortality for annual screening was 34.4 versus 35.5% for the 3-year group[13] probably because extra cancers found by more frequent screening are counterbalanced by extra-interval cancers found in the 3-year cycle.

The optimum screening interval remains variable throughout the Western world, without consensus. The American Medical Association, American Cancer Society and American College of Radiology have recommended two-view films every year for all women over the age of 40. This would not be a practical proposition in the UK.

Screening younger women

There has been considerable debate regarding the benefit of screening women under the age of 50. The so-called 'forties' trial examined this question, but as yet there are no data that have been released. There has been a lack of enthusiasm for seeing the trial completed owing to political, economic and organisational issues because screening this age group has greater demands on quality control. Screening in this age group is more difficult as the breasts tend to be denser and the natural incidence of cancer is lower. The cancer detection rate is smaller and the cost per cancer detected and life saved higher. Balanced against the greater potential for saving lives by screening older women, screening women under 50 has few champions. In 1995, 53 000 women were screened under the age of 50 and 156 cancers were found, a detection rate of 2.9 per 1000.

National results from the forties' trial will not be available for a further 5 years so the subject remains controversial. Nonetheless, results of the Trial of Early Detection of Breast Cancer controlled study and the Edinburgh randomised trial have suggested major benefits for screening women aged 45 to 49.[14,15] Other centres in the UK have not found as many cancers as in the pilot sites. Difficulties in identifying cancers in the dense breasts of these women are highlighted in **Figs 2.3, 2.4** and **2.5**.

Screening older women

The Forrest programme adopted an upper age limit of 64 despite the fact that the incidence of breast cancer continues to rise as women get older. This age limit causes concern in pressure groups for elderly women and brought criticism of an ageist stance being adopted by the screening programme. This was further emphasised by a higher screening age limit in other parts of Europe, varying between 69 and 74 years. Chen *et al.* reported that breast screening was just as effective in reducing mortality in women aged 65 to 69 as it was in women aged 50 to 64.[16] Currently women over the age of 64 are entitled to self-refer every 3 years, but after pressure to extend the screening up to the age

Figure 2.3
Craniocaudal mammograms of patient from prevalent round of forties' screening trial. The breast contains vague densities; however, there was multifocal grade 3 cancer extending for 11 cm, which does not image well, and the patient had more than 10 positive nodes and liver metastases at presentation.

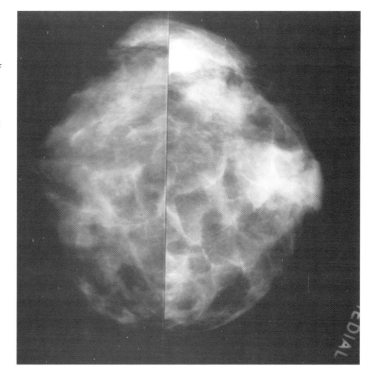

Figure 2.4
Prevalent round forties' trial showing rounded density in the upper part of the left breast, but both breasts are dense and difficult to define. Patient had mastectomy and immediate reconstruction chemotherapy and tamoxifen for a grade 2 cancer with four positive nodes. She is disease free 7 years later.

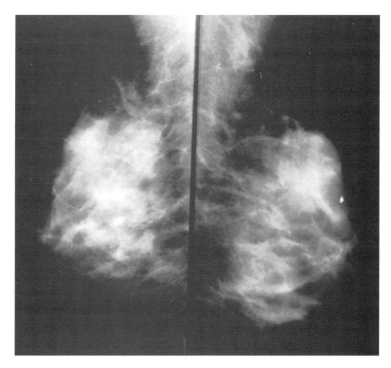

Figure 2.5
Forties' screening trial, images of 1992 (left) and 1993 (right). 1993 shows subtle multifocal calcification suggestive of ductal carcinoma in situ (DCIS), which is difficult to see. Patient had mastectomy and immediate reconstruction and had 6 cm of high-grade DCIS with microinvasion. Five years later she developed widespread distant metastases indicating that the microinvasive component was biologically aggressive.

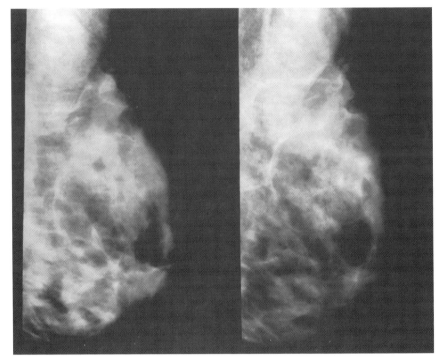

of 70, a pilot study will examine the issues. Rubin *et al.* reported that more than 70% of women took up the extra invitations and, that screening was likely to be successful.[17] The House of Commons Select Committee on Breast Cancer will make judgement and recommendations based on these results.

The number of women aged 65 and over attending for screening in 1997/98 increased by almost 30% compared with the previous year and reflects the increasing awareness of older women. The statistics for the 86 240 women screened in 1997/98 showed that only 5.4% were recalled for assessment compared with 5.3% in the 50–64 age group, but the cancer detection rate was 10.7 per 1000 compared with 5.9 in the younger group.[7] The NHSBSP launched a video in June 1998 in conjunction with Age Concern to encourage women over 65 to attend for screening.

Changes in practice

Pathology

The same pathological entities found in patients with symptoms were also found by the screening process, but the 'lead-time' effect meant a shift in prognostic features to the better end of the spectrum. An increased number of non-invasive and special types of cancer of a less aggressive nature may account for the so-called 'lag-time' bias.

Radial scars

Radial scars or complex sclerosing lesions are one of the commonest benign entities found by the screening process. The radiological features that distinguish them from stellate cancers is the presence of the long radicals radiating from the central core. Characteristically they are seen better on one mammographic view than another. They are almost always asymptomatic, and sometimes the mammographic features can be alarming. Some are associated with more serious pathology. In a series of 43 radial scars, 35% were associated with cancer and a further 12% with atypical ductal hyperplasia. When cancer was present it was either ductal carcinoma in situ (DCIS), tubular cancer or infiltrating duct cancer that was grade 1 and node negative.[18] It is difficult to know whether these are cancers in evolution or involution. At present there is still no reliable mammographic or cytological sign to distinguish the benign from the more aggressive types of radial scar, and it remains a current national recommendation that these should be removed. Attempts to understand radial scars using core biopsy have not proved totally satisfactory. An example of a radial scar taken from the forties' trial is shown in **Figure 2.6**.

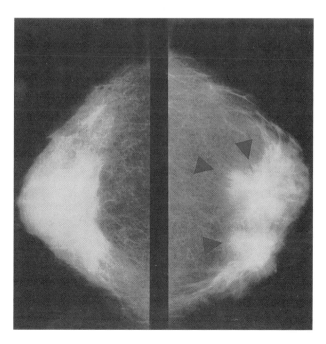

Figure 2.6
Complex sclerosing lesion (radial scar) detected in the prevalent round of the forties' trial. Craniocaudal views showing dense left breast, with arrowed spiculated densities in right breast. Histology showed radiating ducts with florid epithelial hyperplasia but no atypia.

Axillary lymph nodes

A key component to prognosis is the pathological status of axillary nodes, removed either by sampling or clearance. It is one of the three fundamental parameters of the NPI. Node positivity in symptomatic breast cancers ranges from 25 to 55%, but in screen-detected disease the rate is much lower at 15–25%.[19] The current recommendation from the quality assurance programme is that lymph nodes should be removed in all patients with invasive cancer, but not patients with DCIS alone. Despite these recommendations there is considerable variation in the practise of surgeons dealing with this issue (**Fig. 2.7**). Failure to remove nodes may lead to a false sense of security and underutilisation of appropriate adjuvant treatments. The Manchester group found that in the prevalent round very small cancers were highly unlikely to be associated with positive nodes and, therefore, a lymph node procedure could theoretically be omitted. However, they have found that the rate of lymph node positivity is higher in the incidence rounds than in those from the first round.[20] The national figures for the year ending 1998/99 show that 90% of women with screen-detected invasive cancer had lymph node status recorded, and overall 23% had node-positive disease.[21] The use of sentinel lymph node assessment looks promising in the context of screen-detected cancers because it is particularly accurate for small cancers and in younger women.[22] The combined approach utilising preoperative scintigraphy, peroperative gamma-probe localisation of radio-active nodes and intraoperative mapping with Vital V blue dye is recommended. An example of a screen-detected cancer with sentinel node mapping is shown in **Figure 2.8**.

Figure 2.7
Lymph node status by region for invasive cancers detected in 1997/98. In a total of 6427 invasive cancers, 22% were node positive, 65% were node negative, 13% had an unknown nodal status and 9% had <4 nodes retrieved.

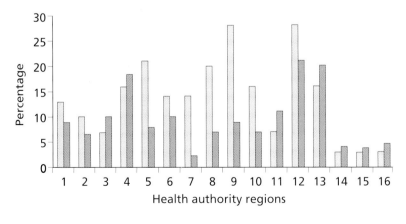

□ Nodal status not obtained
▨ <4 nodes obtained

TMN

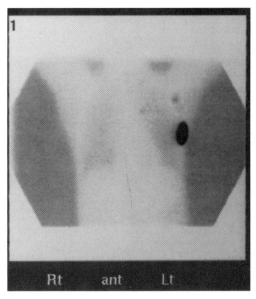
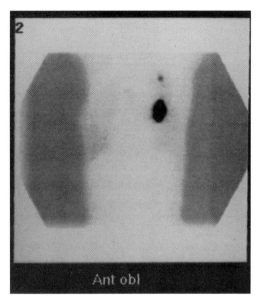

Figure 2.8
Scan of a sentinel node in a 37-year-old woman with a 10 mm invasive ductal carcinoma and both an internal mammary sentinel node and an axillary sentinel node. Both nodes were hot, and the axillary node was blue. The nodes were free from metastases.

DCIS

In symptomatic breast cancer, DCIS accounts for 4% of all cancers, but in screen-detected disease it is present in up to 20%. This increase in numbers of non-invasive cancers has led to a reclassification of this pathological entity according to cell type and necrosis rather than pure morphological features. An example of screen-detected DCIS is shown in **Figure 2.9**. When DCIS is widespread the treatment of choice is a mastectomy. This may come as a shock to a patient who has no symptoms, and such women should be offered immediate breast reconstruction whenever possible to lighten the psychological trauma. The role of sentinel node assessment in patients with extensive DCIS remains controversial but may be an important future staging procedure. When DCIS is more localised, initial surgical treatment of choice is wide local excision by needle localisation biopsy (NLB). Having obtained local control it may be prudent to consider the use of both radiotherapy and tamoxifen as providing optimum protection against further similar change in the future. Trials have been completed in America, Europe and the UK (see below).

Within the screening context DCIS is almost always impalpable, and the diagnosis depends on image-guided procedures. Not infrequently more than one procedure will be required as the extent of the disease is commonly underestimated by mammograms. Silverstein has proposed a useful working classification and prognostic index which looks at cell type, presence of comedo necrosis, the extent of the change and the margins of surgical resection.[23] Patients with the highest scores are best managed by subsequent mastectomy,

Figure 2.9
Magnification views of a central area in the left breast of a 65-year-old woman with ductal carcinoma in situ (DCIS). The appearances show typical calcifications without density. This was the patient's second invitation for screening and she was asymptomatic and the calcification had been absent 3 years previously. Histology showed a 10 mm zone of large cell comedo DCIS with secure margins. Patient was randomised to adjuvant treatment with tamoxifen as part of DCIS trial.

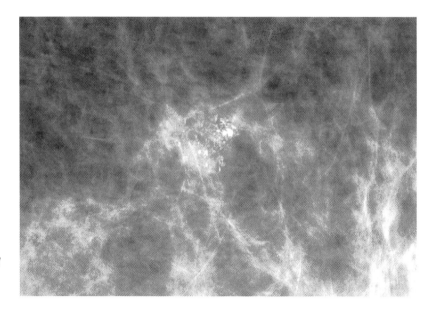

those with intermediate scores by radiotherapy with or without tamoxifen, whereas those with the lowest scores require surgery alone.

Special types

Special types of breast cancer are found with much greater frequency in screened populations and include tubular, tubular mixed, cribriform, mucoid and papillary cancers as well as small infiltrating grade 1 duct tumours. The quality assurance target mandates that these should account for more than 30% of all invasive cancers detected by screening, and it is expected that more than 50% of invasive cancers will be less than 15 mm in diameter. Patients with these special type cancers are suitable to be entered into the British Association of Surgical Oncology (BASO) 2 trial (see below).

Techniques for diagnosis

In symptomatic breast clinics the diagnosis of cancer is established utilising clinical examination, mammography, ultrasonography and FNAC or core needle biopsy. These tests can usually be conducted as a one-stop process, with the advantage that the patient can be counselled and have a care plan formulated at the initial visit.[24] The main difference in screen-detected cancer is an increased number of impalpable lesions. Thus in 1997/98, 2150 palpable cancers were diagnosed by screening versus 5510 impalpable ones. This places a greater emphasis on new techniques for evaluating and diagnosing impalpable lesions.

FNAC

Until 1994 the commonest method of obtaining a diagnosis from an impalpable lesion involved image-guided cytology using stereotactic mammography or ultrasonographic guided sampling. A computerised device is added to a conventional mammographic unit and this calculates the co-ordinates of the impalpable lesion. Using a 21 gauge needle, cytology samples are taken by 7–10 passes in a single plane.[25] An example is shown in **Figure 2.10**.

Cytology has a high sensitivity (55–80%) and specificity (56–80%), a high positive protective value (99%) and a low false negative rate (0–19%).[26] The inadequacy rate is anything up to 26%.

The main complications are vasovagal attack and haematoma formation. Cytology lends itself to the one-stop process, with diagnosis the same day. The main problem is the inadequacy rate and the impossibility of differentiating between invasive cancer and DCIS. The technique demands an experienced cytologist. Cytology can also be used to predict grade and hormonal receptor status.[27] Ultrasonographic guided FNAC is quicker and easier to perform provided the lesion is visible by sound waves. It enables real-time positioning of the needle, so that the size of the sampling area is reduced (**Fig. 2.11**). The method is not practical for lesions consisting of microcalcification alone or mild architectural distortion.

Core biopsy

Since 1994 stereotactic core biopsy has considerably improved the preoperative diagnostic rate. Local anaesthetic is used to infiltrate around the core placement site, and for optimal results five passes are made using a 14 gauge needle fired from an automated biopsy gun. Preoperative diagnosis can increase to 90% with such techniques, leading to a 64% reduction in the need for

Figure 2.10
Stereotactic fine needle aspiration biopsy. Arrow shows zone of microcalcification without density with right and left parallax images showing the needle within the zone of interest.

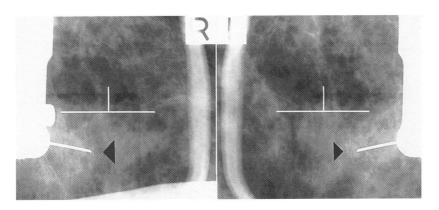

Figure 2.11
Ultrasound-guided fine needle aspiration (FNA) biopsy and localisation in a 60-year-old woman without breast symptoms. (a) Ultrasound-guided FNA biopsy needle tip (NT) shown in real time within cancer (C). (b) Ultrasound image prior to excision. (c) Specimen radiograph showing adequate margin of resection. The histology showed an 8 mm infiltrating duct cancer grade 1 (subscore 3), negative nodes and no DCIS or vascular invasion. Prognostic index score 2.2, no further adjuvant therapy.

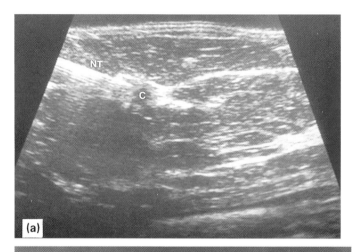

(a)

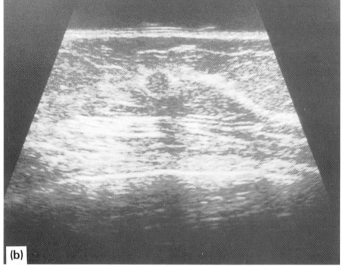

(b)

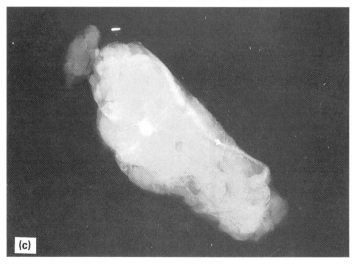

(c)

diagnostic open biopsies.[28] It is particularly useful in the preoperative assessment of lesions thought to be pure DCIS. This in turn improves the management of operating lists and surgical decision making.

In summary, for palpable lesions either cytology or core biopsy should prove successful in up to 90% of women. For impalpable lesions that are present on mammograms as calcifications alone, stereotactic core biopsy is now the preferred method. Impalpable lesions visible by ultrasonography can have guided FNAC or core biopsy. In 1997/98, 71% of impalpable breast cancers were diagnosed preoperatively whereas only 73% of those with a palpable lesion had a preoperative diagnosis.

Vacuum-assisted mammotomy

A recently developed method of minimally invasive breast biopsy involves the use of a directional vacuum-assisted instrument. The Mammotome (Ethicon Endo-Surgery, Berkshire, UK) works on an entirely different principle from an ordinary core biopsy gun. Instead of a tru-cut-style needle that collects tissue in a sample notch and that must be withdrawn after each passage, the instrument uses vacuum to retrieve tissue and therefore the probe does not have to be withdrawn each time. Larger amounts of tissue can be removed as the probe is rotated while in the breast. Once the target lesion has successfully been biopsied a metallic clip can be placed down the instrument to mark the biopsy site, which is useful for further assessment and surgical procedures. The suction aspect of the device ensures that there is little haematoma. A variety of vacuum-assisted biopsy guns can be used in conjunction with upright or prone table mammographic units or jury-rigged ultrasound machines (**Fig. 2.12**).

Ultrasonography

High frequency ultrasound (13 MHz) enables the detection of nearly all screen-detected mass lesions of the breast. When high frequency ultrasonography is used in conjunction with colour flow Doppler technology there is a greater reliance on the differentiation between benign and malignant lesions. The European Group for Breast Cancer Screening (EGBCS) felt that although ultrasonography was a useful adjunct to mammography it was by itself an unsuitable screening tool.[29, 30]

Magnetic resonance imaging

Magnetic resonance imaging (MRI) of the breast is an exciting new sophisticated diagnostic tool. Screening by MRI is free of ionising radiation and can be combined with intravenous non-specific extracellular gadolinium contrast based

Figure 2.12
*A mammotome.
Under stereotactic
or ultrasound
guidance the
probe is
positioned in the
breast to align the
aperture with the
lesion. Tissue is
gently vacuum
aspirated into the
aperture and the
rotating cutter is
advanced forward.
The cutter is
withdrawn,
transporting the
specimen to the
tissue collection
chamber while the
outer probe
remains in the
breast. With
permission
from Ethicon
Endo-Surgery,
Bracknell,
Berkshire.*

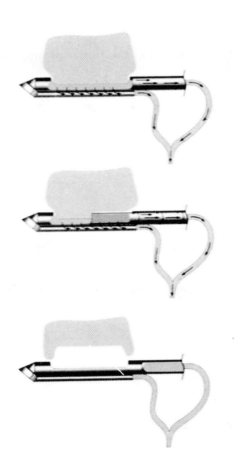

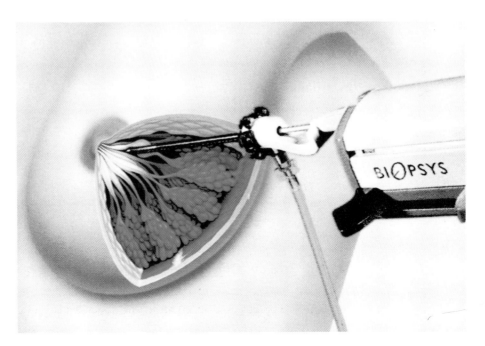

agents.[31] MRI may be better at detecting multicentric tumours than conventional mammograms and provides the highest spatial resolution of a breast cancer, by greatly enhancing lesion conspicuity. The sensitivity varies between 95 and 100%.[32] MRI may be especially useful, albeit costly, in the screening of women with increased genetic risk of breast cancer.

Digital mammography

Digital mammography is currently under evaluation as a means to improve the diagnostic accuracy of conventional mammography. It allows more flexibility with exposures, amplification of contrast and reduction of exposure areas and allows easier storage on optical disks of the computerised digital images. There is no difference between digital and conventional mammography regarding microcalcification assessment. At present the main disadvantage is the high cost of introducing digital machines as well as the time taken to both screen and read the digital image, even though it is in real time.[31]

Scintimammography

Scintimammography using 99Tc-sestamibi and allied agents has a high sensitivity and specificity for the detection of breast cancer, but only for large lesions. The sensitivity for tumours less than 1 cm is not good enough for this technique to be used in screening at the present time.[33]

Computer-aided diagnosis

Computer-aided diagnosis is a promising new area that could substantially decrease the cost of screening by taking away manpower requirements. It may be particularly useful with digital mammography in the detection of cancers situated within a dense breast. Computer-aided diagnosis is very successful in identifying microcalcifications.[34]

New surgical procedures

As the screening process moves from the prevalent to the incident rounds more of the abnormalities detected will be asymptomatic and impalpable. The majority of screen-detected cancers are suitable for breast conservation surgery. The technique of needle localisation allows two primary aims of breast conserving surgery: satisfactory tumour control and good cosmetic appearance. The surgeon is responsible for orientating the specimen for accurate pathological assessment.

Figure 2.13
Needle localisation biopsy. (a) Hawkins 2 needle inserted from above with needle tip close to microcalcifications (arrowed). Calcifications were new on second screen having been absent 3 years previously. Stereotactic cytology was positive for cancer. (b) Specimen radiograph confirming excision of calcifications (arrowed). Note ligaclips used to orientate specimen. Histology showed 10 mm zone of large cell comedo ductal carcinoma in situ (DCIS) with 5 mm margins. Patient was randomised to receive tamoxifen as part of DCIS trial.

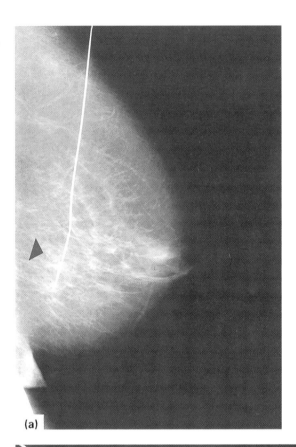

(a)

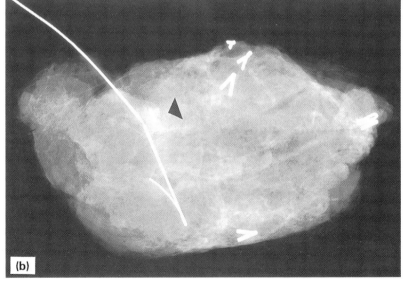

(b)

Needle localisation biopsy

Needle localisation biopsy requires close cooperation between surgeon and radiologist. A needle is placed into the breast with the aid of ultrasonography, or

X-ray control using a stereotactic machine, grid system or ultrasound probe. A variety of different needles with fixation devices can be used. An example is shown in **Figure 2.13** with a Hawkins 2 needle, which has a hook that flicks into position after accurate placement at the target. Needles are usually inserted from either a superior or a lateral aspect. It is not always necessary to follow the pathway of the needle during surgery. Thus it is possible to calculate the position of the needle tip and plan to intercept it close to the target lesion.[35] The aim of needle localisation biopsy is to remove a ball of tissue with the needle tip and target at its centre. If the procedure is being done for diagnostic purposes the weight of the specimen should not exceed 20 g and the time taken for the specimen check radiography to be back in theatre should not exceed 10 minutes.[36] If the procedure is being done for therapeutic reasons then a larger weight of tissue is usually excised to give a minimum of 10 mm margins. Two-view specimen radiography is preferred, and if one of the margins seems too close, further tissue should be taken immediately. If a diagnosis of cancer has not been previously established the use of frozen section is discouraged, particularly if the target is microcalcification alone. More than 80% of marker wires should be within 10 mm of the target in any one plane, and more than 95% of impalpable lesions should be correctly removed at the first localisation biopsy. The best images of the removed specimen are obtained by radiography of the specimen on the mammographic unit with maximum compression. This will sometimes reveal extra radiological abnormalities that were not appreciated on ordinary mammographic films. Factors involved with successful needle localisation are related to the experience of the surgeon and the size of the target lesion.[37]

One-stage surgery

The primary aim of the screening service is to reduce the number of unnecessary biopsies to a minimum. The increased use of preoperative cytology and core biopsy means that most patients with impalpable cancer do have a positive diagnosis prior to their first surgical intervention. If the target is microcalcification alone there is a strong possibility that this represents non–invasive disease, and a day–case procedure can be undertaken without need to disturb the axilla. If subsequent definitive histology shows the presence of invasive disease then lymph nodes are removed at a second intervention. A second surgical procedure is also required if the margins around the cancer are less than 5 mm (preferably 10 mm).

When the diagnosis of cancer is established in an impalpable lesion with features of either asymmetric density, spiculate density or a complex lesion, then a one-stage surgical procedure involving removal of the cancer and lymph nodes can be carried out with the assumption that this is an invasive tumour. Quality assurance guidelines suggest that in 90% of patients where a preoperative diagnosis is established no further surgery should be required for incomplete excision. Once the learning curve has been negotiated all centres should report improved usage of one-stage surgery. The Avon screening service reported a 77% inadequate surgical clearance rate during a learning curve, but only in 19% of these was the preoperative diagnosis of cancer established.[38] Increasing the preoperative diagnostic rate decreases the need for second operations, although problems commonly persist with DCIS as X-ray films underestimate the extent of microscopic change. The national average for preoperative diagnosis of impalpable cancers was 80% (range 70% to 89%). In the screening year 1998/99, 6449 cancers had a positive preoperative diagnosis, and 84% of these were removed in a single operation because of that. Fifteen percent required two operations and 1% three or more procedures. Image-guided biopsy is now such an accurate procedure that only 1.3% of impalpable lesions require more than one operation.

Care of the specimen

It is a surgeon's responsibility to ensure the correct orientation of the specimen for pathological assessment. A variety of systems have been devised to ensure this. The safest is placement of metal clips in a set pattern.[39] This aids identification of margins during the operation and subsequent studies in the pathology laboratory. A series of ligatures can be placed in set directions, and these can be colour coded or of different lengths according to the margin concerned. Other systems utilise pinning the specimen on a template or board. Specimens should be sent as quickly as possible to the pathology department where the margins are marked with India ink or organically coloured gelatines.[40] The stains show up on subsequent histology slides and in this way an accurate estimation of the margin can be made.

Pathology report

The minimum dataset includes the type of cancer, maximum diameter, grade, presence of DCIS, presence of vascular invasion and lymph node status. This in turn provides all the information required to construct a prognostic index and thus plan adjuvant therapy. A new addition to the minimum dataset is immunohistochemistry assessment for oestrogen receptor. In addition progesterone receptor and receptors for HER NEU oncogenes are increasingly important for directing optimum adjuvant strategy.

Therapeutic trials

DCIS trial

The DCIS trial was set up in 1990 to address adjuvant treatment after complete local excision of a small focus of DCIS. Patients were randomised on a two-by-two factorial basis comparing surgery with either tamoxifen or radiotherapy or tamoxifen and radiotherapy. The trial closed in 1998, with 1694 patients randomised. The majority of women came from the UK and one 10th from Australasia. The results of this trial are awaited. One of the key issues not addressed by this trial has been the width of safety required after a local excision but the results will be matched against trials from America (NSABP B-17) and Europe (EORTC 10853). The American trial at 8 years follow-up showed that the addition of radiotherapy to surgery for localised DCIS reduced invasive recurrence from 13.4 to 3.9% and further DCIS from 13.4 to 8.2%, concluding that radiotherapy was an essential component.[41] The European trial has recently reported its results from 4 years and shown a reduction of invasive recurrence from 8 to 4% and of non-invasive recurrence from 8 to 5%.[42] The UK DCIS trial will answer questions on the interaction of tamoxifen and radiotherapy and complement these other results.

BASO 2

A similar randomisation on a two-by-two factorial basis was used in the BASO 2 trial for patients with cancers with a good prognosis, including the various special types of cancer, which carry an expected survival prospect of more than 90%. The outcome of this trial will help decide whether radiotherapy can safely be withheld in certain groups with a good prognosis, be associated with a significant reduction in the cost of treatment and reduce potential side effects. Unlike the DCIS trial it is recommended that patients entering the BASO 2 trial have a minimum of 1 cm clear tissue around each cancer. This trial is still recruiting and will eventually be reporting preliminary results in the year 2003. So far 956 patients have been entered.

Outcomes of the programme

Two undoubted strengths of the screening programme are the quality assurance measures and the enthusiasm of the staff. Through these it is possible to get results of the screening process and to record the treatments being carried out. Initially only surrogate measures of breast cancer mortality were produced in the form of a prognostic index measurement. The NPI divides patients into groups of good, medium and poor prognosis according to a scoring system.[43] This has been validated in groups of patients from 1983–87 and 1988–92. A score of less than 3.4 represents an excellent prognosis with a 10-year survival prospect of more than 85%, whereas a prognostic score of greater than 5.4 is associated with a poor prognosis with a survival prospect of below 20%. In patients with symptomatic breast cancer, 34% have a good prognosis, 52% a moderate prognosis and 14% a poor prognosis. In contrast, in a screening context 71% have a good prognosis, 25% a moderate prognosis and only 4% a poor prognosis. This shift may be preliminary evidence of breast screening obtaining its expected targets or it may represent lead-time bias. These figures only apply for invasive disease. There has also been an increase of non-invasive disease from 4% up to 1987 rising to 24% in the patients with screen-detected cancers up to 1992. Some of these patients with non-invasive disease may have progressed to invasion had they not been dealt with at this earlier stage. As well as surrogate measures of outcome the quality assurance programme has now been able to provide real evidence of 5-year survival for a cohort of women screened in the years 1992/93 and 1993/94 (see below).

Quality assurance programme

The quality assurance (QA) guidelines for surgeons involved in breast cancer screening were first published in 1992 and revised in 1996 as the first guideline document in the UK for any aspect of surgery and the first in the world for breast cancer screening.[36] The quality criteria are set out in four main domains as summarised in Table 2.2. The general performance criteria are largely dependent on the radiological process of screening and assessment and are not surgeon dependent. Biopsy quality objectives are much more surgeon oriented and also depend on cooperation between surgeon, cytologist and radiologist. Technical aspects are under scrutiny here. The treatment-related objectives are fairly loose without many specific targets. Of all the objectives the waiting times are the most contentious since it does not seem possible to admit 90% of patients with screen-detected cancer within 3 weeks of being informed of the diagnosis, owing to resource limitation.

QA inspections

Good assessment of performance of each unit is easily obtained in each screening centre. Considerable variation in performance is noted. Data from one screening centre can be broken down further to see whether specific members of that team are performing outside the guidelines.

Avoiding mistakes

Errors in the screening process occur and the QA team should identify these, clarify the problem, take corrective action and ensure that similar events are avoided. In radiology there is always a balance between sensitivity and specificity, which means a trade-off between an acceptably low recall rate and an acceptably low missed cancer rate. Missed cancers may appear as interval cancers and it is, therefore, important that surgeons involved with screening should flag any interval cancer back to the radiological QA team.

Once a patient comes to surgery, it is the surgeon's responsibility to try and make sure that all the evidence for the diagnosis of cancer is concordant. Postoperative checks that mammographically identified lesions that were impalpable have been totally removed must occur. This may be by specimen radiography or, if in doubt, early check mammography.

Changes in practice

The QA programme can produce worthwhile changes in practice at local and national levels. An example at local level would be the correction of surgical practice outside the guidelines, e.g. if the surgeon did not remove lymph nodes in patients with invasive cancer.

As far as national surgical standards are concerned, the targets set in 1996 were more stringent that those set in 1992, and these are due for further revision in the year 2000. In the old guidelines the reoperation rate was supposed to be less than 30% but is now less than 10%; the preoperative diagnostic rate was more than 60% but is now more than 70%; and the \special type of cancer rate was more than 20% and is now more than 30%. Radiological changes in standards have included the transformation from one-view to two-view mammography on the first screen, and less than 7% recall to less than 5% for the prevalent round and 5 to 3% in the incident round.

A working party has recently reported on aspects of surgical quality assurance and produced eight recommendations. It was recognised that there was no clinical oncology input to any part of the QA process, and an oncologist is now to be included in the personnel on the QA team. It is best practice to carry out QA visits on an annual basis, and QA professionals from outside should be invited to avoid stagnation and nepotism. The format of the visit should include data questionnaires completed beforehand and review of hospital case notes chosen at random by the QA reference centre. Each surgeon would have the notes of five patients with cancer and one with a benign lesion open for scrutiny to make sure that quality standards had been achieved. After a QA visit the surgical QA professional prepares a report submitted direct to the regional coordinator who in turn forwards it to the regional director of public health. Criticisms of individual breast screening surgeons are made, and surgeons are given an opportunity to comment on their performance. Attendance at multidisciplinary meetings should be mandatory and, where possible, the QA professional should make planned or unplanned visits to the multidisciplinary meeting. When shortcomings in performance have been identified solutions must be sought.

These changes to QA assessment methods have occurred as a result of failure of some screening teams e.g. Exeter 1997.[44]

National results

In the earlier years of screening the only results available were those related to the screening process rather than to measures of performance and outcome.

With the advent of robust QA systems there is a mandate for the compilation and presentation of results, culminating in two events each screening year. Each autumn the NHSBSP publishes screening results in general and in the spring there is a meeting to audit surgical performance.

Screening process data

The number of women screened in 1998/99 was 1.3 million, with an uptake of about 75% and just over 5% being recalled for assessment. The overall cancer detection rate is currently 5.8 per 1000 women screened. During 1998/99, 8028 cancers were detected, with 3381 of these being less than 15 mm in size. Data regarding the screening process is summarised in Tables 2.3 and 2.4 and the uptake, recall and cancer detection rates have remained stable over the past 6 years. As screening experience has increased the biopsy rate for benign disease has decreased and the preoperative diagnosis rate has increased.

An overall preoperative diagnostic rate of 80% was achieved in the last screening year and represents a 9% increase from the previous year, probably owing to an

	1994/95	1995/96	1996/97	1997/98
Invited (×000s)	1507	1517	1559	1668
Uptake (%)	76.7	75.8	75.2	75.1
Recall (%)	5.3	5.1	4.9	5.3
Breast biopsy	6334	6496		
Benign breast biopsy	2000	2472	3268	2212
Cancer detection rate/1000 (%)		6.3	5.6	5.9
Cancers	6500	6664	7141	7932
Small invasive cancers (<15 mm)	2660	2807	3156	3381

Table 2.3 UK national screening results (1994–98)

	Prevalent round		Incident round	
	1996/97	1997/98	1996/97	1997/98
Uptake (%)	72.5	73	87	86.6
Recall (%)	7.6	7.8	3.6	3.8
Invasive carcinoma/1000 (%)	4.8	5.0	3.7	3.8
Ductal carcinoma in situ (%)	20	23.9	19	20.9
Invasive <15 mm (%)	54	48.9	56	55.2

Table 2.4 UK national screening results (1996–98)

increased use of preoperative core biopsy. Improved performance for preoperative diagnosis was achieved for impalpable as well as palpable lesions.

Surgical performance data

Surgical data were available in the last screening year for 8028 patients with screen-detected cancer of which 79% were invasive, 20% non-invasive and 1% microinvasive disease. The proportion of non-invasive disease was higher than the 10.6% experienced in the Swedish two counties trial. This may reflect a genuine difference between the two populations.

Overall, 429 surgeons were involved in the treatment of patients with screen-detected cancer, with an average number of 20 patients each, (range 1–134). Forty-one percent of screening surgeons treated less than 10 patients a year because there is evidence from other quality targets that surgeons treating more than 50 patients a year had the best results, and 66% of women with screen-detected disease were being treated by surgeons with more than 30 patients per year. This critical number has been shown to be the threshold for which overall survival is not compromised.[45]

Nodal status was known in 90% of patients with invasive disease, reflecting a steady increase year on year from when screening first started. Sixty percent received a clearance and 34% a sampling procedure. In 6.7% of the sampling procedures less than four nodes were retrieved and the process may have been, therefore, an underestimate of true nodal activity. Twenty-seven percent of women had a mastectomy for DCIS and 28% for invasive cancer, with the number decreasing to 19% for cancers less than 15 mm in maximum dimension. The mastectomy rate for DCIS varied from region to region from 20 to 41% it is unknown how much the availability of immediate breast reconstruction affects the frequency of mastectomy.

The screening project recommends tough targets for waiting times for either a diagnostic or a therapeutic operation. The standard for a diagnostic procedure was supposed to be 14 days or less, but only 39% of women admitted for diagnostic surgery achieved this standard. The NHSBSP is also failing to deliver a waiting time of 21 days or less for therapeutic surgery, which is only achieved in 74% of patients. The reasons for failing to achieve these targets are lack of theatre time and surgical staff, clinical delay to give neoadjuvent systemic therapy or patient choice.

Survival

A total of 4864 women with invasive breast cancers detected in the screening year 1992/93 were examined in a case-specific analysis with 5 years of follow-up. This pilot study aimed to combine data retrieved from the breast screening programme with that recorded by regional cancer registries. Overall,

92.5% of the population survived to 5 years post-diagnosis without problems. The best survival rates were identified for patients with small, grade 1, node-negative tumours. This pilot study has shown that survival analysis at a national level is possible through collaboration between screening surgeons and the data managers. The pilot study confirmed the prognostic index score as an accurate reflection of eventual outcome.

Individualising results

The national picture contains variations between regions, and a regional picture can hide variations between different screening centres and in turn differences in policy by different surgical teams. Moritz *et al.* looked at 600 women with screen-detected disease presenting during 1991–92 in one region.[46] There was broad agreement on the use of adjuvent tamoxifen in 94% of women but only 2.5% received chemotherapy. Nineteen percent of patients having breast conservation failed to have radiotherapy, including a significant number of patients with adverse local features. This suggested that some of the screening teams were not working in a true multidisciplinary manner.

Problems

Data collection

Various domains of data retrieval are easy, whereas others are more difficult to obtain. There is good quality information now consistently available from the screening process. Treatment information is much better than it has been in the past, but there are still some regions where data are incomplete. More funding for this activity is now urgently required.

Interval cancer

For the screening project to be successful mammography must detect small cancers which, if left, would be capable of killing the patient. At the same time the number of cancers presenting in the first, second and third years after a normal screen must be kept to a minimum. True interval cancers are those that were definitely present on review of previous screening mammograms. False negatives are those presenting between screens where review of the previous mammograms shows that the cancer had been missed. Any cancers presenting between screens are not easily classifiable because either they are occult, have minimal signs or the mammography was not carried out at the time of symptomatic presentation (probably uncommon nowadays). Woodman described 297 interval cancers from a screening population of 140 000 women screened between 1988 and 1992. The results were compared against a cancer detection rate found by a screening of 59 per 10 000 women and the assumption that the background overall cancer rate was 18.3 per 10 000 (as calculated from the Swedish two counties study). The results showed an interval cancer rate per 10 000 women at a much higher level than had been anticipated, with 5–7.5 in the first year after screening, 9.3–10.5 in the second year and 13.5–18.0 in the third year.[47] This increased level of detection of interval cancer was acceptable in the first 2 years, but in the third year the level was very close to the expected background rate without screening. It was thus thought that the screening interval of 3 years was too long.

The data from this region were similar to those from Nijmegen and Stockholm but higher than those from the Swedish two counties study. Values from other screening units in the UK have confirmed that interval cancer rates are disconcerting. For example, the results from the Avon screening service from 1989–92 showed rates per 10 000 women of 7 for the first year, 12.5 for the second year and 14 for the third year. Values from the South West Thames region for the same period (excluding DCIS) were similar with rates per 10 000 women of 4.7 for the first year, 12.9 for the second year and 14.2 for the third year. New national QA targets for interval cancer rates per 10 000 women have been set: up to 12 for the first two years and less than 13 for the third year.[48]

The problem of interval cancers can be tackled in a variety of ways, all of which are aimed at decreasing the false-negative rate. These include the introduction of two-view mammography for every screen, the concept of films being double read independently by two trained radiologists or radiographers, the increases in the mean optical density of the films and improved and increased staff training, especially in the appreciation of subtle mammographic signs. The problem of true interval cancers was addressed in the randomised trial comparing 1- versus 3-year screening. It had been hoped that more frequent screening would decrease the true interval cancer rate but preliminary results suggest that this is not necessarily the case.

Background cancer rate

The success of screening therefore depends on the balance between background cancer rate, the screening detection rate and the interval cancer rate. Many of the targets of the programme have been based on knowing what the background cancer rate is, but this has usually been based on other studies. The cancer registry information may have underestimated the number of cancers in the population, and the interval cancer data, therefore, may not be quite so disconcerting. One of the primary targets for breast screening was a reduction in mortality at the beginning of this century by 25%. The background mortality from breast cancer is in a state of flux, which had started to change prior to the introduction of screening, and this may be due to the introduction of more effective systemic therapies. The death rate from breast cancer in England and Wales stopped increasing in the late 1980s and has now started to decrease. This means approximately 10% less cancer deaths in 1993 compared with 1985 to 1989 in the age range 20 to 79 years.[49] This decline appeared too soon to be influenced by the implementation of the screening project, but it is hoped that screening will accelerate this decrease. A similar reduction in breast cancer mortality has been reported for Scotland.[50] This decrease in deaths from breast cancer may be an indirect 'spin-off' for the improved services delivered to women that has come about since the introduction and reorganisation of the service mandated by the screening project as a whole.

The patient

For most women who attend breast screening, the process is a positive experience. Questionnaire studies have shown a high level of satisfaction, with many encouraging comments regarding its organisation, professionalism and communication. Nonetheless it is well recognised that it also induces considerable anxiety and that for every 1000 women attending for screening 995 will not have cancer but may experience potentially negative experiences while awaiting the results. Indeed some 65 per 1000 women will have been recalled for further assessment and for some form of biopsy for what proves to be benign disease. Additional concerns have been voiced about the hidden dangers of screening mammography, particularly in women less than 50,[51] including overdiagnosis of irrelevant lesions, particularly DCIS (lag-time bias) or small invasive cancers resulting in treatment at a time when women are asymptomatic (lead-time bias), and potential increased cancer formation due to repeated exposure to radiation, particularly in women carrying the ataxia–telangiectasia gene.

The health economics research group at Brunel University has conducted studies into the effects of screening on the psychological profile of women in the relevant age band. A total of 219 detailed healthcare questionnaires were obtained from women aged 40–44 and 231 from women aged 50–64 years. The assessments concentrated on aspects of the breast screening process such as a clear screen result, assessment, a cancer and an interval cancer as well as aspects of treatment such as mastectomy, tamoxifen and breast conservation with radiotherapy. Compared to a value of 1.0 for good health, a clear screening result description was valued at 0.92 and all other remaining descriptions were at values of 0.66. There was no exception between the younger and the more mature women except for breast conservation. Of the women attending screening 20% said they felt more anxious than usual when they received their invitation, 16% said they were more anxious while waiting for the appointment on the day, but only half of these said they were extremely anxious. About 30% felt more anxious than usual while waiting to be assessed and 42% more anxious than usual while waiting for their results, half of these again being extremely anxious. The main finding was that not only does screen-detected breast cancer have an adverse effect on the woman's quality of life but so does that of a clear screening after assessment and the development of an interval cancer. The value obtained for a clear screening result was very close to the value for good health, suggesting that screening as a whole does not have an adverse quality of life effect.

The decision for a woman to participate in screening is complex and influenced by social, demographic and economic factors. It has been argued that psychological factors also impact on recruitment, compliance and regular attendance and are thus essential to the success of all organised screening programmes.[52] The whole area of psychological distress associated with breast screening has been subject to a review by Steggles *et al.*[53] The greatest distress seems to be in the women requiring further investigation, and this is understandable. Many of the efforts to determine the degree of psychological morbidity associated with screening are bedevilled by difficulties in measuring distress and finding control groups for comparison. Many have been carried out retrospectively.

Targeting poor attenders

The NHSBSP believes that once a woman is fully informed about breast screening she has the right not to attend. However, there are certain groups that are being targeted to improve attendance owing to their known previous poor compliance. Women from ethnic minorities have been a problem in the past as in some cultures breast cancer is taboo and the idea of breast screening culturally unacceptable. Women who do not speak English may feel disadvantaged. The screening programme produces leaflets and tapes in several different languages, particularly for women from the Indian subcontinent, and is actively recruiting these women. Wheelchair access proved to be a problem on the mobile breast screening units for the physically disabled. In Scotland all the units are fitted with wheelchair access. In England, however, women who use wheelchairs are invited to attend a static unit. Two tapes are available for blind women, 'Be breast aware' and 'NHS Screening—the facts.' Deaf women can receive a video with subtitles explaining the screening process. Mencap examined the uptake of eligible women with learning difficulties who attended for screening in 1998. Only 50% attended compared with the national average of 65%. There are often difficulties on taking films of these women as poor compliance by the client can lead to inadequate or poor quality films. Women who are financially constrained, often living in the inner city with more pressing health and economic problems, often do not attend screening. This is irrespective of ethnic background or language difficulties. Uptake in some inner city areas is as low as 40%, and such women are being specifically targeted with new initiatives by the NHSBSP.

Hormone replacement therapy

The prevalence of women taking hormone replacement therapy (HRT) has increased substantially since the introduction of the UK screening programme. In 1988 less than 5% of the population were receiving HRT and these were usually women with an early menopause. In 1998 this had increased to over 30%, with many women going through a normal menopause going on to take HRT. It is estimated that one third of women who are attending breast screening are now taking HRT. It has been known for some time that HRT increases the mammographic background density in approximately one third of women, and that cysts and fibroadenomas continue to grow in the postmenopausal woman taking HRT.[52] Women with high mammographic densities have worse sensitivity and specificity and HRT use affects the whole process and increases the number of women likely to be recalled.[53]

The 'million women' study is a joint project between the Imperial Cancer Research Fund and the screening programme to examine the relationship between HRT and other women's health issues. Most of the breast screening units in the UK are taking part in this study, which aims to recruit one million women over the next 5 years. The study intends to answer the key question of how HRT affects women's breasts, whether women on HRT are at greater risk of having breast cancer diagnosed at screening and how HRT affects the ability of mammograms to detect breast cancer. Initial reports from 26 733 women from four regions shows that 14% of women had previously taken HRT and 33% were currently taking HRT. There is no significant difference in the recall rate between past users and never users. Dose or type of HRT had not affected the recall rate. There was an apparent variation in HRT by screening round, with a significant increase in false-positive recalls at the incident round compared with the prevalent round. The estimate was that there may be 6000 extra unnecessary recalls due to the effect of HRT on the breast. The original Swedish trial was randomised between 1977 and 1980 when the use of HRT was rare. By the time the NHSBSP was introduced HRT usage was much higher and this may mean real differences between comparing the NHSBSP project to the original Swedish trials from which it was derived. Rosenberg *et al.* have shown a 7% decrease in the sensitivity of screening mammograms in HRT users compared to non-users. This was particularly marked and largely confined to women with mammographically dense breasts.[54] However, other studies from Sweden have shown that HRT did not affect the screening process.[54] These apparent differences may be owing to different types of HRT in usage.

Genetic screening

Over the past 5 years it has been well documented that up to 9% of breast cancer has an association with an inherited familial predisposition. Furthermore specific mutations on several chromosomes have now been identified, including *BRCA1*, *BRCA2*, *ATM* gene, *PTEN* (Cowden's disease) and *p53* (Li-Fraumeni syndrome). Other less frequently occurring genes include the androgen receptor gene, *HNPCC* genes and possibly the oestrogen receptor genes.

Women either carrying or at increased predisposition of such genes have not only an increased risk of breast cancer but tend to form breast cancers at an earlier age. Part of the surveillance includes use of mammography at an age earlier than the routine screening project. This poses problems with the increased density of the breast of that age. Guidelines for screening women at increased risk of breast cancer have still to be published. In general terms women at increased risk should be enrolled in mammographic surveillance programmes starting at an age 5 years younger than their youngest first-degree relative with breast cancer. Breast cancer units with a family history service have screen detection rates of between 5 and 6 new cancers per 1000, which is a rate similar to that found in the screening programme for women between the ages of 50 and 64. This may be two to three times the background incidence of women in the younger age group. It is uncertain whether repeat mammograms starting at an earlier age cause any injurious effects to the breast and promote the development of cancer. This may be of particular relevance in women carrying the ataxia–telangectasia gene. In the future, specific programmes may be designed for specific populations. Thus there is a much higher frequency of *BRCA1* mutations in the Ashkenazi Jewish population of the UK, which may be as high as 1%. The total population of Ashkenazi Jews in the country is 500 000, and specific breast screening programmes for this group of women may be designed in the future.

The possible advantage of MRI in the detection of breast cancer in women with high genetic risk is currently being evaluated in a multicentre trial comparing MRI versus mammography on an annual basis.[56] As with women in the 'forties' trial, strict attention to detail is required and mammograms need to be repeated on an annual basis. The interface between genetic risk and mammographic surveillance is likely to change quite rapidly in the next few years. Having identified women at increased risk their screening activity should take place in a small number of nationally designated screening units.

Breast screening in Europe

There is a considerable variation in breast screening programmes within Europe. Only the UK, the Netherlands and Sweden have had programmes of significance that have been running for some time and reached the whole population.

During an international workshop in December 1998 representatives from 11 countries met to design a process for the development of information on screening programmes and specifications for a uniform database to assess the effectiveness of screening.[57] This laid the ground work for the International Breast Cancer Screening Network (IBSN). This organisation surveyed countries that were involved in breast screening, firstly in 1990 and then again in 1995. The IBSN wanted to know what the funding and organisational programmes were and which women were being targeted. They were also interested to compare cancer detection rates and interval cancer rates between countries. The objectives of the programme were to produce policy statements to allow funding and administration and comparison of results across the European nations.

The European Community initiated the Europe against Cancer programme in 1990 to compare this problem further.[58] Guidelines to compare the screening projects in different countries were drawn up and lead clinicians appointed from working party groups. The initial European network was established in Belgium, Ireland, France, Spain, Portugal and Greece and later Italy, Denmark, Luxembourg and Germany. The target population was women aged 50–64, with flexibility given to individual countries to alter the age. Close links were then developed between the IBSN and the European network and the information from both was published in a survey in 1995 (**Tables 2.5 and 2.6**).[59] These give information on the structure of breast cancer screening in each country and the guidelines used. Since the 1995 study, two countries have decided to implement nationwide breast screening programmes. Ireland started its programmes in the year 2000. Women aged 50–64 will be offered free mammography and will be screened biennially, with each mammogram being read independently by two radiologists.[60] In 1997 the Danish national board of

Country	Year organised programme began	% Target population covered by organised programmes	Year national coverage expected	Type of system	Facility used	Funding
Finland	National 1985	100	1989	C	MC	Government
Iceland	Regional 1987	100	1989	C	MC M GR	Government
Italy	Regional 1990	<25	Not planned	DC	MC	Government
Netherlands	National 1988	76–100	1997	PC	MC M	Government
Sweden	National 1986	100	1997	PC	MC	Government
UK	National 1988	100	1996	PC	MC M	Government
European network pilot projects						
Belgium	Regional 1992	<25	Not planned	D	GR (non-dedicated) MC	Government
Denmark	Regional 1992	<25	2004	PC	GR	Government
France	Regional 1992 National 1994	30–40	2004	D	MC GR M	National Health Assurance
Germany	Three projects in process of installation		First project to start late 2000			
Greece	Regional 1989/91	60; <25	2000	D	MC GR M	Europe Against Cancer
Ireland	Regional 1989	<25	Not planned	PC	MC M	Government
Luxembourg	National 1992	36	Not planned	C	GR (non-dedicated centre)	Union of Sickness
Portugal	Regional 1990	25–50	Not planned	PC	Mobiles and screening centre	Government
Spain	Regional 1989	<25	Not planned	N/A	Mobile units and screening centre	Government

C, centralised system with national policy and administration; PC, partially centralised system with same characteristics as central systems except programmes are administered regionally; DC, decentralised systems that have a national policy, but regional funding and administration. MC, dedicated mammographic screening centre; M, mobile screening unit; GR, non-dedicated general radiology department.

Table 2.5

health announced its official recommendations for a national screening project to be implemented by the year 2002. The Danish plan aims to recruit women from 50 to 69, with screening biennially. The cost was estimated to be US$10 million a year and hoped to save between 1100 and 1200 women over

International Breast Screening Network	Age group covered		Screening interval years		Detection method
	Lower	Upper	Age 40–49	Aged ≥50	
Finland	50	59	NA	2	Mammography
Iceland	40	69	2	2	Mammography/clinical
Italy	50	69	NA	2	Mammography
Netherlands	50	69	NA	2	Mammography
Sweden	40–50 (depends on county)	64–74	1.5	2	Mammography
UK	50	64 (or older if they so request)	NA	3	Mammography
European Network pilot projects					
Belgium	50	69	NA	2	Mammography
Denmark	50	69	NA	2	Mammography
France	50	65–69	NA	2–3	Mammography
Germany	50	69	NA	2	Mammography
Greece	40	65	2	2	Mammography/breast self-examination/clinical
Ireland	50	65	NA	2	Mammography
Luxembourg	50	65	NA	2	Mammography/clinical
Portugal	40	None	No recommendations given in national guidelines	2	Mammography
Spain	45	64	2	2	Mammography

Table 2.6

10 years, mainly through early detection. Currently, screening is only performed in the counties of Funen and Copenhagen.[61]

Conclusions

Trials have shown that screening mammography can reduce breast cancer mortality. In the UK a bold plan of screening for the whole nation has been adopted in an effort to help reduce the high mortality from the disease. The results will be particularly interesting as the overall survival rate from breast cancer has started to improve just at the same time breast screening was introduced. This is probably from the widespread application of systemic therapy for breast cancer. This may make it more difficult to measure the true impact of screening. National programmes currently exist in Australia, Holland and Sweden and have recently been introduced in other European countries. The UK programme has successfully implemented a nationwide screening process. Furthermore it has both defined and refined quality standards and guidelines for the programme. Initially the programme was only able to give surrogate measures of its achievements as far as mortality is concerned. Now real 5-year survival data are coming through and look very encouraging indeed. There is no doubt that the NHSBSP will reduce mortality, and it has already improved the services delivered for the diagnosis and treatment of breast cancer as a whole.[62,63]

Phenotypic drift

The 5-year survival statistics produced nationally for the years 1993 and 1994 show that more than 90% of patients with screen-detected cancer were alive at that time. These are very encouraging data. It is important to further speculate what will happen to these patients at the 10-year mark. In the Swedish two counties trial, Tabar found that very small cancers of 10 mm or less were associated with a 12-year survival of 95%, and this was independent of the usual prognostic factors such as nodal status or grade. Furthermore for tumours less than 15 mm there was a 90% survival at this time for both grade 1 and grade 2 lesions.[64] Tabar concluded that breast screening arrests the disease and prevents phenotypic drift towards grade 3 lesions, which would otherwise occur. The cancers need to be found as small as possible before phenotypic drift occurs. This means that it is not the pure number of interval cancers that is important but the actual size and biological potential of the interval lesions. Klemi has focused on the concept of phenotypic drift and has maintained that although screening can find biologically favourable cancers at very small size, it is important not to overtreat them.[65] The concept of phenotypic drift interfaces with the optimum interval screening period. One would imagine that it should be as short as possible. Hakama put forward the alternative explanation that phenotypic drift did not occur because the DNA content of tumours did not change throughout the screening rounds.[66] This would go along with the preliminary data from the trial of 3-year versus 1-year screening detailed above. As standards for screen-detected cancer improve it is also necessary to improve services for diagnosing patients with minimal symptoms who may be presenting with faster growing, aggressive interval lesions. Thomas has emphasised the need to improve services for these women who should take precedence over a decreasing screening interval.[67]

Costs

When screening was set up there were many critics who thought the whole process would not be worthwhile in human terms. The debate has moved forwards into the financial arena. Kattlore made a detailed analysis of the costs and benefits of screening and the treatment of early breast cancer.[68] The recommendation was that screening mammography had benefit only for women aged 50–69. This is an expensive luxury compared with the benefits of adjuvant therapy and the abandonment of routine follow-up. Baum, extracting data from this paper, commented that there may be a price tag of £1 million for each women who benefits from screening. Others put the cost of a life saved more in the region of £100 000. Nonetheless, as Baum comments, 'it is invidious to put a price on a woman's life.'[69]

The future

Sometime in the future a better test than mammography may be devised as a means to screen populations with high and natural incidence of breast cancer. Until such time the UK screening programme continues to gather pace. It is producing high quality data and is filled with a sense of enthusiasm and achievement as well as healthy self-criticism. It is already known that two-view mammography in all the rounds of screening is better than one. More information will also become available on how to treat DCIS. There is a benefit for screening 40 year olds although the cost–benefit ratio is high. Screening annually rather than every 3 years may not be as worthwhile as originally thought.

The population of women eligible for screening in the UK is continuously increasing, and it is estimated that it will increase by 30% over the next 20 years. In 1992 the screening population was just under 4 million, but by the year 2020 it will be over $5\frac{1}{2}$ million. As the programme has exceeded all targets by comparison with the Swedish two counties study on which it was based, there is pressure from the screening professionals to widen the programme. The most effective and most politically advantageous change would be to increase the upper limit of the screening age to 69. To reduce the age to 40 is much more expensive in terms of the cost of each life saved and is unlikely to gain favour. On the latest information shortening the 3-year cycle to two or less is unlikely to be introduced. However, two views at each screen will become standard. A major problem is the lack of radiologists with a specific interest in breast screening. The Department of Health will be looking at other healthcare professionals to fill this gap, with film reading being carried out by suitably trained radiographers. Nonetheless, some critics believe that the extra money this would cost would be better spent on treating symptomatic breast cancer.[70]

The important issues for the next 5 years centre on who will take the films, who will read the films, who will assess the women and who will make the clinical treatment decisions. Technology is rapidly advancing and maybe the new millennium will bring better forms of imaging and digital mammography; this is certainly around the corner although expensive for a nationwide programme. The NHSBSP must keep on improving current standards, balancing confidence in screening with realistic expectations. The goals should be to provide an honest screening service that is readily accessible to all who choose to use it.

References

1. Breast cancer screening report to the health ministers of England, Wales, Scotland and Northern Ireland by working group chaired by Professor Sir Patrick Forrest, 1986, London: Her Majesty's Stationery Office.

2. Nystrom L, Lutquist RLE, Wall S *et al*. Breast cancer screening with mammography: overview of Swedish randomised trials. Lancet 1993; 341: 937–8.

3. Kertilowske K, Grady D, Rubin S *et al*. Efficacy of screening mammography, a meta analysis. JAMA 1995; 273: 149–54.

4. Gotzsche P, Olson O. Is screening for breast cancer with mammography justifiable? Lancet 2000; 355: 129–34.

5. De Koning HJ. Assessment of nationwide cancer screening programmes. Lancet 2000; 355: 80–1.

6. Statement by the NHS breast screening programme in response to the paper in the Lancet (8 Jan, 2000). Is mammographic screening for breast cancer justified? Press release, Julietta Patnick (National Co-ordinator) NHSBSP 6 Jan, 2000.

7. Patnick J (ed). NHS breast screening programme review 1999. Meeting new challenges. Sheffield: NHSBSP, 1999.

8. Wald NJ, Murphy P, Major P *et al*. UKCCR multicentre randomised controlled trial of one and two view mammography in breast cancer screening. BMJ 1995; 311: 1189–93.

9. Bird DL, Fox JN, Ashley S *et al*. Results of the first year of breast cancer screening in a district hospital. Br J Surg 1992; 79: 922–4.

10. Blanks RG, Given-Wilson RM, Moss SM. Efficiency of cancer detection during routine repeat (incident) mammographic screening: two versus one view mammography. J Med Screen 1998; 5: 141–5.

11. Blanks RG, Wallace MG, Given-Wilson RM. Observer variability in cancer detection during routine repeat (incident) mammographic screening in a study of two versus one view mammography. J Med Screen 1999; 6: 152–8.

12. Galea MH, Blamey RTW, Elston CW *et al*. The Nottingham prognostic index in primary breast cancer. Breast Cancer Res Treat 1992; 22: 207–19.

13. Blamey RW, Day N, Duffy S *et al*. The MRC trial of frequency of breast screening. Breast Cancer Res Treat 1999; 57: 59 (Abstract 214).

14. 16-year mortality from breast cancer in the UK trial of early detection of breast cancer. Lancet 1999; 353: 1909–14.

15. Alexander FE, Anderson TJ, Brown HK *et al*. 14 years of follow-up from the Edinburgh randomised trial of breast screening. Lancet 1999; 353: 1903–8.

16. Chen H-H, Tabar L, Faggerberg G *et al*. Effect of breast cancer screening after age 65. J Med Screen 1995; 2: 10–4.

17. Rubin G, Garvican L, Moss S. Routine invitation of women aged 65–69 for breast cancer screening: results of first year of pilot study. BMJ 1998; 371: 388–9.

18. Kissin MW, Cooke J, Kissin C *et al*. Radial scars—a screen detected lesion that must be removed. Proceedings of the Nottingham EORTC Joint Breast Cancer Meeting, 1993: 1.

19. Holland PA, Walls J, Boggis CRM *et al*. A comparison of axillary node status between cancers detected at the prevalence and first incidence breast screening rounds. Br J Cancer 1996; 74: 1643–6.

20. Walls J, Boggis CR, Wilson M *et al*. Treatment of the axilla in patients with screen-detected breast cancer. Br J Surg 1993; 80: 436–8.

21. NHS Breast Screening Programme and British Association of Surgical Oncology. An audit for screen detected breast cancers for the year of screening April 1998 to March 1999. BASO Specialist Group Meeting, Apr 2000.

 22. Veronesi U, Paganelli G, Galimberti V et al. Sentinel-node biopsy to avoid axillary dissection in breast cancer with clinically negative lymph-nodes. Lancet 1997; 349: 1864–7.

 23. Silverstein MJ, Lagios MD, Craig PH et al. A prognostic index for ductal carcinoma in situ of the breast. Cancer 1996; 77: 2267–74.

24. Gui PH, Marygold-Curling O, Allum WH et al. One-step diagnosis for symptomatic breast disease. Ann R Coll Surg Engl 1995; 77: 24–7.

25. Guidelines for cytology procedures and reporting in breast cancer screening. Cytology sub-group of the National Coordinating Committee for Breast Cancer Screening Pathology. NHSBSP Publication No 22; Sheffield: 1993.

26. Ciatto S, Cariggi P, Bulgraesi P et al. Fine needle aspiration cytology of the breast. A review of 9533 consecutive cases. Breast 1993; 2: 87–90.

27. Robinson IA, McLittle G, Nicholson S et al. Prognostic value of cytological grading of fine-needle aspirates from breast carcinomas. Lancet 1994; 343: 947–9.

28. Litherland JC, Evans AJ, Wilson ARM et al. The impact of core-biopsy on pre-operative diagnosis rate of screen detected breast cancers. Clin Radiol 1996; 51: 562–5.

29. Teh W, Wilson ARM. The role of ultrasound in breast cancer screening. A consensus statement by the European Group for Breast Cancer Screening. Eur J Cancer 1998; 34: 449–50.

30. Kopans D. Breast cancer screening with ultrasonography. Lancet 1999; 354: 2096–7.

31. Greco N, Agresti R, Giovanazzi R. Impact of the diagnostic methods on the therapeutic strategies. QJ Nucl Med 1998; 42: 66–80.

32. Heywang-Kobrunner SH, Veiweg P, Heinig A et al. Contrast enhanced MRI of the breast: accuracy, value, controversies, solutions. Eur J Radiol 1997; 24: 94–108.

33. Scopinaro F, Mezi S, Ierardi M et al. 99mTc MIBI prone scintimammography in patients with suspicious breast cancer: relationship with mammography and tumor size. Int J Oncol 1998; 12: 6612–4.

34. Jiang Y, Nishikawa RM, Wolverton DE et al. Malignant and benign clustered microcalcifications: automated feature analysis and classification. Radiology 1996; 198: 671–8.

35. Querci Della Rovere G, Benson JR, Morgan M et al. Localisation of impalpable breast lesions—a surgical approach. Eur J Surg Oncol 1996; 22: 478–82.

36. Quality assurance guidelines for surgeons in breast cancer screening. Prepared by the national co-ordination group for surgeons working in breast cancer screening NHSBSP. Publication No 20; Sheffield: 1996.

 37. Dixon JM, Raviseker O, Cunningham M et al. Factors affecting outcome of patients with impalpable breast cancer detected by breast screening. Br J Surg 1996; 83: 997–1001.

38. Chinyama CN, Davies JR, Rayter Z et al. Factors affecting surgical margin clearance in screen detected breast cancer and the effect of cavity biopsies on residual disease. Eur J Surg Oncol 1997; 23: 123–7.

39. Dixon JM, Raviseker O, Walsh J et al. Specimen orientated radiography helps define excision margins of malignant lesions detected by breast screening. Br J Surg 1993; 80: 1001–2.

40. Armstrong JS, Weinzwieg IP, Davies JD. Differential marking of excision planes in screened lesions of organically coloured gelatins. J Clin Pathol 1990; 43: 604–7.

41. Fisher B, Dignam J, Wolmark N et al. Lumpectomy and radiation therapy for the treatment of intraductal breast cancer: findings from National Surgical Adjuvant Breast and Bowel Project B-17. J Clin Oncol 1998; 16: 441–52.

42. Julien JP, Bijker N, Fentiman IS et al. Radiotherapy in breast-conserving treatment for ductal carcinoma in situ: first results of the EORTC randomised phase III trial 10853. Lancet 2000; 355: 528–33.

43. Todd JH, Dowle C, Williams MR et al. Confirmation of a prognostic index in primary breast cancer. Br J Cancer 1987; 56: 489–92.

44. Calman K. Breast cancer services in Exeter and quality assurance for breast screening. Report to the Secretary of State. Department of Health Publications, Wetherby; 1997.

 45. Richards M, Sainsbury R, Kerr D. Inequalities in breast cancer care and outcome. Br J Cancer 1997; 76: 634–8.

46. Moritz S, Bates T, Henderson SM et al. Variation in management of small invasive breast cancers detected on screening in the former south east Thames region: observational study. BMJ 1997; 315: 1266–72.

47. Woodman CBJ, Dowle C, Williams MR et al. Confirmation of a prognostic index in primary breast cancer. Br J Cancer 1987; 56: 489–92.

48. Field N, Michelle NJ, Wallis MGW *et al.* What should be done about interval breast cancers? Two view mammography and possibly a shorter screening interval. BMJ 1996; 310: 203–4.

49. Beral V, Hermon C, Reeves G *et al.* Sudden fall in breast cancer death rates in England and Wales. Lancet 1995; 345: 1642–3.

50. Brewster D, Everington V, Hakness E *et al.* Incidence of and mortality from breast cancer since the introduction of screening. BMJ 1996; 312: 639–40.

51. Dickersin K. Breast screening in women aged 40–49 years: What next? Lancet 1999; 353: 1896–7.

52. Fallowfield LJ, Rodway A, Baum M. What are the psychological factors influencing attendance, non-attendance and re-attendance at a breast screening centre? J R Soc Med 1990; 83: 547–51.

53. Steggles S, Lightfoot N, Sellick S. Psychological distress associated with organized breast cancer screening. Cancer Prev Control 1998; 2: 213–20.

52. Cyrlak D, Wong CH. Mammographic changes in post menopausal women undergoing hormone replacement therapy. Am J Roentgenol 1993; 161: 1177–83.

53. Litherland JC, Evans AJ, Wilson ARM. The effect of hormone replacement therapy on recall rate in the nation health breast screening programme. Clin Radiol 1997; 52: 276–9.

54. Rosenberg RD, Hunt WC, Williamson MR *et al.* Effects of age, breast density, ethnicity and estrogen replacement therapy on screening mammographic sensitivity and cancer stage at diagnosis: review of 183,134 screening mammograms in Albuquerque, New Mexico. Radiology 1998; 209: 511–8.

55. Thurfjell EL, Holmberg LH, Persson I. Screening mammography: sensitivity and specificity in relation to hormone replacement therapy. Radiology 1997; 203: 339–41.

56. Leech MO, Padhani AR, Eales RA *et al.* A multi-centre trial of MRI as a method of screening women who are at high genetic risk of breast cancer. Medical Research Council and NHS Research and Development ongoing trial. The Royal Marsden Hospital, London.

57. Shapiro S. Report on the international workshop on information systems in breast cancer detection. Cancer Suppl 1989; 64: 2645–50.

58. Jensen O, Esteve J, Miller H *et al.* Cancer in the European Community and its member states. Eur J Cancer 1990; 26: 1167–256.

59. Shapiro S *et al.* Breast cancer screening programme in twenty two countries: current policies, administration and guidelines. Int J Epidemiol 1998; 27: 735–42.

60. Payne D. Ireland announces national breast screening programme. BMJ 1999; 318: 1025.

61. Skormand K. Danes to start national breast screening. Lancet 1997; 350: 196.

62. Winstanley JHR, Leinstern SJ, Wake TN *et al.* The value of guidelines in a breast screening service. Eur J Surg Oncol 1995; 21: 140–2.

63. Birch D, Chia Y, Payne M *et al.* Good prognosis tumours in breast cancer screening. Ann R Coll Surg Engl 1995; 77: 185–7.

64. Tabar L, Fagerberg G, Day ME *et al.* Breast cancer treatment and natural history: new insights from results of screening. Lancet 1992; 339: 412–4.

65. Klemi PJ, Joensuu A, Toikkanen S *et al.* Aggressiveness of breast cancers found with and without screening. BMJ 1992; 304: 467–9.

66. Hakama M, Holli K, Isola J *et al.* Aggressiveness of screen-detected breast cancers. Lancet 1995; 345: 221–4.

67. Thomas BT. Population breast cancer screening: theory, practise, and service implications. Lancet 1995; 345: 205–7.

68. Kattlore H, Liberati A, Keller E *et al.* Benefits and costs of screening and treatment for early breast cancer. JAMA 1995; 273: 142–8.

69. Baum M. Screening for breast cancer, time to think—and stop? Lancet 1995; 346: 436–9.

70. Baum M. Money may be better spent on symptomatic women. BMJ 1999; 318: 398.

3 Treatment of early stage breast cancer and breast reconstruction

Richard Sainsbury

Breast cancer

Breast cancer remains one of the commonest solid epithelial neoplasms, with an annual incidence of about 20 000 new patients per year in the UK. The estimated worldwide incidence is of a million women per year. The prevalence is some five times higher, so for a unit seeing 100 new patient per year there will be approximately 500 women alive with the disease at any one time.

Breast cancer accounts for 50% of all cancers in women between 40 and 55 and thus remains a major health problem. The modal age of presentation is 58. The incidence is rising,[1-3] but the mortality rate in the UK seems to have fallen in the past few years.[4]

Comparisons with European data show a poorer outcome (5-year survival rate) for patients treated in the UK by about 5–10%.[5] The reasons for this are unclear but may include greater use of adjuvant therapies in mainland Europe. After reports from the British Breast Group[6] and the British Association of Surgical Oncology (BASO)[7] (which now acts as a central group for breast surgeons in the UK), a consensus as to how breast cancer will be managed is emerging. It is envisaged that patients with breast cancer will be managed locally, provided a multidisciplinary breast team is functioning and that there are enough patients to make such a team viable.

There is evidence that the patients of clinicians with a special interest in the disease or those who treat larger numbers of patients have improved outcomes.[8,9] In recent years larger numbers of women with breast cancer are being treated by fewer surgeons, and this trend is to be welcomed.

The breast care team should consist of surgeons with dedicated sessions, both out-patient and operative, radiologists, pathologists and breast care nurses. Regular, documented meetings with clinical and/or medical oncologists are essential, although the necessary radiotherapy may well be provided off site.

Dedicated in-patient beds and facilities for chemotherapy should be provided locally with suitable supervision. Protocols of care will be essential as will regular audit. A suitable computer program for such audit has been developed (BASO 2 database). Access to psychological support, and reconstruction methods is also essential.

Most patients with breast cancer still present with a lump as the dominant symptom. In the 50–65 age group (for whom screening is available), the percentage of screen-detected cancers rose through the first years of screening to about 45% but has fallen back now that the prevalent cases have been detected (**Fig. 3.1**). Other symptoms (in descending order of frequency) include lumpiness, distortion of the breast, nipple discharge and breast pain, although the last is uncommonly associated with malignancy. **Figure 3.2** shows the typical numbers of women attending a breast clinic serving a population of 212 000.

The Department of Health issued guidelines on referral of patients with breast symptoms to all general practitioners in 1999 to reduce the number of inappropriate referrals.[10] This has had the opposite effect and resulted in more patients being referred! The ratio of women with benign to malignant disease averaged about 10:1 but has now risen to 15:1 in some practices. The introduction of the '2-week rule' in April 1999, whereby patients have to be seen by a specialist breast surgeon within 2 weeks of an urgent referral has further distorted the work pattern of breast clinics. There is *no* evidence that diagnosing a woman within 2 weeks will impact on survival. Women waiting longer than this who have a cancer detected may legitimately feel let down. Large numbers

Figure 3.1
Percentage of screen-detected cancers 1992–98 for women aged 50–65.

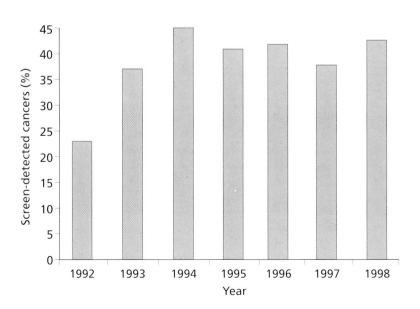

Figure 3.2
Relative proportion of referred symptoms to breast clinic (consultations about family history excluded).

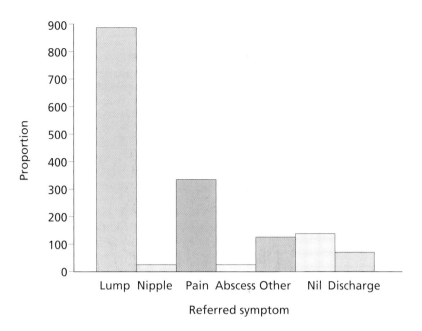

of 'worried well' women are being referred and approximately 20% of women with breast cancers, unrecognised by general practitioners, are being delayed.

Aetiology

The cause of breast cancer remains unknown. It is rare before the age of 25, but the incidence increases with age until the menopause, when there is a slight levelling off (the menopausal hook of Clemmenson) before the incidence again rises, although at a reduced rate compared with the premenopausal years. The incidence is increasing worldwide despite screening, and currently involves about 1 million women a year. The average age at diagnosis is 58.

There is a marked geographical variation in the incidence and mortality of breast cancers between countries. The level of fat consumption has been implicated. Immigrants from a country with a low incidence of breast cancer to one of higher incidence experience an increase in incidence to levels just below that of their adopted country within three generations. Breast cancer is more common in women of higher than lower socioeconomic status.[11,12]

Risk factors

Women who have more menstrual cycles (i.e. an early menarche and late menopause) have an increased risk. Women whose menopause is before 45 have half the risk compared with those whose menopause occurs after 55. Those who have had an oophorectomy under 35 have a 40% reduction in the risk of breast cancer compared with those who have had a natural menopause.

Nulliparity and late age at first birth both increase the lifetime incidence of breast cancer. Women who have their first child after age 35 seem to have a risk higher than that associated with nulliparity. Breast feeding was thought to reduce the risk of breast cancer, but this view has recently been challenged. Use of the contraceptive pill, especially if before the birth of a child, increases the risk slightly but this risk seems to disappear within 5 years of stopping treatment.

Family history is important. The extent of the risk depends on the number and relationship of relatives affected, the age at onset of the disease and relations with multiple sites of cancers. Fewer than 10% of all breast cancers are due to autosomal dominant susceptibility genes, which may be transmitted through either maternal or paternal lines.[13,14] The main characteristics of an inherited susceptibility are:

- Early age of onset
- Bilateral disease
- Multiple primaries in the same woman
- At least two different affected first-degree relatives

Referral to a genetics service may be appropriate to discuss risk and to see whether testing for *BRCA1* or *BRCA2* or *p53* abnormalities is indicated.[15] There is now evidence that testing of populations at extra risk with known defects (such as Ashkenazi Jews who have a deletion at amino acid 185 in the *BRCA1* gene) is worthwhile. Other risk factors include obesity in the post-menopausal woman, previous radiation to the breast and a previous biopsy that has shown proliferative disease (especially if combined with a positive family history). There may be a small risk for prolonged use of hormone replacement therapy (HRT), but this may well be outweighed by its protective effect for osteoporosis and cardiovascular disease.

There are conflicting data as to whether patients with breast cysts large enough to require aspiration are at increased risk. Different authors use different definitions of cystic disease. The overall increase in risk ranges from 1.7 to 7.5 times that of the normal population but seems to be highest in those presenting under the age of 45. All the above factors play upon the incidence of no more than 30% of breast cancers.[16]

Screening

Screening by regular mammography has been shown to reduce the risk of death from breast cancer for populations aged 50–65 by approximately 29%.[17] There is no evidence from randomised trials that screening the 40–50 age group is cost effective, but screening those aged 65–70 detects significant numbers of cancers and may yet be introduced into national programmes.

In the UK, women at risk are identified by their general practitioners and are screened every 3 years using two views of each breast (from 1995). The films are usually read by a single radiologist, although double reading picks up an additional 5–10% of abnormalities.

On the basis of studies in Scandinavia many feel that 2 years would be a more appropriate screening interval. This is being prospectively studied as a trial within the UK National Screening Programme. Preliminary results suggest that a non-significant number of extra cancers are detected.

Screen-detected cancers are likely to be of better histological grade or special type and are less likely to be node positive than symptomatic cancers of the same size. Ductal carcinoma in situ (DCIS) is detected in about 30% of women compared with less than 2% of women with symptoms. The move away from investigation of screen-detected abnormalities by fine needle aspiration cytology to core biopsy has significantly increased the accuracy of preoperative diagnosis and thus reduced the number of open, stereotactic-guided biopsies.

Objectors to the programme point out the large costs involved in screening (about £42 million per year), the uncertainty of whether screen-detected disease would ever cause the patient harm and whether the anxiety generated by screening is worthwhile. It is, however, the only proven technique currently available of reducing mortality and is unlikely to be halted.

Prevention of breast cancer

Effective ways of reducing the incidence of breast cancer (although not preventing it totally) include prophylactic mastectomy or oophorectomy before 35 years of age. Neither has been considered generally acceptable, although more women are asking for these operations if judged to be at increased risk on the basis of a family history. A study of high-risk women undergoing prophylactic mastectomy between 1960 and 1993 at the Mayo Clinic showed a reduction from a predicted 37 cancers to an actual occurrence of 4 (89% reduction, $P<0.001$).[18] Such surgery should only be performed at centres that have close cooperation with a geneticist. Psychological support is often needed. Breast reconstruction is nearly always undertaken at the same time.

There is a UK trial of prevention of breast cancer with tamoxifen, which has been shown to reduce the incidence of contralateral breast cancer when used as adjuvant treatment.[19] This trial aims to recruit 10 000 women worldwide who will be randomised to either tamoxifen or placebo for 5 years. Concerns about the effects of tamoxifen on the uterus have slowed trial entry, which is due to close in mid-2000. The National Surgical Adjuvant Breast and Bowel Project trial on tamoxifen (NSABP-P1) was stopped early at the request of the data monitoring committee. In this trial 13 388 women at increased risk of breast cancer were randomised to tamoxifen 20 mg day^{-1} or placebo. There was a highly significant 49% reduction in the risk of invasive breast cancer for those treated with the active agent.[19] The trial entry criteria for the US study were different from the UK, with women over the age of 60 being allowed to participate as well as those with lobular carcinoma in situ. Those with an increased risk as judged by the Gail model (a multivariate logistic regression model in which combinations of risk factors are used to predict the probability of occurrence of breast cancer with time) formed the largest entry group. The Gail model over-estimates the risk as it uses the number of previous benign biopsies as a risk factor. The P1 study had the secondary aims of examining the effect of tamoxifen on fatal and non-fatal myocardial events and also on whether there would be a reduction in bone fractures. Both these questions were rendered unanswerable by the early stopping of the trial.

Other possible preventative interventions include dietary manipulation with reduction of fat intake or the use of vitamin A analogues such as the retinoids.[20,21] The introduction of compounds such as specific oestrogen receptor modulator (SERM), for example raloxifene, has led to alternative strategies in prevention. Raloxifene (a benzothiophene) was shown to reduce the risk of breast cancer (by 76%) in a trial of its use to prevent osteoporotic fractures (where the women were at lower risk than in the NSABP-P1 study). The percentage reductions look large but relate to relatively few events. It is now being compared to tamoxifen in a prevention trial in the USA (STAR) and is rapidly recruiting the 22 000 necessary participants.

Options available for women at high risk of breast cancer are shown in **Table 3.1**.

Diagnosis and investigations

Optimal treatment for patients with breast cancer is a multimodality activity requiring an input from surgeon, radiologist, pathologist, medical and clinical oncologist, general practitioner, breast care nurse and the woman herself. There is evidence that women treated by specialists seeing sufficient workloads to maintain such teams have a better outcome.[9] All primary care doctors in England and Wales have been circulated with updated guidelines on referral practice prepared on behalf of the Department of Health.[10]

The patient should be encouraged to participate in any decisions (but not forced to against her wishes). Psychological distress may be reduced by informed discussion prior to treatment.[22]

Option	Advantages	Disadvantages
Screening	May avoid breast loss Allows further interventions	Does not prevent disease May miss chance of cure Compliance unknown
Prophylactic mastectomy	Reduces breast cancer risk Tissue specific intervention	Loss of breasts Irreversible Major surgical intervention Overtreats those who would not develop disease
Prophylactic oophorectomy	Reduces breast cancer risk Preserves breasts	Premature menopause Replacement hormones may carry risks Overtreats those who would not develop disease
Tamoxifen (and other specific oestrogen receptor modulators)	Probably reduces risk Preserves breasts Allows other options	Undesirable systemic effects Magnitude of effect in high risk women unclear Duration of effect unclear Overtreats those who would not develop disease

Table 3.1 Options for women at high risk of breast cancer

To achieve the above, a preoperative diagnosis of breast cancer is essential, and this is achieved through a history, clinical examination, imaging and cyto-histological confirmation (the triple assessment).

History

The history includes details of age of menarche, number of children and breast feeding, oral contraceptive use, family history, age of menopause, use of HRT and current medications.

Clinical examination

Both breasts and nodal drainage areas (axilla and supraclavicular fossa) should be carefully examined by palpation after a visual inspection. This should be performed with the patients placed in a good light across the room. She should raise her arms above her head and return them to her side. This allows minor degrees of distortion or skin tethering to be seen as well as more obvious lumps.

Clinical examination is not completely reliable (over 55% of screen-detected cancers are impalpable; in younger women the sensitivity of clinical examination is even lower with only 37% of cancers being detected).[23]

Detection of axillary nodes is difficult and, on examination, is accurate in only 50% of patients.[24] Ultrasonography, mammography and radioantibody scanning fare not much better, and histological examination of resected tissue remains the only reliable method for determining axillary nodal status. The inception and validation of sentinel node biopsy may allow selective axillary surgery to be performed with reduced morbidity.

Imaging

Mammography remains the commonest imaging tool for detecting breast cancer. The breast is compressed between two plates, and usually two exposures of each breast are made. These are in the oblique and craniocaudal positions, although a true lateral view, axillary extended views and magnification views can all be obtained. If an abnormality is detected, further techniques such as paddle magnification can be performed. These are often combined with core biopsy sampling. If a screen-detected lesion is impalpable, it may be localised by mammography and a wire placed to mark the site of the lesion. The patient can then have the area resected, and a check X-ray film will show complete removal.

A mammogram is important even with a clinical diagnosis of breast cancer, as it allows assessment of the contralateral breast as well as showing multifocal disease. For women with DCIS, mammography is better than clinical examination at determining the extent of the disease, but, even so, often underestimates the full extent of the malignant change.[25] Mammography may not detect all breast cancers. HRT does increase the density of the breast and may reduce the sensitivity of mammography. It is not currently a recommendation that women commencing HRT undergo mammography.

Ultrasonography is good at distinguishing between solid and cystic lumps. It is useful for assessment of tumour size and may be more useful than mammography in demonstrating the margins in young women or those with denser breast.[26] It can be used to provide serial measurements of tumours being treated by induction chemotherapy or long-term endocrine therapy and is increasingly being used to localise impalpable disease prior to biopsy. Technological developments, with the production of high frequency probes (up to 21 MHz), have improved resolution. The use of false colour Doppler ultrasonography allows estimation of blood flow into an area of interest and may improve the ability to differentiate between malignant and benign lesions or lymph nodes.

Not all breast cancers are detectable by mammography and ultrasonography. Persistence of a lump or other clinically suspicious area necessitates further investigation. The common pitfall is the lobular type of breast cancer that may present as diffuse lumpiness rather than a discrete lesion.

Biopsy techniques

FNAC (or biopsy) has been used for many years to confirm a diagnosis of palpable breast cancer.[27] In addition, it may be used to help prove that a clinically benign lump is such. The accuracy of FNAC is high when the operator is experienced and the cytologist is expert. It is reported on a 0–5 scale (see table), and a C5 report in conjunction with clinical and radiological evidence of a carcinoma is sufficient to proceed to definitive surgery.[28] False positives have been reported, but these tend to be where the cytology has given a discordant result from mammography and/or clinical findings. In such a case either an open or core biopsy needs to be taken. An acellular specimen may be appropriate if a random cytology of a fibrous area has been performed, but it should not be accepted if a discrete solid lesion is being aspirated and needs repeating.

It is possible to determine hormone receptor status on specimens obtained by fine needle aspiration. Core biopsies are now taken using a 14 gauge spring-driven device. The skin is infiltrated with local anaesthesia and a scalpel used to nick the skin to allow passage of the core needle. Many women find this more comfortable than FNAC. It allows a core of tissue to be examined histologically thus allowing architectural detail to be shown. It can be used on impalpable disease by guided localisation.[29] The cores should be radiographed if microcalcifications were present on the original X-ray film. Core biopsy should not be used instead of FNAC, but it is a valuable adjunct.

Newer diagnostic—and to some extent therapeutic—interventions include the Mammatome and ABBI systems. The patient lies prone with her breast hanging dependently through the table top. Large cores are taken after infiltration with local anaesthesia. Proponents claim greater diagnostic accuracy with this technique and the ability to completely remove small lesions and areas of microcalcification without the need for conventional open biopsy. Opponents point out that completeness of excision cannot be guaranteed and that orientation of specimens is difficult.

The use of FNAC and core biopsies should allow most breast cancers to be diagnosed preoperatively, thus allowing an informed discussion with the patient about treatment options and and the type of definitive surgery to be performed. The combination of FNAC, mammography and clinical examination provide the highest diagnostic yield and the lowest risk of diagnostic error. The accuracy of the different investigations is shown in **Table 3.2**.

There is a tendency for all the above investigations to be provided at the time of the patient's first visit (the one-stop clinic) thus allowing repetition of FNAC should the result be inadequate. Whether the results are given to the patient the same day is a matter of local practice. A breast nurse should be present when the results are given as should a companion of the patient.

Open biopsy is occasionally needed if FNAC and a core biopsy have failed to provide a diagnosis. This can be carried out as a day-case procedure. A biopsy is not a definitive procedure but is a diagnostic tool and should not be confused with a treatment procedure such as a wide local excision (although sometimes,

	Clinical examination	Ultrasonography	Mammography	Fine needle aspiration cytology
Sensitivity	88	85	88	95
Specificity	91	88	90	95
Positive predictive value	95	92	94	99.8

Sensitivity = % of cancers considered malignant.
Specificity = % of lesions diagnosed benign that are benign.
Positive predictive value = % of lesions diagnosed malignant that are cancer.

Table 3.2 Accuracy of investigations

for a small lesion, the two may be the same). Frozen section is seldom used now but may have an occasional place to confirm a suspicious cytology test result. The lesions that are difficult to diagnose on FNAC and core biopsy may also be difficult to diagnose histologically. In these cases the pathologist is often better off with properly fixed tissue that has undergone routine processing than poorly fixed frozen sections with an impatient surgeon awaiting an answer.

Other preoperative investigations

For early stage breast cancer (stages 1 and 2) there has been a move away from a panoply of staging investigations that have repeatedly been shown to give little useful information.[30]

Currently, a full blood count, liver function tests and chest radiography are all recommended, along with investigation of specific complaints such as bone pain. For larger cancers where there is a higher chance of metastatic disease, a bone and liver ultrasound scan should be added. Tumour markers such as carcinoembryonic antigen (CEA) or CA 15.3 may be helpful in monitoring response to treatment[31] but are generally non-specific and unreliable.

The above advice may change if the preliminary results of skeletal MRI are confirmed. There is some evidence to show a correlation between bony lesions detected by MRI (in asymptomatic women) and early symptomatic relapse in bone. Another diagnostic tool is bone marrow aspiration and examination for tumour cells. Patients with circulating tumour cells have earlier relapses and a greatly reduced chance of 5-year survival.

Pathology

Breast cancer arises in the terminal duct-lobular unit. The terminology used continues to change, moving away from descriptive terms. Most cancers are of no special type (NST)—also known as invasive ductal cancer or ductal NOS (not otherwise specified), and these account for about 70% of unselected cases. Tumours with specific features that allow characterisation are associated with a better prognosis. Carcinoma cells that have not yet broken through the basement membrane and are thus confined within the terminal ductolobular units are termed carcinoma in situ. Again, these were historically broken down into ductal (DCIS) and lobular (LCIS) types. DCIS was described according to architectural features such as comedo or cribriform, but this has given way to cytological features such as high grade and low grade, which has improved prognostic significance.

Pathological examination of the resected specimen is not just used to provide a diagnosis but also to confirm completeness of excision and to provide extra management information such as hormone receptor status.

If breast conservation has been performed the resected specimen should be oriented either by clips or sutures, and if the margins are involved a re-resection should be performed. Some try to avoid the need for this by performing cavity shavings and only return the patient to theatre if the shavings are involved.[32]

The pathology report should include the size of tumour, its type and grade (the Bloom and Richardson grading system is used for NST tumours), clearance of resection margins, presence and absence of tumour multifocality, the presence of DCIS in and around the tumour, lymphovascular invasion and axillary node positivity. This should be given as both numbers of nodes retrieved and number involved. In addition, hormone receptor status (oestrogen receptor (ER) and progesterone receptor (PR)) should be performed. Other markers such as erb B-2, epidermal growth factor receptor (EGFr), cell cycle kinetic or proliferative markers can be estimated. Most of the proliferative markers have yet to be proven to give additional prognostic information, although with the introduction of anti-erb B-2 antibody (Herceptin) and the development of tyrosine kinase inhibitors these may be of therapeutic value.

Staging and prognostic factors

The TNM (primary tumour, regional nodes, metastasis) classification is still used but is not well suited for this purpose. It was designed to be used clinically; the nodal status and size frequently change when the pathological measurements are given, and there is thus little conformity as to which groups of patients are being compared. The International Union against Cancer staging encompasses the TNM system and is still widely used. Of more importance is the full pathological description that allows patients to be compared in a meaningful manner. Various pathological measurements have been reproducibly shown to influence prognosis, either individually or in combination. Nodal status is the single most

Prognosis	Index score	15-year survival (%)
Good	<3.4	80
Moderate	3.4–5.4	40
Poor	>5.4	15

Table 3.3 Nottingham Prognostic Index and survival

important factor, with an increasing loss of life expectancy with number of involved nodes. Grade, size, presence of lymphovascular invasion, S-phase fraction, Ki-67 staining, EGFr, ER and PR all have prognostic significance. The combination of tumour size, grade and nodal status (the Nottingham Prognostic Index)[33] has good discriminant function (**Table 3.3**). Patients can thus be separated into a group whose survival mirrors the normal population, a group whose outcome is so poor that either no therapy or very aggressive therapy will be needed. The intermediate group may well be important since it may be possible to influence the course of the disease by means of chemotherapy.

Management options

Surgery

The aim of surgery is to achieve local control by eradication of the primary tumour. From screening studies it is clear that surgical intervention of early disease affects outcome although there are no randomised control studies of surgery against other treatment modalities. Because of its ability to influence local control, surgery remains the first treatment modality for patients with early breast cancer.

Surgical treatment has evolved into two methods: breast conservation by wide local excision (WLE) or mastectomy. Both should be combined with an axillary procedure. WLE consists of removal of the tumour with about 1 cm of surrounding normal tissue (and skin if necessary). It is essential to achieve clear resection margins otherwise a high incidence of local recurrence is seen. This procedure is suitable for unifocal tumours generally smaller than 4 cm (although overall breast size modifies this).[34] An increasing incidence of local recurrence occurs with increasing tumour size. Patients with extensive intraductal component (EIC) are best treated with mastectomy as are patients where the cosmetic result is likely to be poor (such as with large central tumours). Skin incisions should be planned with both cosmesis and the need for postoperative radiotherapy in mind. If the scar is a long way from the tumour bed, the clinical oncologist must be informed as the scar is often used to plan any top-up boost.

Postoperative radiotherapy is part of conservation treatment and should be given unless part of a trial for specific groups of patients, such as those with small, special types of tumours (the BASO 2 trial). It is important to orientate the lumpectomy specimen for the pathologist, and the AIM technique is recommended (one suture, or metal clip, **A**nteriorly, two **I**nferiorly and three **M**edially).

Many randomised controlled trials have shown equal survival benefits after WLE combined with radiotherapy and mastectomy (when both have included axillary dissection).[35–37]

The incidence of local recurrence in a conserved breast is of the order of 1% per year[38] compared with 0.5% per year after a mastectomy.[39]

About 70% of cancers detected by mammography and 50% of those that produce symptoms are suitable for conservation therapy.[40]

Mastectomy is appropriate for those with multifocal disease, ill defined margins, EIC or where the tumour directly involves the nipple or central skin or the patient chooses such an operation. Mastectomy requires removal of all the breast tissue, with conservation of the pectoral muscles and dissection of the axilla. Radiotherapy is not needed to the axilla after dissection but may be used to the mastectomy flaps if the tumour was large, of high grade or had extensive lymphovascular invasion.

It was once thought that conservation therapy reduced the risk of anxiety and depression postoperatively, but it now seems that being offered a choice is more important than the procedure actually performed.[41] Many women who need a mastectomy can have a reconstruction either as an immediate or delayed procedure (see below).

Timing of surgery for premenopausal women may be important. Some reports have shown a survival benefit for patients operated on in the luteal phase (second half) of the menstrual cycle. The theory behind this is that operating when unopposed oestrogens are present allows dissemination and implantation of malignant cells. Other centres have been unable to find such an effect and others an opposite effect, with improved survival in the follicular phase! A prospective non-randomised study (the intervention, timing and survival study) is currently underway to answer this question. Recruitment is complete and analysis will follow.

Axillary dissection

Axillary dissection is either performed in continuity with a mastectomy or through a separate incision with a WLE. It aims to allow assessment of the nodal status for prognostic purposes, eradication of metastatic disease within the nodes and assessment of nodal status to determine adjuvant treatment. There is as yet no reliable method of determining nodal status without surgical resection of nodes. Clinical examination of the axilla is unreliable. Sentinel node biopsy has been proposed as a more sensitive method of staging the axilla and is widely practised in the USA. The Medical Research Council sponsored ALMANAC trial, underway in the UK, had an audit phase where surgeons had to carry out 40 procedures before going on to the randomised phase, where patients are randomised to further axillary surgery after a sentinel node biopsy. The argument over whether injection of a blue dye is better than a radioactive tracer (based on the gamma emitter technetium (99mTc)) is gradually being settled. There is still work to be done on the best size of carrier molecule and detection system, but on the whole the technique is proving reliable.

An axillary sample is an operation favoured by some who pick out the four largest nodes in the axilla, but neither allows full staging nor treats the axilla properly.[42] Both the numbers of nodes retrieved and the number involved should be reported. The former is also a function of the pathologist as well as the surgeon. Surgery should not be combined with axillary radiotherapy as an unacceptable incidence of lymphoedema occurs.[43] As radiotherapy has been associated with brachial neuropathy and frozen shoulder, many teams favour an axillary clearance.

After an axillary clearance, the axilla should be empty—the axillary vein should be clear and the nerve to serratus anterior and the thoracodorsal trunk should be preserved. The intercostobrachial nerve may have been divided, although some try to preserve it—this may defeat the object of an oncological clearance. Even when preserved, the nerve may not function well (presumably because it has been stripped of its blood supply). All women undergoing axillary surgery should be warned of the risk of an area of altered sensation below the axilla. The interpectoral nodes (Rotters) need attention as do the very lowest nodes that may be inadvertently left if too low an incision is made, as may occur if the axilla is being cleared as a separate procedure. Pectoralis minor may need formal division to allow access to the highest nodes, although if the arm is rotated above the head it can be retracted medially to allow access to level III nodes.

Patients may present with palpable nodes and no obvious primary tumour. If the primary is breast cancer (lymphoma is the second commonest pathology), 70% will be found on mammography, ultrasonography or MRI. If no primary tumour is found, then the patient should be treated by axillary clearance, breast radiotherapy and systemic chemotherapy with tamoxifen if the tumour is ER positive. An alternative is to proceed straight to mastectomy, but this has to be a decision made with the patient. Post-treatment the patients seem to fall into two groups: those who behave as any other node-positive patient and those who do much better than expected.

Paget's disease

This condition of the nipple is associated with DCIS or invasive carcinoma in the majority of patients. A mammogram may show microcalcifications under the nipple. If there is no associated mass then wide excision of the nipple and underlying breast tissue followed by radiotherapy is appropriate. An alternative is mastectomy, which may be more appropriate if there is an associated mass. Paget's disease can be found in 2–3% of all mastectomy specimens even if not clinically apparent. It is important to perform a biopsy in patients with suspected Paget's disease and to avoid the overdiagnosis of nipple eczema, although the two conditions can usually be differentiated by clinical examination. Nipple eczema is treated by 0.5 or 1% hydrocortisone applied twice daily.

Adjuvant treatment

Radiotherapy

Radiotherapy is an essential part of the treatment of breast cancer if conservation therapy has been performed and is used selectively after a mastectomy. Failure to give radiotherapy after WLE exposes patients to an increased risk of local recurrence and the need for subsequent mastectomy.[44] The need for radiotherapy after small tumours of special type detected through screening is debated, and there is a trial currently running (BASO 2) that addresses this problem. The need for a boost to the site of surgical resection is also debated. Radiotherapy after mastectomy was given as a standard treatment, but the results from several trials have shown that the routine addition of radiotherapy gave no additional benefit over a watch policy, with radiotherapy used at the time of local recurrence.[45] In addition, simple mastectomy and radiotherapy gave results equivalent to mastectomy and axillary dissection. Techniques for giving radiotherapy have changed since the early trials, and the excess of cardiac deaths seen for left-sided tumours have subsequently disappeared.[46] There was a move away from radiotherapy after mastectomy in the 1980s as a result of the above studies, but it has become clear that there are patients at high risk of local (flap) recurrence. These could be identified as those who have large tumours that were node positive and of high grade and those with marked lymphovascular invasion.

Two papers have shown a survival benefit for patients with node positive tumours who received radiotherapy in addition to chemotherapy.[47,48] These studies have increased the demand for radiotherapy post-mastectomy.

Radiotherapy is associated with complications that occur either early (redness and soreness of skin which normally resolve within a few weeks) or late. Some are dose and fraction dependent, and good skin care is an important part of the management of these patients. The rare complications of brachial plexopathy, second malignancy, lymphoedema and small degrees of pulmonary fibrosis still occur.[49] The clinical oncology team gives radiotherapy, which is usually based at cancer centres where the necessary technology is available. The quality of radiotherapy delivery is important in avoiding complications. A survey of fraction size and total dose given showed wide variation in practice across UK centres. There is an uneven distribution in radiotherapy machines across the country, with some regions having insufficient resources to provide adequate timely treatments.

Newer techniques of giving radiotherapy (such as intensity modulated treatment) and better planning systems may further decrease the morbidity from breast cancer, but there are currently insufficient machines available to render this possible.

Radiotherapy after the local excision of DCIS has been shown to reduce the risk of both recurrent DCIS and invasive disease, but this may be overtreatment for a significant numbers of patients.[50]

Systemic adjuvant therapy

This includes hormonal treatments as well as cytotoxic chemotherapy and is normally started immediately after the surgical episode, with the aim of reducing the micrometastatic burden and thus improving overall survival.

 It is now clear that adjuvant systemic therapy with multi-agent chemotherapy, tamoxifen[51] or ovarian ablation (in those under 50)[52] will reduce the risk of recurrence and death for both node positive and node negative women.

The effects of systemic adjuvant treatment are reviewed every 5 years, where all trials utilising these agents are combined and subject to meta-analysis.[51]

 This has shown a highly significant improvement for both recurrence-free and overall survival (8.4% and 6.3%, respectively at 10 years) (**Table 3.4**). These effects were twice as large for women under 50 as for those over 50.

There is some evidence that anthracycline-based regimens are more effective than the traditional cyclophosphamide, methotrexate and fluorouracil (CMF) regimen. The exact details of chemotherapy regimens will not be discussed here. Adjuvant chemotherapy has little effect on local control and should not therefore be substituted for radiotherapy, where the risk of local regional recurrence is high.[53] Dose intensity is important,[54,55] and reduction of doses may merely breed out clones of resistant cells. The use of high-dose chemotherapy in the adjuvant setting has been investigated and was not shown to have a survival advantage.[56] The only paper purporting to show a survival benefit in a randomised trial was subsequently shown to be fraudulent.

Age	% Reduction in annual odds of recurrence (SD)	% Reduction in annual odds of death (SD)
<40	37 (7)	27 (8)
40–49	34 (5)	27 (5)
50–59	22 (4)	14 (4)
60–69	18 (4)	8 (4)
All ages	23 (8)	15 (2)

Table 3.4 Reduction in recurrence and death by age in trials of chemotherapy

The role of taxanes is still under investigation. These drugs were originally derived from extracts of the Pacific yew tree, but are now synthesised. They work by a different mechanism than conventional chemotherapy, stabilising the cell microtubular system. There has been a move to give adriamycin and a taxane as standard adjuvant therapy in the USA. The data to support this remain scanty, and further follow-up is awaited.

Chemotherapy has well known side effects including nausea, vomiting, alopecia and tiredness.[57] The sickness can be reduced by the use of the 5-HT$_3$ antagonists such as ondansetron. Chemotherapy may induce amenorrhoea that may be temporary or permanent if the patient is perimenopausal. There are suggestions that some, if not all, of the effects of chemotherapy may be mediated through ovarian suppression. Prolonged or high doses of anthracyclines may be associated with congestive cardiac failure. Scalp cooling can reduce the alopecia associated with some drugs but requires appropriate equipment and patience as the cooling cap has to remain in place for some time after the infusion finishes. Reported concerns over an increase in scalp metastases seem to be unfounded.

Tamoxifen

Tamoxifen was developed as a possible contraceptive but was not selective enough in its actions. It is now classed as one of the first selective-oestrogen receptor modulators (SERM) and has both agonist and antagonist actions. Many individual trials as well as the overview analyses have shown the benefit for women who take tamoxifen post-surgery.[51] The optimum duration of exposure seems to be about 5 years, but trials continue to determine if longer than this gives additional benefit. It is clear, however, that a minimum of 2 years' dosing gives a reduction in odds of death of approximately 27% for postmenopausal women. Data from the Cancer Research Council over 50's trial and other studies suggest that 5 years' tamoxifen gives prolonged survival. That longer duration of treatment may be deleterious was hinted at in the NSABP B-14 trial, but these results require confirmation. There are both laboratory and clinical observations that tamoxifen may stimulate the growth of some breast cancers with prolonged exposure, and withdrawal responses have been seen.

The beneficial effect of tamoxifen seems to be greater in women whose tumours were ER positive, although a beneficial effect was also reported in 5–15% of ER-negative women. The methodology used to determine ER status at that time was not that currently used (immunohistochemistry), and re-examination of the original tumour blocks has not shown an effect for ER-negative patients. Some early data suggest that patients with ER-negative tumours undergoing chemotherapy have a worse prognosis if given tamoxifen.

The major side effect of tamoxifen that has emerged is the oestrogenic effect on the endometrium, causing hyperplasia and, rarely, neoplasia. The beneficial effects of tamoxifen on reduction in deaths from breast cancer and reduction in the incidence of contralateral breast cancer[51] outweigh the risk from endometrial carcinoma.

The role of tamoxifen in younger women has been re-evaluated. It was thought that tamoxifen was only effective in postmenopausal women, where it did not have to compete with higher levels of ovarian hormones. It is now clear that there is a significant disease-free and overall survival for patients with ER-positive tumours both below and above age 50.

Tamoxifen is currently undergoing investigation as a preventative agent in women at increased risk of breast cancer (as judged by family history). The UK placebo controlled trial is still recruiting 10 000 women worldwide. The rationale for this is the finding of a 25% reduction in the incidence of contralateral breast cancers in women taking tamoxifen in the adjuvant setting.[58]

Newer selective ER modulators include a pure antioestrogen (Faslodex), which seems to have few side effects, and drugs such as raloxifene (Evista), a compound originally developed for the prevention of postmenopausal osteoporosis. Work continues on their efficacy and side effects.

Aromatase inhibitors

The development of third-generation aromatase inhibitors based on non-steroidal triazole derivatives (letrazole, anastrazole and vorazole) or the steroidal examestane has allowed an alternative endocrine approach. The parent compound, aminogluthimide, blocked conversion of cholesterol-based precursors into sex steroids. The compound was unselective and had to be given with hydrocortisone. Second-generation compounds blocked the conversion of androstenedione to oestrone and oestradiol but had to be given by injection. The third-generation drugs are given orally and reduce postmenopausal oestrogen synthesis (in peripheral tissues such as muscle and fat and perhaps in the tumour itself). Anastrazole has been shown to be effective in advanced breast cancer, with a survival advantage when compared with patients treated with megoestrol acetate, and both it and letrazole cause rapid shrinkage in large, ER-positive breast cancers. A large trial (Armidex, Tamoxifen, Alone and in Combination; ATAC) comparing anastrazole with tamoxifen, either alone or in combination, has finished recruiting participants, and an interim analysis is expected in late 2000. These compounds are used in clinical practice as second-line endocrine agents but are more expensive than tamoxifen.

Ovarian ablation

Stopping ovarian secretion in premenopausal women confers long-term benefit; a reduction of 25% for mortality and 26% for recurrence—results similar to those achieved by polychemotherapy.[52] There is debate over how much of the chemotherapy effect is achieved by ovarian suppression—over 50% of patients have a menopause induced by chemotherapy. There is less information about the combination of ovarian ablation with chemotherapy, but this is being addressed by the ABC trial currently under way.

Ovarian ablation can be achieved by radiotherapy (usually three fractions), open surgery or laproscopic surgery. In the short term a luteinising hormone-releasing hormone (LH-RH) analogue will achieve similar effects, but these are expensive and currently have to be given by injection. Trials of LH-RH super-agonists against CMF chemotherapy for patients with node-positive disease have been performed, and the results show equivalence for ER positive patients but superiority for chemotherapy in those who were ER negative.

Trials currently available

The major national trials under way can be divided into those addressing issues of dosage (both intensity and density), combinations of treatments and duration of treatments. Quality of life measurements and economic evaluations are now essential parts of most studies.

The Oxford group performs an overview analysis of trials of chemotherapy, endocrine therapy and endocrine ablation every 5 years. Using the techniques of meta-analysis, small, individual trials can be combined to allow firm conclusions to be drawn.[51]

Clinical trials remain important in guiding the future management of patients with breast cancer. Even small differences in treatment arms may be significant because of the large number of women with the disease. Large numbers of patients are needed to provide such answers, but the randomisation rate remains low. Less than 10% of eligible patients are entered into studies in the UK and this may be owing to the time taken to talk to patients about studies, and lack of support staff. Provision of support such as research nurses and data managers allows an increase in recruitment and should be part of the funding stream for breast units.

Breast reconstruction

The aim of breast reconstruction is to restore the normal shape and, to some extent, consistency of the breast after excisional or ablative surgery. It is commonly associated with mastectomy, but the realisation that a quadrantectomy or a large WLE can lead to a major cosmetic defect has also led to techniques for filling such defects.[59]

Reconstruction after mastectomy is performed either at the time of initial surgery or as a delayed procedure. The advantages of the former include the patient having only to undergo one operation. Many patients do not wish to come back into hospital for further surgery 6–9 months after the time of their mastectomy, when their lives are getting back to normal and so do not take up the offer of a delayed reconstruction. There is evidence that the psychological benefit is greater after immediate reconstruction,[60] and the techniques used do not prevent giving adjuvant chemotherapy or hormone therapy. Disadvantages of immediate reconstruction include the time taken and the need for cooperation between breast and plastic surgeon (although more breast surgeons are being trained in such procedures).

The simplest form of reconstruction is an external prosthesis worn within the bra. This is, however, unsatisfactory for many as it feels unnatural and may move. Newer techniques include adhesive prostheses, where a shaped plaster is stuck to the chest wall and a prosthesis attached to the plaster with velcro. Coloured prostheses are available for those whose skin is not white.

Tissue expansion allows stretching of the skin and muscle at a mastectomy site by means of placement of a temporary expander. This is an inflatable bag usually placed under the pectoralis major muscle, with a short connecting tube to an injection port that is usually placed laterally over the ribs. Some prostheses have integral injection ports, which require care when inserting the needle used for inflation in case the main prosthesis is ruptured. Gradual inflation allows a pocket to be created into which a definitive (usually silastic) prosthesis can be placed. Care must be taken to site the expander and prosthesis correctly—it must not be allowed to sit too high or laterally towards the axilla. Dissection under the upper part of the rectus musculature may be necessary. Newer prostheses, such as the Becker expander/mammary prosthesis (Mentor Medical Systems, Oxford, UK), can combine both functions and reduce the need to return the patient to theatre for a change of expander to prosthesis although they are more expensive. This consists of a pocket filled with injections of saline surrounded by a silicone gel outer envelope. The gel provides a more natural feel whereas injections of saline allow adjustment of size. The port can be removed under local anaesthetic after final volume has been achieved. A period of relative over expansion of the expander is recommended as it allows some postoperative shrinking to occur without deforming the outline of the new breast. Both speed of expansion and time of over-expansion are variable, with some practitioners carrying this out relatively quickly and others taking several months to achieve a similar result. Complications include extrusion of the prosthesis, haematoma, infection, pain and capsular contracture. The incidence of capsular contracture has decreased since textured (rough) prostheses have been introduced.[61] Late rupture can occur as can damage if fine needle aspiration is inappropriately performed. The current technique of choice for proving capsular rupture is MRI. Ultrasonography can be helpful if MRI is not available but is less sensitive.

Silastic prostheses were thought to be associated with new cancers or autoimmune diseases but subsequent research has shown no increased incidence of either condition, and they are now judged to be safe.[62,63] A newer prosthesis fill material, soya oil, was marketed as a safer option if capsular rupture occurred, but this has subsequently been withdrawn from sale. Polyurethane prostheses gave good shapes with less capsular contracture, but degradation products were shown to be carcinogenic to rats and the prostheses were subsequently withdrawn. Saline fill prostheses were popular with patients concerned by the scares over silastic but did result in 20% deflation after insertion. This incidence has reduced with newer shells, and they are currently undergoing a resurgence of popularity.

The usual shape of implant is round but implants with more of an anatomical pear shape are available.

Tissue expansion and silastic implants can provide an adequate breast mound, but the degree of ptosis commonly associated with the normal breast may be difficult to mimic. Such reconstructive methods are best suited to women with small volume requirements and non–ptotic breasts. The procedure is, however, relatively quick and does not require a large investment of time or trouble for the patient. Tissue expansion is often difficult to achieve after radiotherapy and tissue transfer is preferred. It has a place after bilateral standard mastectomy, as symmetry is easy to achieve.

Flap reconstruction (autogenous tissue reconstruction)

Flap reconstruction provides fresh skin, fat and muscle. The imported tissue can withstand adjuvant treatments such as radiotherapy and chemotherapy. Flaps can be used to create a much more normal looking breast, with ptosis and filling in both the axillary portion and infraclavicular area.

The commonest flaps are the latissimus dorsi myocutaneous (LD) and the transverse rectus abdominis myocutaneous (TRAM), although superior gluteal and inferior gluteal flaps are also used. The LD flap is based on the thoraco-dorsal vessels and provides skin and muscle but little fat. It is useful to cover chest wall defects but often requires a supplemental silastic prosthesis to provide a realistic breast. It can be used to fill upper outer quadrant defects associated with lumpectomy or quadrantectomy. The blood supply is generally forgiving, and the flap can be used after radiotherapy. It can be used when relative contraindications to a TRAM flap exist. LD flaps are regaining popularity, with endoscopic harvesting techniques being used to reduce the scar on the back that contributed to morbidity.

The TRAM flap can be swung on a pedicle based on the superior epigastric vessels or transferred as a free flap with a microvascular anastamosis between inferior epigastric and intercostal or axillary vessels. The blood reaches the skin and fat by means of perforator vessels, which have to be carefully preserved during the operation. Large amounts of subcutaneous tissue can be moved with a TRAM flap thereby allowing shaping and formation of a more normal breast. The donor site is closed with a long transverse scar as in an abdomino-plasty, and the secondary effect of a 'tummy tuck' is appealing to many patients.

Pedicled TRAM flaps can utilise either one or both rectus abdominis muscles (or be split to provide bilateral reconstructions). A free TRAM flap is time consuming and requires an expertise in microvascular surgery that is usually beyond the remit of the breast surgeon.

Complications are more common with free flaps and include loss of part (uncommonly all) of the flap. Blockage of venous drainage rather than problems with arterial inflow result in impaired circulation within the flap. Areas of fat necrosis may occur in poorly vascularised portions of the flap, leaving hard areas of tissue that can be confused with local recurrence. The donor site may cause problems; an unsightly, stretched scar can occur after transfer of part of latissimus whereas herniation through the rectus sheath can occur after a TRAM flap.

A TRAM flap is the current 'gold-standard' reconstruction but is time consuming and requires much commitment from patient and surgeon. Results are less good in patients with an impaired microvasculature such as smokers, obese patients or diabetics, and such patients are excluded in some centres. The latest variation in TRAM flap reconstruction is the free deep inferior epigastric perforator flap (DIEP). This leaves the muscle intact and relies on two or three perforators from the deep inferior epigastric artery. Because the muscle and fascia are left and only fat and skin moved, there are no problems with abdominal wall closure nor is there a need for synthetic mesh to buttress any closure.

Postoperative mobilisation is therefore quicker and the procedure less painful for the patient although it is longer for the surgeon. It is currently only available in specialist units.

Other free flaps requiring microvascular anastomosis exist and tend to be used in those who have insufficient back or abdominal tissue or have had extensive surgery to those donor areas. They include superior and inferior gluteal flaps (from the respective arteries).

Skin-sparing mastectomy can be combined with the above techniques and reduce the amount of tissue needed for transfer. The inframammary crease is also preserved, making for increased symmetry. The nipple is usually removed, although some surgeons retain it as long as biopsies from the terminal ducts are free from cancer cells. A subcutaneous mastectomy with immediate placement of a subcutaneous prosthesis is no longer indicated, as the results are poor.

Whether breast reconstruction is performed at the time of mastectomy or as a delayed procedure depends on local circumstances including the presence of appropriately trained staff. There does not seem to be a significant risk of increased local recurrence after either delayed or immediate reconstruction,[64] nor does immediate reconstruction delay commencement of adjuvant therapies. The use of radiotherapy does, however, have a negative impact on the appearance of a prosthetic reconstruction, with an increased rate of capsular contracture.[65] TRAM flaps seem to tolerate radiotherapy better than tissue expansion or other forms of reconstruction, although there is still an effect that may require revisional surgery.

Nipple reconstruction is possible but the number of alternative techniques is testament to none having an outstanding claim to success. Free grafts can be taken from a wide range of sites including labia, opposite nipple, ear or toe. Local flaps are commonly used but tend to be carried out as a delayed rather than immediate procedure. This is because of concerns that both the blood supply to the newly created main flap and the position chosen may not be ultimately appropriate after the flap settles. A local flap often requires tattooing to provide a colour match.

An artificial nipple may be created by taking a plaster cast of the opposite nipple and constructing a colour-matched silastic prosthesis.[66]

Surgery to the contralateral breast is commonly needed and should be discussed at the outset. This usually takes the form of a mastopexy or breast reduction, although occasionally an implant may be required. The need for future mammographic surveillance needs to be considered and techniques used that avoid creation of fat necrosis or microcalcifications, which may mimic new malignant disease.

Whether reconstructive surgery is the domain of the plastic surgeon or the breast surgeon is debatable. Provided that appropriate training in the techniques involved as well as a full awareness of how to avoid (and get out of) trouble are in place then the surgery may be performed by a breast surgeon.

References

1. Ewert Z, Duffy S. Incidence of female breast cancer in relation to prevalence of risk factors in Denmark. Int J Cancer 1994; 56: 783–7.

2. Holford TR, Roush GC, McKay LA. Trends in female breast cancer in Conneticut and the United States. J Clin Epidemiol 1991; 44: 29–39.

3. Persson I, Bergstrom R, Sparen P et al. Trends in breast cancer incidence in Sweden 1958–1988 by time period and birth cohort. Brit J Cancer 1993; 68: 1247–53.

4. Hermon C, Beral V. Breast cancer mortality rates are levelling off or beginning to decline in many western countries: analysis of time trends, age-cohort and age-period models of breast cancer mortality in 20 countries. Br J Cancer 1996; 73: 955–60.

5. Coleman MP, Esteve J, Damiecki P et al. Trends in cancer incidence and mortality. International Agency for Research on Cancer Scientific Publications 1993; 121: 411–32.

6. Report of a working party of the British Breast Group. Provision of breast services in the UK: the advantages of specialist units, 1994.

7. The Breast Surgeons Group of the British association of Surgical Oncology. Guidelines for surgeons in the management of symptomatic breast disease in the United Kingdom. Eur J Surgical Oncol 1995; 21 (suppl A): 1–13.

8. Gillis CR, Hole DJ. Survival outcome of care by specialist surgeons in breast cancer: a study of 3786 patients in the West of Scotland. BMJ 1996; 312: 145–8.

 9. Sainsbury JRC, Haward R, Rider L et al. Survival from breast cancer. Influence of clinician workload and patterns of treatment on outcome. Lancet 1995; 345: 1265–70.

10. Austoker J, Mansel R, Baum M et al. Guidelines on referral of patients with breast cancer symptoms. London: Department of Health, 1999.

11. Williams J, Clifford C, Hopper J et al. Socioeconomic status and cancer mortality and incidence in Melbourne. Eur J Cancer 1991; 27: 917–21.

12. Fleming NT, Armstrong BK, Steiner HJ. The comparative epidemiology of breast lumps and breast cancer. Intl J Cancer 1982; 30: 147–52.

13. Newman B, Austin MA, Lee M et al. Inheritance of human breast cancer: evidence for autosomal dominant transmission in high risk families. Proc Natl Acad Sci USA 1988; 85: 3044–8.

14. Iselius L, Slack J, Little M et al. Genetic epidemiology of breast cancer in Britain. Ann Hum Genet 1991; 55: 151–9.

15. Bishop DT. BRCA1, BRCA2, BRCA3 … a myriad of breast cancer genes. Eur J Cancer 1994; 30A: 1738–9.

16. Seidman H, Stellman SD, Mushinski MH. A different perspective on breast cancer risk factors: some implications of non attributable risk. Clin J Cancer 1982; 32: 301–13.

 17. Nystrom L, Rutqvist LE, Wall S et al. Breast cancer screening with mammography: overview of Swedish randomised trials. Lancet 1993; 341: 973–6.

 18. Hartmann LC, Schaid DJ, Woods JE et al. Efficacy of bilateral prophylactic mastectomy in women with a family history of breast cancer. N Engl J Med 1999; 340: 77–84.

19. Powles TJ. The case for clinical trials of tamoxifen for prevention of breast cancer. Lancet 1992; 340: 1145.

20. Hursting SD, Thornqvist M, Henderson MM. Types of dietary fat and the incidence of cancer at five sites. Prev Med 1990; 19: 242–8.

21. Willett WC, Hunter DJ. Vitamin A and cancers of the breast, large bowel and prostate: epidemiologic evidence. Nutrl Rev 1994; 52: S53.

22. Fallowfield LJ, Hall A, Maguire GP et al. Psychosocial outcome of different treatment policies in women with early breast cancer outside a clinical trial. BMJ 1990; 301: 575–80.

23. Ashley S, Royle GT, Corder A et al. Clinical, radiological and cytological diagnosis of breast cancer in young women. Brit J Surg 1989; 76: 835–7.

24. Davies GC, Millis RR, Hayward JL. Assessment of axillary node status. Ann Surg 1980; 192: 148–51.

25. Holland R, Hendriks JHCL, Verbeek ALM *et al.* Extent, distribution and mammographic/histological correlates of breast ductal carcinoma in situ. Lancet 1990; 335: 519–22.

26. Hirst C. Sonographic appearances of breast cancers 10 mm or less in diameter. In: Madjar H *et al.* (eds). Breast ultrasound update. Basel: Karger, 1994: 127–39.

27. Furnival CM, Hocking MA, Hughes LE. Aspiration cytology in breast cancer: its relevence to diagnosis. Lancet 1975; ii: 446–9.

28. Sterrett G, Harvey J, Parsons RW *et al.* Breast cancer in Western Australia in 1989: III. Accuracy of FNA cytology in diagnosis. Aust NZ J Surg 1994; 64: 745–9.

29. Parker SH, Lovin JD, Jobe WE *et al.* Non-palpable breast lesions: stereotactic, automated large core biopsies. J Radiol 1991; 180: 403–7.

30. Del Turco R, Palli D, Carridi A *et al.* Intensive diagnostic follow-up after treatment for primary breast cancer: a randomised controlled trial. JAMA 1994; 271: 1593–7.

31. Ward BG, Joy GJ, Ramm LE *et al.* Comparative study of mammography and mammary serum antigen estimation for breast cancer screening. Med J Aust 1992; 157: 161–4.

32. MacMillan RD, Purushotham AD, Mallon E *et al.* Breast conserving surgery and tumour bed positivity in patients with breast cancer. Br J Surg 1994; 81: 56–8.

33. Galea M, Blamey RW, Elston CE *et al.* The Nottingham Prognostic Index in primary breast cancer. Breast Cancer Res Treat 1992; 22: 207–19.

34. Calais G, Berger C, Descamps P *et al.* Conservative treatment feasability with induction chemotherapy, surgery and radiotherapy for patients with breast carcinoma larger than 3 cm. Cancer 1994; 74: 1283–8.

35. Blichert-Toft M. A Danish randomised trial comparing breast conservation with mastectomy in mammary carcinoma. Br J Cancer 1990; 62 (S12): 15.

36. Veronisi U, Banfi A, Slavadori B *et al.* Breast conservation is the treatment of choice in small breast cancer: long term results of a randomised trial. Eur J Cancer 1990; 26: 668–70.

37. Fisher B, Redmond C, Poisson R *et al.* Eight-year results of a randomised clinical trial comparing total mastectomy with or without radiation in the treatment of breast cancer. N Engl J Med 1989; 320: 822–8.

38. Fisher B, Anderson S, Fisher ER. Significance of ipsilateral breast tumour recurrence after lumpectomy. Lancet 1991; 338: 327–31.

39. Fisher B, Redmond C, Fisher ER. 10-year results of a randomised clinical trial comparing radical mastectomy and total mastectomy with or without irradiation. N Engl J Med 1985; 312: 674–81.

40. Collins J. The role of the surgeon. Cancer Forum 1994; 18: 92–5.

41. Fallowfield LJ, Baum M, Maguire GP. Effects of breast conservation on psychological morbidity associated with diagnosis and treatment of early breast cancer. BMJ 1986; 293: 1331–4.

42. Kissin MW, Thompson EM, Price AB *et al.* The inadequacy of axillary sampling in breast cancer. Lancet 1982; i: 1210–1.

43. Bundred NJ, Morgan DAL, Dixon JM. Management of regional nodes in breast cancer. BMJ 1994; 309: 1222–5.

44. Gelber RD, Goldhirsch A. Radiotherapy to the conserved breast: is it avoidable if the cancer is small? J Natl Cancer Inst 1994; 8: 652–4.

45. Stewart HJ. Controlled trials in the treatment of 'early' breast cancer: a review of published results. World J Surg 1977; 1: 309–13.

46. Cuzick J, Stewart HJ, Peto R *et al.* Overview of randomised trials of postoperative adjuvant radiotherapy in breast cancer. Recent Results Cancer Res 1988; 111: 108–29.

47. Overgaard M, Hansen PS, Overgaard J *et al.* Post-operative radiotherapy in high-risk premenopausal women with breast cancer who receive chemotherapy. Danish Breast Cancer Cooperative Trial. N Engl J Med 1997; 337: 949–55.

48. Ragaz J, Jackson SM, Le N *et al.* Adjuvant radiotherapy and chemotherapy in node-positive premenopausal women with breast cancer. N Engl J Med 1997; 337: 956–62.

49. Pierquin B, Mazeron JJ, Glaubiger D. Conservative treatment of breast cancer in Europe: report of the Groupe Europeen de Curietherapie. Radiother Oncol 1986; 6: 187–98.

50. Julien J-P, Bijker N, Fentiman IS *et al.* Radiotherapy in breast-conserving treatment for ductal carcinoma in situ: first results of the EORTC randomised phase III trial 10853. Lancet 2000; 355: 528–33.

51. Early Breast Cancer Trialists' Collaborative Group. Systemic treatment of early breast cancer by hormonal, cytotoxic or immune therapy. 133 randomised trials involving 31,000 recurrences and 24,000 deaths among 75,000 women. Lancet 1992; 339: 1–15, 71–85.

52. Early Breast Cancer Trialists' Collaborative Group. Ovarian ablation in early breast cancer: overview of the randomised trials. Lancet 1996; 348: 1189–96.

53. Fisher ER, Leeming R, Anderson S *et al.* Conservative management of intraductal carcinoma (DCIS) of the breast. J Surg Oncol 1991; 47: 139–47.

54. Wood WC, Budman DR, Korzun AH *et al.* Dose and dose intensity of adjuvant chemotherapy for stage II, node-positive breast cancer. N Engl J Med 1994; 330: 1253–9.

 55. Bonadonna G, Valagussa P. Dose–response effect of adjuvant chemotherapy in breast cancer. N Engl J Med 1981; 304: 10–5.

56. Peters WP, Ross M, Vredenburgh JJ *et al.* High-dose chemotherapy and autologous bone marrow support as consolidation after standard-dose adjuvant therapy for high-risk primary breast cancer. J Clin Oncol 1993; 11: 1132–43.

57. Coates AS, Abraham S, Kaye SB *et al.* On the receiving end—patient perception of the side effects of cancer chemotherapy. Eur J Cancer Clin Oncol 1983; 19: 203–8.

58. Fisher B, Constantino J, Redmond C *et al.* A randomized clinical trial evaluating tamoxifen in the treatment of patients with node-negative breast cancer who have estrogen receptor-positive tumors. N Engl J Med 1989; 310: 479–84.

59. Yelland A, Rainsbury D. The use of the latissimus dorsi musculocutaneous flap for immediate correction of the deformity resulting from breast conservation therapy. Br J Plast Surg 1999; 52: 420–1.

60. Dean C, Chetty U, Forrest APM. Effect of immediate breast reconstruction on psychosocial morbidity after mastectomy. Lancet 1983; i: 459–61.

61. Malata CM, Feldberg L, Coleman DJ *et al.* Textured or smooth implants for breast augmentation? Three year follow-up of a prospective randomised controlled trial. Br J Plast Surg 1997; 50: 99–105.

62. Brooks PM. Silicone breast implantation: doubts about the fears. Med J Austral 1995; 162: 432–4.

63. Fisher J. The silicone controversy: when will science prevail? N Engl J Med 1992; 326: 1696.

64. Rosenqvist S, Sandelin K, Wickman M. Patients' psychological and cosmetic experience after immediate breast reconstruction. Eur J Surg Oncol 1996; 22: 262–6.

65. Dickson MG, Sharpe DT. The complications of tissue expansion in breast reconstruction—a review of 75 cases. Br J Plast Surg 1987; 40: 629–35.

66. Sainsbury JRC, Walker V. A better nipple prosthesis. Ann R Coll Surg Engl 1991; 73: 67–9.

4 Treatment of advanced stage breast cancer

Richard Sainsbury

Advanced stage breast cancer

Patients with breast cancer may present with advanced disease or may acquire this as part of the natural history of their disease progression. A working definition of advanced stage breast cancer is that which is no longer curable by local treatments. As such this stage requires systemic therapy, although surgery may still have an important place as part of a multidisciplinary team approach.

The standardised mortality for breast cancer remains approximately 50%, with a median survival of 8 years. Most patients go through one or more recurrences before death; these episodes may span many months and the management of this phase is important. Even after dissemination, the median survival is 14–20 months.[1] Breast cancer can recur at the site of previous surgery (local recurrence), in the area of the chest wall and lymph nodes (locoregional recurrence) or as disseminated disease. Each of these types of recurrence may present in isolation or in combination.

It is common to stage or restage a patient on presentation with recurrent disease as this may provide information that affects management. Staging at the time of initial treatment has been shown to be unhelpful and costly, at least for T1 and T2 tumours.[2] Normally chest radiography, bone scan, liver function tests and a full blood count will suffice, although tests specific to any local complaint may also be necessary such as a liver scan or radiography of a painful bony area.[3] The role of tumour markers to assess disease recurrence remains unclear, although they may be useful in monitoring progression or response to therapy.[4] The combination of tumour markers such as CA 15.3 and carcinoembryonic antigen (CEA) seem to give better discrimination.

The diagnosis of recurrent disease may cause the patient and family more distress than that experienced at the time of the original diagnosis. This can arise for several reasons, including the realisation that the disease has not been cured and is likely to prove terminal. Appropriate support to the patient and her family is vital as patients frequently express that whereas the initial diagnosis and management was good, the delivery of the news of recurrence and its subsequent management was less so. Although multidisciplinary working is increasing it is still common for the onset of recurrence to mark a change in the personnel caring for the patient as the surgeon transfers care to a clinical or medical oncologist. This can be a difficult time for both physician and patient. Involvement of the palliative care team at this stage is often beneficial. Recurrent disease may be difficult to diagnose. It is more common for the patient to represent with new symptoms than for signs to be detected at routine follow-up, and the role of large follow-up clinics run by junior staff is increasingly questioned and, indeed, actively discouraged in the NHS Clinical Outcome Group guidelines. Nurse-led follow-up clinics with protocols for referral to the oncology clinics are increasing in popularity.

Presentation

There are a group of patients who present with large, locally inoperable cancers in whom radical local surgery (Halstead radical mastectomy) or chest wall resection would once have been the only treatment option. Long-term survivors from this condition confirm the non-metastatic nature of this form of disease in some patients. Most, however, quickly experience extensive local recurrence. Some of these patients have had their tumours for a long time and have concealed them. In these, estimation of oestrogen receptor (ER) status by fine needle aspiration cytology or core biopsy and treatment with tamoxifen may be worthwhile since ER-positive response rates of greater than 60% can be expected and may be of prolonged duration. Subsequent changes of endocrine therapy and even withdrawal of tamoxifen alone can give further responses. The introduction of oral third-generation aromatase inhibitors has extended the options for endocrine treatment.

Younger patients, those with ER-negative tumours and those in whom the disease is progressing rapidly are now treated with neoadjuvant (up front or primary) chemotherapy. After diagnosis and staging, induction chemotherapy is given. Response is then assessed, and patients who fail to respond have radiotherapy and second-line chemotherapy.[5] Their outlook is generally poorer. Those who respond either go on to surgery then radiotherapy and further chemotherapy or radiation therapy and chemotherapy alone. Although clinical response rates are high (up to 80% in some series) the histological complete response rate is much lower (7–20%). Resection of the original tumour site is therefore indicated, although this may be difficult if the tumour has 'disappeared.' The survival rates for patients having neoadjuvant therapy are not significantly better than those for standard therapy, and the technique is now generally reserved for those with tumours too large for conservation therapy to render this possible.

Inflammatory cancers are a special subgroup of advanced tumour and present as an indurated, reddened breast with peau d'orange from lymphatic blockage. Once universally fatal within a short time they are now treated with chemotherapy and radiotherapy, with surgery being used to resect any residual disease. Response rates over 70% are now seen, with 5-year survival rates of between 10 and 55% reported.[6] Further increases in response rates may be expected with the use of high-dose chemotherapy and stem cell transplantation, although the early promise of longer survival has not been proven in clinical trials.

Aims of treatment

Advanced stage breast cancer is, by definition, incurable, but worthwhile symptom control and extension of survival are achievable. Such concepts should be discussed with the patient and her family, especially if toxic treatments are being proposed. If cure is no longer possible, quality of life becomes of paramount importance and should be formally assessed both before and during treatment. There are validated formal measures of quality of life, but one simple method is to ask patients if they feel better at the end of treatment, if they think the treatment was worthwhile and whether they would undergo it again.

Local recurrence

After conservation therapy

The ideal management of local recurrence after conservation treatment is prevention! This means selection of patients for whom this treatment is appropriate and the use of radiotherapy as part of the treatment. The choice of conservation treatment does not, by itself, influence survival. It is important to recognise that some patients are unsuitable for conservation and should be advised to have a mastectomy. This applies to both invasive and non-invasive cancers as there is now recognition of subtypes of ductal carcinoma in situ (DCIS), with increased rates of local relapse. Although DCIS may be reduced by radiotherapy, there is still a high enough incidence to warrant primary treatment by mastectomy (with the addition of immediate reconstruction should the patient wish).

Resection margins must be clear of disease (by 0.5–1 cm) and the axilla should be surgically treated (for patients with invasive disease) to provide staging information and to prevent the need for radiotherapy to the axilla. High-grade, node-positive tumours with extensive lymphovascular invasion are more likely to be associated with recurrence. Appropriate chemotherapy is also necessary, although it is not clear to what extent this affects local recurrence rates.

Radiotherapy is needed after conservation for invasive cancers and reduces local recurrence. The evidence whether it influences long-term survival is less strong. One randomised trial found no beneficial effect,[7] whereas others report an improved long-term survival for those treated with radiotherapy, especially in the node-positive subgroup.[8] Critics of the latter paper point out the relatively low amounts of chemotherapy used in these studies and suggest that had the patients been treated with optimum chemotherapy the effect of radiotherapy on survival would disappear.

Whether radiotherapy is needed for all types of cancers is debatable. The British Association of Surgical Oncology trial (BASO 2) is examining this. Patients with small, well differentiated node-negative tumours are randomised to radiotherapy or none and/or tamoxifen or none. This is an important area, as the number of patients with such lesions has increased greatly following the introduction of the NHS breast screening programme. Early results do not show an increased local failure rate for those having surgery alone, although follow-up is currently short.

Detection of recurrence in the conserved breast is not always easy. Clinical examination may be difficult as radiotherapy may lead to fibrosis. Mammography has a lower sensitivity and specificity, and cytology may produce cells that look abnormal. Completion mastectomy should not be planned on the basis of cytology alone, and core, or open, biopsy is essential to avoid mis-diagnosis. Magnetic resonance imaging (MRI) seems to be useful but needs a special breast coil and is not readily available.[9] Newer techniques using gadolinium contrast and short acquisition times seem to give improved results. The current recommendation for surveillance monitoring is for mammography every 18–24 months.

If an isolated local recurrence is detected the options may include further local excision or completion mastectomy. If radiotherapy has already been given, it is not repeated, and chemotherapy or a change in hormone therapy is not usually indicated. Recurrence at the original tumour site is probably due to inappropriate or inadequate initial therapy and, therefore, the greatest care must be taken initially in the evaluation of the extent of the disease and in the choice of treatment.

After mastectomy

Large aggressive tumours predispose to local recurrence, which is more often of the locoregional type. It is, unfortunately, still possible to find a true local recurrence after mastectomy if the operation has left large amounts of breast tissue behind or after involved posterior margins. A mastectomy may not be an easy operation in a woman with large breasts, especially if unequal skin flaps are needed. Attention to detail over axillary surgery and radiotherapy to the flaps are important when recurrence is likely.

A spot recurrence in the flaps in the absence of disseminated disease is best treated by local resection. Although further skin nodules are to be expected, there is a group of (often elderly) women who can be dealt with by repeated local excisions. A change in hormone therapy is often tried and may slow down the development of more nodules. Multiple spot recurrences can be dealt with by a wide excision and either primary closure under tension or by means of a skin graft or rotation flap. Radiotherapy to the area should be employed if it has not already been used. Occasionally a second treatment may be employed if the original adjuvant radiotherapy occurred some time previously, using a different technique such as electrons. Skin changes such as telangectasia are then to be expected. Newer treatments include photodynamic therapy, where laser light is used to destroy cancer cells that have been sensitised by the oral administration of certain compounds. This technique seems to be successful for small isolated recurrences.[10]

The role of systemic chemotherapy in the management of local recurrence is not clearly defined. In the absence of proven systemic spread, many would reserve it for later use and try a change of hormone treatment initially. The range of hormonal manipulations has increased, and the use of the new generation of oral aromatase inhibitors and a pure anti-oestrogen (Faslodex) has given extra options.

Chemotheraputic agents have been tried topically but do not seem particularly active. Regional chemotherapy with infusion of agents into the feeding vessels to the chest wall has been used with some success. It requires cannulation of the internal mammary and lateral thoracic arteries or infusion into the subclavian artery, depending on the extent of the infusion required.[11] This was initially performed as an open operation but is now carried out via the femoral route by interventional radiologists. High doses of drug are delivered locally, with good responses if the vascular supply is intact. Unfortunately, the blood supply has often been compromised by previous surgery and radiotherapy, and so little drug reaches the affected area after a standard intravenous administration. In addition, previous adjuvant chemotherapy may have selected out a clone of resistant cells. If untreated, such patients can go on to develop cancer-en-cuirasse—a particularly distressing form of the disease. The cancer remains in the subcutaneous plane and often does not metastasise elsewhere. The benefits of regional chemotherapy are best when previously untreated disease is being treated, when clinical response rates of 80% are common.

Continual infusion of 5 fluorouracil via a Hickman or peripherally inserted central catheter seems to be effective in controlling local recurrence. This can be given alone[12] or in combination with boluses of cisplatin and an anthracycline, as in the epirubicin, cisplatin and infusional 5-fluorouracil (ECF) regimen.

Locoregional recurrence

Disease recurring in the ipsilateral axillary nodes can be treated by axillary clearance if this has not been previously performed, although the risks of lymphoedema are high. If the nodal disease is fixed or growth has occurred into the surrounding fat, then local radiotherapy or chemotherapy may be more appropriate.

Nodal recurrence in the supraclavicular fossa represents systemic spread, as does recurrence in the jugular chain. Occasionally a node may need to be biopsied to confirm the nature of the recurrence but radiotherapy and not surgery is the main therapy. Patients with a high proportion of positive axillary nodes often receive a supraclavicular field as part of the primary radiotherapy to try and prevent recurrence at this site.

Systemic recurrence—dissemination

Systemic recurrence marks the onset of disease that is incurable but still very treatable. There are distinct types of recurrence with different outcomes. Recurrence in bone and soft tissue is associated with a longer survival and is more responsive to treatment than disease in liver, lung or brain. There are many case reports of metastatic breast cancer presenting in odd places, but this is more a reflection of how common the disease is rather than a propensity for metastases in unusual sites. The length of time to dissemination after original presentation is important, and patients with a longer disease-free interval tend to respond better to subsequent therapy.

Restaging with bone and liver scans, chest radiography, full blood count, liver function tests, bone biochemistry and tumour markers and investigation of any specific patient signs are indicated.[3] A treatment plan needs to be agreed between the patient and relevant specialists as part of the multidisciplinary team. Support from breast nurse specialists/counsellors is also essential. Various treatment strategies can be used depending on the site and speed of relapse. An isolated painful bony metastasis can, for instance, be treated by a single fraction of radiotherapy with or without a change in endocrine therapy, whereas rapidly progressive disease in the liver requires chemotherapy.

An indication of how patients may respond to treatment can be obtained from the disease-free interval; those who relapse quickly after primary treatment are less likely to respond to hormone therapy and should probably start on chemotherapy.

Endocrine treatment

Oophorectomy was the first hormonal manipulation attempted and was performed in 1896 by Beatson, whose first two (of six) patients with advanced disease responded to surgical removal.[13] This response rate of 30% is typical of endocrine treatments in unselected patients. Surgical oophorectomy is still used if histology is needed or if scanning has shown any evidence of ovarian abnormality, otherwise a radiation menopause using 3 fractions of radiotherapy can be performed. Adrenalectomy and hypophysectomy have ceased to be performed as medical endocrine manipulations have evolved. The endocrine agents currently available are shown in **Table 4.1**. Tamoxifen remains the commonest treatment in the adjuvant setting but is being used less for advanced disease as patients increasingly have already been exposed to it. Rechallenge with tamoxifen is possible after time off treatment. Most oestrogens in postmenopausal women are made in peripheral fat and muscle by aromatisation of steroid precursors. A similar effect also occurs in the tumour itself. Inhibition of peripheral aromatisation lowers circulating oestradiol concentrations and is associated with clinical response. Aminoglutethimide was the first aromatase inhibitor but was non-specific in its action and had the side effect of adrenal suppression, requir-

Specific (o)estrogen receptor modulators (SERMs)
Tamoxifen
Raloxifene
Toremifine
Faslodex

Aromatase inhibitors
Injectable
   4 Hydroxyandrostenedione
Oral
   Anastrozole
   (Vorozole)*
   Letrazole
   Formestane—a steroidal agent

Luteinising hormone releasing-hormone agonists
   Leuprorelin
   Goserelin

Others
   Medroxyprogesterone acetate
   Megestrol acetate

* Not available in market place

Table 4.1 Current endocrine therapies in clinical use

ing patients to take supplemental hydrocortisone. It also caused a rash and is now no longer used. The second-generation aromatase inhibitors had to be given by injection but the third-generation compounds such as letrazole and anastrozole are orally available and their use is increasing. They have displaced medroxyprogesterone acetate and megestrol acetate as second-line endocrine agents. There are recent reports that there may be a survival advantage for patients taking aromatase inhibitors compared with other second-line agents.

Oophorectomy remains an option for treatment for premenopausal women but in the advanced disease setting is usually achieved by radiotherapy or chemical means. The luteinising hormone releasing-hormone agonist Zoladex (goserelin) provides effective castration but requires monthly injections.

Endocrine treatments are more likely to be effective in patients whose tumours were ER-positive (approximately 60% response rate). It was thought that there might be a 5–15% response rate in those with ER-negative tumours but this is questioned with better methods of estimating ER status. There are even recent suggestions that patients with ER-negative tumours have a lower survival if treated with tamoxifen (at least in the adjuvant setting). If response to one endocrine agent is obtained than a second agent should be tried at relapse as long as the disease is not progressing rapidly.

Table 4.2 shows the options for endocrine treatments.

Chemotherapy

Combination chemotherapy is given in a similar manner to adjuvant therapy, although different regimens may be used. There is no evidence that treating patients with asymptomatic metastases improves overall survival, and chemotherapy should be reserved for those patients with symptomatic disease that can not be controlled by other means.

Premenopausal
  Oophorectomy
    Surgical
    Radiotherapy
    Luteinising hormone releasing-hormone agent

Postmenopausal
  Tamoxifen unless previously received, otherwise
  Oral aromatase inhibitor
  Pure antioestrogen
  Medroxyprogesterone acetate
  Megestrol acetate

Table 4.2 Endocrine options for patients with advanced breast cancer

Aggressive disease or recurrence in sites likely to progress (liver and lung) is treated aggressively with anthracycline-based drugs. Patients who have relapsed while taking or after such drugs may be treated with the taxanes.[14] These newer agents work by inhibiting formation of the tubules needed for cell division. They were originally derived from the needles of the Pacific yew tree but are now synthesised. They have different side effects but have some activity in anthracycline-resistant disease. High-dose chemotherapy with bone marrow rescue or support has attracted much attention. Bone marrow can either be harvested prior to a dose of chemotherapy that would ultimately kill the patient, and can be reinfused to rescue the patient. A more modern alternative is to mobilise the marrow stem cells into the peripheral circulation, where they can be extracted and reinfused after treatment. The early mortality (around 10%) has dropped, and this technique gives higher response rates. The early promise has not translated into long-term survival in the current trials, although some researchers still have to report.[15]

A summary of chemotherapy regimens is given in **Table 4.3**. Given that these drugs are being provided for palliation it is important that side effects are minimised and that the full use of supportive measures to reduce nausea and vomiting is in place.

Response rates to chemotherapy for patients with advanced disease is of the order of 40–60%, with a median time to relapse of 8–14 months. Further courses achieve lower response rates (around 25%) and third courses lower still. Trials of palliative chemotherapy against best supportive care are under way to see which provides better quality of life.

Newer agents

End-stage refractory breast cancer is often treated with trial agents. This may be an inappropriate setting as some of the newer biological agents may be better at prevention of relapse rather than treatment of end-stage disease. There has,

---

Single agent
 Mitoxantrone
 Epirubicin
 Adriamycin
 Taxoids (Taxotere and Taxol)

Combination regimens
 CMF—Cyclophosphamide, methotrexate, 5-fluorouracil
 MMM—Mitoxantrone, methotrexate and mitomycin-C
 FEC—5-fluorouracil, epirubicin, cyclophosphamide
 ECF—Epirubicin, cisplatin and infusional 5-fluorouracil

Table 4.3 Current chemotherapy regimens

Telomerase inhibitors
Cytotoxic agents
   New analogues
   New molecular targets

Drug-resistance modulators

Immunological approaches
   Antibodies
     Polyclonal
     Monoclonal
   Immunoconjugates
   Vaccines
   Fusion proteins

Growth factor directed therapy
   Anti-EGFr (C-225)
   Anti-HER-2 (trastuzumab)
   Steroid hormone receptors
   Mammastatin
   Anti-osteoclast

Intracellular signal transduction inhibitors
   Tyrosine kinase inhibitors
   Farnesyl transferase inhibitors

Angiogenesis inhibitors (at least 50 in clinical trials)

Apoptosis

Inhibitors of metastatic pathway
   Adhesion molecules, integrins
   Matrix metalloprotein inhibitors

Table 4.4 New therapeutic strategies under development

however, been much interest in some agents that seem to give response rates in advanced disease. These strategies are based on the identification of specific molecular targets. **Table 4.4** lists some of the therapeutic strategies under development.

Several growth factors and their receptors have been identified in breast cancer. These include the epidermal growth factor receptor family (also known as HER-1, HER-2, HER-3 and HER-4), insulin-like growth factor receptors and the transforming growth factors α and β among others. Monoclonal antibodies to the EGF receptor (HER-1), such as C-225, and to HER-2, such as trastuzumab (Herceptin), are under investigation in clinical trials, with promising results as sole agents or in combination with conventional chemotherapy drugs. Agents that interfere with post-receptor binding events such as signal transduction are also under investigation. The tyrosine kinase inhibitors, farnesyl protein transferase inhibitors, antisense oligonucleotides and dominant negative mutants are all in active development.

p53 is a key gene in normal cell death (apoptosis). Abnormalities are found in 30–50% of breast cancer specimens (usually point mutations) and might prevent appropriate death of cells. Restoration of normal *p53* function is under investigation using different approaches.

Vaccines and fusion proteins are used in clinical trials for advanced disease as are agents aimed at the metastatic process, including matrix metalloprotease inhibitors and inhibitors of angiogenesis (the process whereby tumours attract a new blood supply allowing them to grow beyond about 1 mm and become invasive).

Specific sites of metastatic disease

Brain

Between 15 and 25% of patients with breast cancer develop central nervous system metastases as detected at postmortem examination. They are more common in young women with ER-negative tumours. Headache occurs in half the patients, with focal weakness and fits in another 20%. MRI is the diagnostic test of choice, although computed tomography is more commonly employed in the UK. In 50% of patients with brain metastases these are single, and some, very selected, patients may be helped by metastasectomy.[16] Radiation is the treatment used most often, although 20% of patients fail to complete the course and less than 10% are alive 1 year after completion of treatment. Radiosurgery with stereotactically delivered high-dose focused radiotherapy may be useful for isolated metastases. Steroids are used to control the symptoms and neurological signs, but their use is short lived and their side effects high. Anticonvulsants should also be used if patients have had a fit.[17]

Cord compression

Cord compression is caused by metastasis to the epidural space. Their recognition and early treatment is essential to avoid the complication of paraplegia. Over 90% of patients have symptoms for over a week before diagnosis and most have concurrent bony metastases elsewhere. Pain is the commonest first symptom, but by diagnosis weakness, autonomic dysfunction and sensory loss all occur. Plain radiography, bone scanning, CT and MRI are all used in diagnosis. Corticosteroids reduce oedema. Laminectomy with or without radiotherapy should be used early, although there is debate in which order these should be performed.[18] This condition is a true emergency, and patients with breast cancer who complain of back pain must be investigated appropriately.

Bone

Four fifths of patients with secondary breast cancer develop bony metastases that are most prevalent in the marrow-rich skeleton—the long bones, pelvis and axial vertebral skeleton. Bony secondaries lead to pain, fractures and hypercalcaemia each of which may need treatment.[19] Investigation is by bone scan or plain radiography with, occasionally, MRI.

Localised bony metastases may be dealt with by a single fraction or short course of radiotherapy. Specific sites may require prophylactic orthopaedic surgery to prevent (or treat) fractures.

Specific therapies directed against the skeleton include strontium[89], which is effective in 90% of patients with generalised bone pain.[20] Unfortunately its expense prevents wider use in the UK. The bisphosphonates stabilise bone mineral and are effective treatments for malignant hypercalcaemia as well as allowing healing of some lytic metastases.[21] They are poorly absorbed orally and are given as intravenous infusions. Patients with hypercalcaemia are often dehydrated, and rehydration remains an important part of treatment. Bisphosphonates are increasingly used as prophylaxis in those at risk of metastatic disease. They are then given orally even though absorption is poor, with 98% of the drug being excreted. Newer agents with much higher efficacy are under development.

Bone pain can be distressing, and effective treatment with non-steroidal anti-inflammatory agents with or without opioids should be used. Care needs to be taken over side effects such as constipation.

Pleural effusions

Up to 50% of patients develop a pleural effusion, most of which need no treatment. After a small sample has been removed to confirm the diagnosis, symptomatic tube drainage rather than simple aspiration is indicated as the latter leads to rapid reaccumulation. Pleurodesis with talc, tetracycline or bleomycin after drainage reduces reaccumulation.[22] Drainage by thoracoscopy and instillation of a talc–mitoxantrone mixture under direct vision may provide better results.

Bone marrow

Marrow involvement leads to a leucoerythroblastic picture, with anaemia being common.[23] Chemotherapy and/or endocrine therapy are necessary although the dose of chemotherapy may need to be reduced.

Isolated liver and thoracic nodules

Metastectomy may be indicated for true solitary isolated metastases. Unfortunately on investigation most patients turn out to have multiple sites of disease, and surgery is not possible. Liver metastases from breast cancer respond better to hepatic artery chemotherapy than do colorectal metastases as they have a better blood supply allowing drugs to reach the tumour deposits.

Pain and symptom control

A pain control or palliative specialist is an important contribution to the team. Many patients have pain as part of their illness.[24] This pain may occur in more than one site and may be caused by different mechanisms. The patients perception of the pain depends on their emotional state, and a thorough assessment is necessary. The concept of a ladder of pain control is a good one, and patients can move up and down this ladder as the disease progresses or is treated. Simple measures such as paracetamol may suffice, but opioids should not be withheld if needed. Concomitant administration of drugs with no analgesic component may help—antidepressants and anxiolytics used judiciously may allow reduction in analgesics. Attention to fluid intake and the avoidance of known side effects is also important.

Other symptoms such as nausea, anorexia, headache, breathlessness and constipation all need addressing. The help of specialist teams such as Macmillan and Marie Curie nurses and the hospice movement can make the difference between a death with dignity and a painful, peaceless end (see also Chapter 6, Palliative Care).

References

1. Leonard RCF. Oncology in practice. Palliative chemotherapy for advanced breast cancer. J Cancer Care 1995; 4: 127–30.

2. Del Turco R, Palli D, Carridi A *et al*. Intensive diagnostic follow-up after treatment for primary breast cancer: a randomised controlled trial. JAMA 1994; 271: 1593–7.

3. Glynne-Jones R, Young T, Ahmed A *et al*. How far investigations for occult metastases in breast cancer aid the clinician. Clin Oncol 1991; 3: 65–72.

4. Hayes DF, Kaplan W. Evaluation of patients after primary therapy. In: Harris JR *et al*. (eds). Diseases of the breast. Philadelphia: Lippincott-Raven, 1996; 630–42.

5. Scholl SM, Fourquet A, Asselain B *et al*. Neoadjuvant versus adjuvant chemotherapy in premenopausal patients with tumours considered too large for breast conserving surgery: preliminary results of a randomized trial. Ann Oncol 1991; 30A: 645.

6. Hortobagyi GN, Buzdar AU. Locally advanced breast cancer: a review including the MD Anderson experience. In: Ragaz J, Ariel IM (eds). High risk breast cancer. Berlin: Springer-Verlag, 1991: 382–403.

7. Forrest AP, Stewart HJ, Everington D *et al*. Randomised controlled trial of conservation therapy for breast cancer: 6-year analysis of the Scottish trial. Lancet 1996; 348: 708–13.

8. Arriagada R, Rutqvist LE, Mattsson A *et al*. Adequate locoregional treatment for early breast cancer may prevent secondary dissemination. J Clin Oncol 1995; 13: 2869–78.

9. Dao Th, Rahmouni A, Campana F *et al*. Tumor recurrence versus fibrosis in the irradiated breast: differentiation with dynamic gadolinium-enhanced MR imaging. Radiology 1993; 187: 751–9.

10. Khan SA, Dougherty TJ, Mang TS. An evaluation of photodynamic therapy in the management of cutaneous metastases of breast cancer. Eur J Cancer 1993; 29A: 1686–91.

11. Lewis W, Walker V, Ali HH *et al*. Intraarterial chemotherapy for patients with breast cancer—a feasibility study. Br J Cancer 1995; 71: 605–9.

12. Ng JSY, Cameron DA, Lee L *et al*. Infusional 5 fluorouracil given as a single agent in relapsed breast cancer: its activity and toxicity. Breast 1994; 2: 87–90.

13. Beatson GT. On the treatment of inoperable cases of carcinoma of the mamma: suggestions for a new

method of treatment, with illustrative cases. Lancet 1896; ii: 104–7.

14. Gollins SW, Barrett-Lee PJ. Response and side effects of Taxotere in advanced breast cancer. Breast cancer treatment today—focus on Taxotere (docetaxel). Meeting at the Royal College of Physicians, London, 1996: 12.

15. Myers SE, Williams SF. Role of high-dose chemotherapy and autologous stem cell support in the treatment of breast cancer. Haematol Oncol Clin North Am 1993; 7: 631–56.

16. Hendrickson FR. The optimum schedule for palliative radiotherapy for metastatic brain cancer. Int J Radiat Oncol Biol Phys 1977; 2: 165–8.

17. Galicich JH, French LA, Melby J. Use of dexamethasone in treatment of cerebral oedema associated with brain tumours. Lancet 1961; i: 46–8.

18. Gorter K. Results of laminectomy in spinal cord compression due to tumours. Acta Neurochir 1978; 42: 177–95.

19. Hortobagyi GN, Libshitz HI, Seabold JE. Osseous metastases of breast cancer: clinical, biochemical, radiographic and scintigraphic evaluation of response to therapy. Cancer 1984; 53: 577–82.

20. Robinson RG, Blake GM, Preston DF et al. Strontium-89: treatment results and kinetics in patients with painful metastatic prostate and breast cancer in bone. Radiographic 1989; 9: 271–8.

21. Theriault RL. Hypercalcaemia of malignancy: pathophysiology and implications for treatment. Oncology 1993; 7: 47–51.

22. Fentiman IS, Rubens RD, Hayward JL. Control of pleural effusions in patients with breast cancer: a randomized trial. Cancer 1983; 52: 737–82.

23. Webster DJT, Preece PR, Bolton PM et al. Leukoerythroblastosis in breast cancer. Clin Oncol 1975; 1: 315–7.

24. Portenoy RK, Foley KM. Management of cancer pain. In: Holland JC, Rowland JH (eds). Handbook of psychooncology: psychological care of the patient with cancer. New York: Oxford University Press, 1989: 369–83.

5 Hormones and chemotherapy

J. Michael Dixon
Robert C.F. Leonard

Patients who present with breast cancer can be classified into three groups, those with:

1. Operable breast cancer ($T_0 T_1, T_2, T_3 N_0, N_1 M_0$);
2. Locally advanced breast cancer ($T_4 N_0, N_1, N_2 M_0$);
3. Metastatic disease (any $T N_3 M_0$ or M_1).

Up to 50% of patients with operable breast cancer and over 80% of those with locally advanced disease will ultimately die of metastatic disease even though many of these patients never develop local recurrence. These observations indicate that even in patients with apparently localised disease, most have systemic metastases present at the time of diagnosis. A possible way of improving survival of these patients and those with overt metastatic disease is to give some form of systemic therapy to eradicate or slow down the growth of these metastases. There are two major forms of systemic therapy in common usage, hormonal therapy and chemotherapy.

Hormonal therapy

Oestrogen and progesterone regulate the growth and differentiation of normal breast tissue. Oestrogens are probably involved in the initiation and/or promotion of cancers arising in breast epitheliums. Evidence for this includes a reduced risk of breast cancer in women who have an early menopause[1] and an increased risk in those treated with oestrogen replacement therapy.[2] Oestrogens probably play an important part in the progression of breast cancer which, like progestogens, exert their effects on cells through binding to specific nuclear receptors.[3] The amount of oestrogen receptors (ERs) and, to a lesser extent, progesterone receptors (PgRs) in the cancer cell nucleus determine the responsiveness to endocrine therapy, given either as treatment for locally advanced or metastatic breast cancer or as adjuvant therapy after surgery and/or radio-therapy.[4,5] Patients with ER-rich tumours have a 50–70% chance of responding to hormonal therapy, and this increases to over 70% in patients whose tumours have both ERs and PgRs.[5] There seems to be a direct correlation between the quantity of ER and the probability and extent of response. Tumours with high ER levels are more likely to respond and have a greater quantitative response than tumours with lower ER levels.[6] Absence of ER predicts for early recurrence and poor short-term survival of patients with breast cancer.[7] ER-PgR-rich tumours are more likely to be well differentiated, to be diploid and to have a lower cellular proliferation rate than tumours that are hormone-receptor negative.[8]

Sources of oestrogens

The major source of oestrogens in premenopausal women is the ovary. Circulating oestrogens in postmenopausal women are at about 10% of pre-menopausal levels. They are synthesised peripherally, principally in fat (including breast fat), skin, muscle and liver from androstenedione, which is produced in the adrenal gland. The production of oestrogens requires the presence of the enzyme aromatase (**Fig. 5.1**).

Historical background

Hormonal therapy—or perhaps more correctly anti-hormonal therapy—for breast cancer dates back to 1896 when Beatson treated premenopausal women with metastatic breast cancer by oophorectomy and documented the regression

Figure 5.1
Enzymes involved in oestrogen biosynthesis. (17β-HSD, 17β hydroxysteroid dehydrogenase).

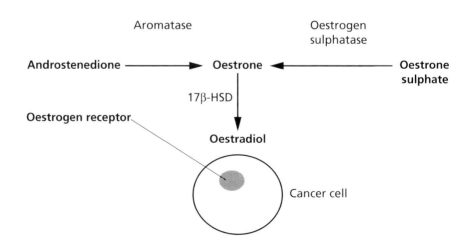

of skin nodules.[9] Subsequently, in 1905, DeCourmelles used ovarian irradiation in patients with breast cancer[10] and recent studies have confirmed the benefit of oophorectomy as a treatment for metastatic breast cancer or as adjuvant therapy after surgery and/or radiotherapy.[11–13]

Oophorectomy is not effective in postmenopausal women,[10] and adrenalectomy was formerly used in these patients as a means of interrupting hormone synthesis.[14] Hypophysectomy has also been used to produce 'total endocrine blockade.'[15] Of the surgical methods, only oophorectomy continues to be used currently, although with the introduction of gonadotrophin-releasing hormone (GnRH) agonists there is a decreasing need for surgical oophorectomy.[14]

Other hormonal agents have been used and include oestrogen preparations such as diethylstilboestrol, ethinyloestradiol and conjugated oestrogen.[11] Exactly how they work is unclear, but they do produce a 20% response rate. Toxicity with high-dose oestrogens was a problem and for this reason they are no longer used. Progestogens continue to be used, although their mechanism of action is unknown.[11,14] Androgens were formerly used in premenopausal women with advanced breast cancer, with an average reported response rate of about 20%,[11] but as with high-dose oestrogens, side effects make them unattractive agents compared with current alternatives.

Hormonal therapies and agents

Oophorectomy

This procedure can now be performed laparoscopically. It increases survival in the adjuvant setting[16] but is rarely used because it has been superseded by GnRH agonists.[13,14]

GnRH agonists

GnRH agonists suppress ovarian hormone production by desensitising pituitary gonadotrophin receptors.[14] Administration of pharmacological doses of these agents stimulates gonadotrophin production initially but an eventual down-regulation of GnRH receptors causes a block to the release of follicle-stimulating hormone (FSH) and luteinising hormone with a marked decrease in production of oestrogen and progesterone and cessation of menstruation. Luteinising hormone-releasing hormone (LHRH) receptors have been demonstrated on the surface of human breast cancer cell lines and in human breast tumours, suggesting that there may be a direct action on breast cancer cells.[18] This does not translate into any benefit for postmenopausal women.[17]

Goserelin is the best known LHRH agonist. It is given as a monthly depot injection subcutaneously in a dose of 3.6 mg. Efforts are underway to produce a three-monthly depot injection. Response rates to goserelin are identical to those of oophorectomy.[19]

Tamoxifen

Tamoxifen is a synthetic partial oestrogen agonist, which acts primarily by binding to the ER. It is the most widely used hormonal treatment for breast cancer. It has a half-life of 7 days and it takes approximately 4 weeks for the drug to reach a steady state in plasma.[20] The standard dose is 20 mg once a day, although at this dose there are wide variations in plasma concentrations between individual patients; there does not seem to be a direct correlation between the level of the drug in plasma and response.[21]

Less than 10% of patients with ER-poor tumours have a response to tamoxifen.[22] Technical problems associated with ER assays and lack of quality control almost certainly account for any apparent response in so-called ER-poor tumours, i.e. they may be ER-rich but the test misclassifies them. Other non-receptor mechanisms of action for tamoxifen have been proposed to explain the very occasional effectiveness of tamoxifen in ER-poor tumours.[10]

Response rates to tamoxifen are similar to those of other endocrine agents, but some tumours develop resistance to tamoxifen. Tumours that have become resistant to tamoxifen do not seem to lose their ER, and overgrowth of ER-negative clones does not explain the development of tamoxifen resistance.[23]

Although tamoxifen seems to be antagonistic to oestrogen in its action on breast cancer cells, it has oestrogen agonist activity at other sites; this accounts for both the benefits and side effects of treatment. Benefits include preservation of bone density,[24,25] decrease in plasma cholesterol concentrations[26] with an associated reduction in cardiovascular morbidity[27] (both agonist effects) and up to a 47% (SD 9) decrease in second primary breast cancers with 5 years' treatment (antagonistic effect).[13] Only 3% of patients given tamoxifen stop taking the drug because of side effects. Hot flushes are among the most common complaints of treatment.[28] Clonidine is occasionally effective in reducing flushing. Evening primrose oil has not been shown to be of any benefit, but megestrol acetate (20 mg twice a day) seems to be effective at reducing this symptom.[29,30] Recent studies have suggested that venlafaxine and fluoxetine may also be effective.[31,32]

Premenopausal women taking tamoxifen can experience decreased vaginal secretions and atrophy and vaginal dryness. This should be treated initially with a non-hormonal cream (such as Replens), but if this is not effective and symptoms are severe, pessaries containing oestrogen should be prescribed.[30] Systemic absorption of oestrogen is a potential concern but seems minimal with agents such as Vagifem. Some postmenopausal women experience vaginal discharge.[31] Tamoxifen has oestrogenic effects on the uterus, which accounts for the two-fold to four-fold increase in the risk of uterine cancer in women taking this drug.[31] The annual effect on risk of uterine cancer is one or two extra cases per 1000 women treated, with the risk being restricted to postmenopausal women. The number of endometrial cancers developing while women are taking tamoxifen is less than the number of contralateral breast cancers that tamoxifen prevents.[13] There is no evidence to suggest that women taking tamoxifen should have regular endometrial screening, but they should be instructed to report all episodes of unexplained vaginal bleeding.[32] Retinal problems have occasionally been reported but are rare.[31] Placebo-controlled trials have not shown an excessive weight gain in women taking tamoxifen, but this is a common complaint of women on long-term treatment.[31]

Dose

The recommended dose of tamoxifen is 20 mg a day, and there is no indication for giving tamoxifen at a greater dose.[10] The optimal duration of treatment is being addressed by current trials but available data suggest it should be given for 5 years.[13]

Role in premenopausal women

Tamoxifen has been used both as an adjuvant treatment and as primary therapy for metastatic breast cancer in premenopausal women.[31] It does not seem to have a major effect on FSH activity and LH concentrations, but oestradiol and oestrone concentrations are increased.[33] Many premenopausal women taking tamoxifen still have regular menses despite some getting menopausal flushes, and it is important to advise these women that pregnancy can occur. Tamoxifen appears as effective in premenopausal as it is in postmenopausal women. It has no apparent effect in ER-negative tumours.

 Tamoxifen produces equivalent rates of response to oophorectomy,[34,35] and in the adjuvant setting it improves survival of premenopausal women with hormone receptor-positive tumours but has no apparent benefit in ER-negative tumours.[13]

Other antioestrogens

Other synthetic antioestrogens or selective oestrogen receptor modulators (SERMs) have been developed and some such as toremifene and raloxifene are in clinical use and others in clinical trials.[10,36] Toremifene and raloxifene has less effect on the uterus but has similar efficacy to tamoxifen on breast cancers. These newer agents retain an agonist effect on bone but have little effect on the uterus. Pure antioestrogens have been developed such as faslodex. Problems with formulation have resulted in this agent being given by a monthly intramuscular injection. In clinical trials it seems to be very effective even after tamoxifen resistance has developed.[36] Recent studies in metastatic disease in patients who have relapsed on tamoxifen have demonstrated that faslodex is as effective as anastrozole in terms of response rate and time to progression.

Aromatase inhibitors

The production of oestrogen requires the presence and activity of the aromatase enzyme (Fig. 5.1). Oestrogen production in postmenopausal women is by peripheral aromatisation of androgens produced from the adrenal glands.[37] Several aromatase inhibitors have been used in the treatment of breast cancer and a number are under development.[38,39]

Aminoglutethimide

Aminoglutethimide is not a pure aromatase inhibitor as it also blocks production of cortisol.[14] This drug was developed as an alternative to adrenalectomy, and in randomised clinical trials produced similar response rates to the surgical procedure. There were problems with toxicity and it has now been superseded by newer aromatase inhibitors.

4-Hydroxyandrostenedione

4-Hydroxyandrostenedione (formestane) is 30–60 times more potent than aminoglutethimide at inhibiting aromatase, and studies indicate that this drug inhibits circulating oestradiol concentrations by 60% in postmenopausal women, but it has little effect on an oestradiol suppression in premenopausal women. Unfortunately, 4-hydroxyandrostenedione has to be given by intramuscular injection (250 mg twice per week).[40] Local pain and/or hypersensitivity reactions at the injection site can be a problem with this agent.

Newer aromatase inhibitors

The new generation aromatase inhibitors include the non-steroidal inhibitors with an imidazole or triazole structure.[38] These agents have a far better specificity for the aromatase enzyme and are much less toxic than aminoglutethimide. Anastrozole and letrozole produce 96.7–98.1% and 98.4–98.9% aromatase inhibition, respectively.[38] Letrozole in a dose of 2.5 mg produced higher response rates than megestrol acetate in a study of its use in the second-line setting in patients with metastatic disease. At the same dose it was associated with a significantly better survival in patients with metastatic disease than was aminoglutethimide. Second-line studies using anastrozole have shown that patients treated with 1 mg survived significantly longer than those treated with megestrol acetate. Toxicity with these new drugs is much less, but the side effects include nausea and lethargy.[38]

A new steroidal aromatase inhibitor, exemestane, given at a dose of 25 mg per day produced a significant survival benefit when compared with megestrol-acetate in the second line metastatic setting after tamoxifen failure.

One theoretical advantage of steroidal aromatase inhibitors is that they act as inactivators of the enzyme and bind to it irreversibly. Exemestane appears to produce clinical responses even after patients have become resistant to anastrozole or letrozole.

Progestogens

Response rates to progestogens are similar to tamoxifen when used as second-line drugs.[10] Medroxyprogesterone acetate (MPA) and megestrol acetate are the best known agents. MPA has been most commonly used as an intramuscular injection. Doses of 500–1000 mg per day for 30 days have been used followed by a maintenance dose given weekly. Between 10 and 15% of patients on MPA develop slight cushingoid features; oedema, uterine bleeding, hot flushes and thromboembolic phenomena have all been observed.[41] In the UK and USA, megestrol acetate is the most commonly used progestogen and as with MPA the main problem with progestogen treatment is weight gain. The mechanism of action of progestogens is unknown, but they may interfere with the binding of oestrogen to the ER, accelerate oestrogen catabolism or interfere with aromatisation of androgens to oestrogens. The main reason these agents are reserved for third-line treatment is that they cause more side effects than the aromatase inhibitors,[42] with evidence from randomised trials of lower efficacy. The standard dose for megestrol acetate is 160 mg once a day.

Antiprogestogens

Synthetic antiprogestogens are currently being studied in clinical trials.[10]

Use of hormonal agents

Hormonal agents have classically been used alone or in combination with chemotherapy. Some studies have assessed the combination of different endocrine agents. The optimal sequencing of hormonal agents is not clear.[10] In postmenopausal women the endocrine agent of choice has traditionally been tamoxifen, but with the advent of the new aromatase inhibitors and the results now available from first line metastatic and neoadjuvant studies this may change. In premenopausal women GnRH agonists, oophorectomy and tamoxifen are all used for adjuvant therapy and treatment of metastatic breast cancer.[41] More recent studies have suggested that combining GnRH agonists and tamoxifen is more effective than one drug alone.[43]

Chemotherapy

Many active agents are available for the treatment of breast cancer and numerous combination chemotherapy regimens have been reported. Certain groups of drugs form the cornerstone of treatment.

Anthracyclines

Doxorubicin

Anthracyclines have long been considered to be the most active agents in the treatment of breast cancer. The antitumour antibiotic doxorubicin (adriamycin) is the most widely used of these agents. When used as a single agent ($50-75$ mg/m^2 weekly) in untreated patients with metastatic breast cancer, the response rate ranges from 40 to 50%.[44,45] When combined with other agents the response rates are much higher. Although doxorubicin is usually given as a bolus once every 3 weeks, weekly administration allows some intensification of dosage and possibly reduces cardiac toxicity. Other side effects include myelosuppression and mucositis. Doxorubicin produces alopecia in most patients.[10]

Epirubicin

This is a semisynthetic doxorubicin stereoisomer. Its single agent response rate is comparable to that of doxorubicin and is dose dependent and ranges from 25% in previously treated patients to 62% in untreated patients.[46] It is associated with less cardiac toxicity, the risk of clinical cardiac impairment rising rapidly at doses of 900 mg/m^2 or above, compared with a cumulative toxic dose of 550 mg/m^2 for doxorubicin.[47] It is used most often in combination regimens such as EC (with cyclophosphamide three times weekly) or FEC (with 5-fluorouracil (5-FU) and cyclophosphamide three times weekly) or in some schedules weekly.

Mitoxantrone

Because the cumulative dose and dose rate of doxorubicin are limited by cardiac toxicity, other anthracycline analogues have been developed to circumvent this problem. Although mitoxantrone is reported to produce less cardiac toxicity than doxorubicin, clinical trials have demonstrated cardiac effects with increasing cumulative doses.[48] Response rates when used as a single agent vary from 17 to 35%.[46] Side effects are similar but less severe than those with doxorubicin. In particular, severe alopecia is avoided. It produces a lower rate of regression compared with doxorubicin or epirubicin.

Cyclophosphamide

Cyclophosphamide is inert until activated by microsomal enzymes in the liver, which then produces the potent alkylating cytotoxic metabolite phosphoramide mustard.[49] Although cyclophosphamide is an active single agent, it is usually used in combination regimens such as cyclophosphamide, 5-FU and methotrexate (CMF). Response rates in advanced breast cancer with CMF are around 40%. This regimen with several different schedules is the commonest used in the adjuvant setting and is the regimen on which the influential overview data are based.[49] Specific side effects include mucositis and occasionally a chemical cystitis.[10]

5-FU

5-FU is a pyrimidine analogue, which has been used in cancer chemotherapy for more than 30 years. The drug first has to be metabolised and then binds to the enzyme thymidylate synthase, thus inhibiting DNA synthesis.[50] Activity of 5-FU depends somewhat on peak concentrations and, importantly, on duration of exposure so that scheduling may have significant clinical effects. In early trials, 5-FU was given as a bolus, but more recently it has been used as an infusional therapy, initially over 24 hours, then over 5 days and now continuously, sometimes for many months.[50,51] Specific problems with continuous 5-FU include the 'hand foot' syndrome where patients develop erythema and eventually blistering of epithelium over the hands and feet and mucositis. These problems rapidly disappear if the infusion is discontinued for a few days. This regimen lends itself to combinations with pulsed intermittent agents such as doxorubicin (AF) epirubicin and cisplatin (ECF) and even a variant of CMF.[52]

Methotrexate

Methotrexate is an analogue of folic acid and works by indirectly blocking thymidylate synthesis. In breast cancer it is primarily used in the CMF regimen. Debate continues as to whether substitution of doxorubicin or epirubicin for methotrexate increases the efficacy of this combination therapy.[10]

Platinum compounds

Platinum compounds were first used in the treatment of germ-cell tumours. These compounds work by forming adducts with DNA, which inhibit replication.[53] Cisplatin is the most widely used agent.

Toxicity is a problem with the platinum compounds and includes peripheral neuropathy, renal toxicity and ototoxicity.[10] Carboplatin has a similar efficacy to cisplatin but fewer toxic effects. Cisplatin is most often used in combination with epirubicin and infusional 5-FU in the ECF regimen. Response rates over 90% have been reported in patients with large operable or locally advanced breast cancers.

Mitomycin-C

Mitomycin-C is an antitumour antibiotic, which forms covalent cross links with DNA and inhibits DNA, RNA and protein synthesis.[54] Mitomycin-C causes cumulative myelotoxicity. In the UK it is used in combination with mitoxantrone and methotrexate (MMM combination), and although it is a well tolerated treatment,[55] neutropenia, thrombocytopenia and treatment delays can be problems.

Taxanes *yew tree*

Paclitaxel is a novel chemotherapeutic agent derived from the bark of the Western Pacific yew tree. Paclitaxel has been the most widely used taxane. It has a unique mechanism of action and stabilises microtubular assembly.[56] This prevents cell division. Another semisynthetic taxane, docetaxel, has been derived from the leaves of the European yew tree. Dose-limiting toxicity seems to be myelosuppression.

These agents are very active against breast cancer. Initially the main interest was based on observations of effectiveness, particularly of docetaxel, in anthracycline-resistant or refractory disease.[57] Trials have shown effectiveness in the advanced setting, and more recently these drugs have been shown to be effective when added to anthracyclines as adjuvant treatment.[58]

Vinorelbine

Vinorelbine is a semisynthetic vinca alkaloid which, given as a single agent or in combination chemotherapy, is active against breast cancer. Response rates seen with this drug in second- and third-line chemotherapy for advanced disease are similar to those with paclitaxel. A large study showed it to be well tolerated although neuropathy can be a problem and neutropenia in heavily pretreated patients. Common scheduling schemes are day 1 and day 5 every 21 days or day 1 and day 8 as a single agent or in combination with 5-FU infusion. It may be a preferable choice for elderly or less fit patients than the more active but more toxic docetaxel.

Capecitabine

Capecitabine is the first available oral fluoropyrimidine. The full drug is converted to 5-FU after absorption and there may be differential uptake in tumour cells. Apart from its attraction as an oral compound with predictable absorption patterns, it does not cause hair loss and may be combined with other drugs as it has a low risk of myelotoxicity. It can cause severe mouth ulceration and/or diarrhoea in some patients, who seem to be unduly sensitive to its effects owing to an enzyme deficiency. Usual scheduling is to give it twice daily for 14 of every 21 days.

Trastuzamab (herceptin)

Trastuzamab (herceptin) has caused great interest among the public after media reports. It is a non-cytotoxic humanised (i.e. considered by the body to be human and therefore not rejected) antibody that is directed against the HER-2 oncoprotein. The HER-2 oncoprotein is over-expressed in about 20% of breast cancer cells and is particularly associated with ER-negative aggressive clinical behaviour. The antibodies are active as a single agent in heavily pretreated patients, but interest lies in combining them with cytotoxic chemotherapy in cancers expressing HER-2. Used in these circumstances, a survival gain over the same chemotherapy without the antibody has been shown in a randomised controlled trial either combined with anthracycline or with paclitaxel. The main problem with herceptin is a seemingly synergistic toxic interaction with anthra-cyclines, which accentuates cardiac toxicity. Further studies are needed, but it can be safely combined with taxanes provided that the patient has not had extensive previous treatment with anthracyclines.

Cost constraint

Cost constraint is a major factor influencing the use of newer agents in the treatment of breast cancer. The taxanes, vinorelbine, capecitabine and herceptin continue to be investigated in trials in patients with metastatic disease, locally advanced disease and early disease in the adjuvant setting.

General side effects of chemotherapy

Although hair loss is the most common concern of patients before starting chemotherapy, 80% report fatigue and lethargy as the most troublesome side effect. Alopecia with some chemotherapy regimens may be reduced by scalp cooling. Patients should be measured for a wig before they lose their hair and should be reassured that it does regrow after treatment. Nausea and vomiting are unpleasant side effects but are well controlled by appropriate anti-emetic drugs given just before and after emetogenic chemotherapy. Most patients receiving emetogenic chemotherapy now have serotonin-3 (5-HT$_3$) antagonists given just before and sometimes just after emetogenic chemotherapy.[37] Typically, patients receive either 5-HT$_3$ antagonists and dexamethasone prior to the chemotherapy and are given metoclopramide or domperidone with or without steroids for 2 or 3 days after chemotherapy. The main argument against the universal use of 5-HT$_3$ antagonists has been cost, but this has significantly reduced over the years. Some patients may develop severe constipation or migraine-like headaches with these drugs.

White count nadirs occur typically 7–14 days from the start of treatment although some may be earlier (e.g. docetaxel) or later (e.g. mitomycin-C). Any chemotherapy can lead to neutropenia-associated infective complications owing to Gram-positive or Gram-negative organisms. Non-specific illness especially fever or influenza-like symptoms demands urgent investigation, including a blood count. A low neutrophil count ($<1 \times 10^9$ l^{-1}) and fever requires immediate antibiotics and monitoring. Neutropenia of less than 0.5×10^9 l^{-1} and fever usually requires hospital admission for intravenous antibiotics and monitoring.[59–61]

For many cytotoxics, extravasation of drug can lead to necrosis and ulceration of the skin and subcutaneous tissues. This is a powerful argument for employing trained teams of nurses to deliver cytotoxic chemotherapy.[59]

Complications of adjuvant chemotherapy may occur many months and years after completion of treatment. The major potential toxicities are cardiac dysfunction, premature menopause and the development of second cancers. Cardiomyopathy due to doxorubicin may occur during treatment, shortly after its completion or many months later. By screening for pre-existing heart conditions (echocardiography or, better, isotope ventriculography to examine left ventricular function) symptomatic complications are rare ($<5\%$). Menopausal symptoms and cessation of periods are common and affect approximately 70% of premenopausal women during treatment (return to normal cycles occurs in many patients). The likelihood of permanent menopause is a function of the intensity of the chemotherapy, the agents used and the patient's age.[61] For CMF, about half of patients in their early 40s will develop permanent menopause, for others even when menstrual periods return, the onset of eventual permanent menopause is brought forward by several years. There is some evidence that after chemotherapy there is an increased risk of second cancers, particularly leukaemias.[61] As with Hodgkin's disease, the risk is probably drug and dose related, being more common with alkylating agents.

The overview follow-up information on late complications is reassuring, and specific investigations of the complication rate of CMF-type regimens for breast cancer suggest that the risk of leukaemia is less than 3% at 15 years. There is a worrying association between acute myeloid leukaemia and intensive exposure to anthracyclines, which was revealed in recent trials of intensive therapy with anthracycline-based polychemotherapy.

Operable breast cancer

Systemic therapy can be given after local surgery and/or radiotherapy—adjuvant treatment. Alternatively, systemic therapy can be given as initial treatment to patients with large operable breast cancers (primary systemic therapy or neoadjuvant therapy) prior to locoregional therapy. Whereas the effectiveness of adjuvant treatment has been demonstrated in clinical trials, there are no clear benefits of primary systemic therapy in improving survival although it reduces the number of women needing mastectomy.

Primary systemic therapy

One potential problem with primary systemic therapy is that if a diagnosis of cancer is made by fine needle aspiration cytology alone, non-invasive disease could be overtreated by chemotherapy (cytology cannot differentiate between invasive and *in situ* disease).[60,61] A biopsy by core needle sample to obtain a histological diagnosis of invasive cancer should therefore be obtained before embarking on primary medical treatment. A major concern with this approach is that axillary nodal status is not known prior to the selection of systemic therapy. This information is the most useful prognostic factor for long-term survival.[61] There is no evidence that leaving a cancer in the breast during primary systemic therapy increases patient anxiety.

Primary systemic therapy was introduced initially as treatment for inoperable and locally advanced disease to make the disease operable.[57] Its use has now been extended to patients with large operable breast cancers in an attempt to avoid mastectomy. Response rates ranging from 62% in tumours larger than 5 cm to 93% in tumours of 3 cm have been reported.[62] There seems to be no significant difference in response rates using different chemotherapy regimens. After chemotherapy, breast conserving surgery (quadrantectomy) was possible in 90% of patients in one series, with just over 73% of patients with tumours over 5 cm becoming candidates for breast conservation. At 36 months, 1 of 201 patients treated by primary systemic therapy, quadrantectomy and postoperative radiotherapy had a local recurrence.[63] Preliminary results have been published from two randomised controlled trials. A French study of 272 women with tumours larger than 3 cm were randomised to primary chemotherapy followed by appropriate local treatment, or mastectomy followed by the same chemotherapy to patients who were node positive or ER negative.[64] Of the patients receiving primary chemotherapy, 63% avoided mastectomy and were treated by breast conservation.

More than 1300 patients were randomised in a National Surgical Adjuvant Breast and Bowel study comparing surgery followed by four cycles of adriamycin and cyclophosphamide or four cycles of adriamycin and cyclophosphamide followed by surgery.[65] The initial response rate to chemotherapy was 80%, including 37% who had a complete clinical response. More than 65% of patients in the primary chemotherapy group underwent breast conservation compared with 57% in the adjuvant chemotherapy group. At surgery, 59% of those receiving primary chemotherapy were node negative compared with 42% in the immediate surgery group.

This study has as yet shown no survival differences between the two treatment groups.[66]

Although most studies have treated patients prior to surgery with chemotherapy, there is increasing interest in treating patients with hormone-sensitive disease with primary hormonal therapy.

The use of primary medical (neoadjuvant) treatment for operable breast cancer has increased over the past decade.[60] A theoretical advantage is the ability to assess response *in vivo*, clinically or by using mammography or ultra-sonography.[67] Ultrasonography seems to be the most accurate of these three methods.[68] Both the primary tumour and lymph node metastases can be seen to respond (**Fig. 5.2**), and invasive cancer seems to be more sensitive to chemotherapy than non-invasive disease. Early detection of resistance to treatment allows the oncologist to discontinue ineffective therapy, which avoids unnecessary toxicity and may facilitate a change to a potentially more effective regimen. Primary systemic therapy also has the theoretical advantage that by treating disease earlier it is less likely that resistant tumour clones will have emerged spontaneously.[67] The advantages and disadvantages of primary systemic therapy are summarised in Table 5.1.

Figure 5.2
Mammograms showing primary cancer involving axillary node (a) before and (b) after primary chemotherapy. At subsequent surgery, the patient was found to have no residual carcinoma in the breast or axilla—a complete pathological response. From Dixon JM. ABC of breast diseases, BMJ Publishing Group, 1995.

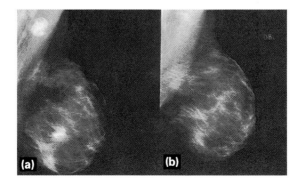

Systemic therapy	Advantages	Disadvantages

Adjuvant	Proved efficacy
	Prognostic information
	  available after surgery
		Uncertainty whether treatment
		  is effective in individual
		  patients

Primary	Allows direct assessment of
	  effectiveness
	Tumour shrinkage may allow
	  breast conservation
	Early treatment of
	  micrometastases
		Loss of prognostic information
		May treat *in situ* disease (if
		  diagnosis made by fine needle
		  aspiration cytology alone)

Table 5.1 Advantages and disadvantages of adjuvant and primary systemic therapy

Chemotherapy

Regimens used for primary chemotherapy have generally been similar to those used for adjuvant treatment, and about 70% of patients show a partial response, 20–30% a complete clinical response and a small number (about 10–15%) achieve a complete pathological response.[60,67] Although evidence indicates that continuous infusional chemotherapy with drugs such as 5-FU combined with intermittent agents such as epirubicin and cisplatin achieve very high response rates (>90%), there has to date been no long-term benefit in survival with infusional chemotherapy.[69]

Primary hormonal therapy

Tamoxifen (20 mg a day by mouth) produces a partial response in up to 60% of elderly patients with hormone-responsive (ER-positive) tumours (Fig. 5.3) and a complete clinical response in 15%.[70] Initial data from non-randomised studies suggested that new aromatase inhibitors may have advantages over tamoxifen in the neoadjuvant setting.[71] This has been confirmed in studies comparing letrozole with tamoxifen in patients who were initially only candidates for mastectomy. Response rate and breast conserving rate were significantly higher with letrozole than tamoxifen.

The use of GnRH analogues (goserelin 3.6 mg monthly given sub-cutaneously or leuprorelin 3.75 mg monthly given subcutaneously or intra-muscularly) as primary medical treatment for premenopausal women with ER-positive tumours has been evaluated.[70] Few patients showed complete pathological response after hormonal treatment, but the side effects are generally much less than with chemotherapy.[70]

Tumours treated with primary systemic therapy are generally treated for to 3–4 months.[60,70] During this period, patients should be monitored carefully using clinical and ultrasonographical assessment of tumour volume. Overall, between 50

Figure 5.3
Patient with large inflammatory cancer of right breast (a) before and (b) after infusional chemotherapy showing a complete clinical response.

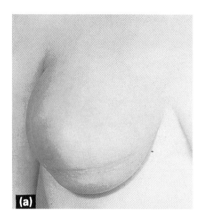

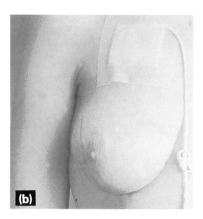

and 70% of patients with large operable tumours will have sufficient tumour regression to avoid mastectomy. Nearly all patients require local treatment (surgery or radiotherapy) after primary systemic therapy. It is acceptable treatment for patients with large operable breast cancers, but the use of primary systemic therapy for other groups of patients cannot be recommended outside clinical trials.[60]

Adjuvant therapy for operable breast cancer

The effectiveness of adjuvant therapy has been shown in clinical trials, but its effectiveness in individual patients cannot be assessed as there is no overt disease to monitor.[60]

Because small randomised trials fail to detect the modest gains in disease-free or overall survival obtained with adjuvant therapy, the benefits of adjuvant treatment only became evident when data from all trials were analysed in an overview or meta-analysis.[13,72]

The large numbers of patients included in such analyses provide great statistical power and allow detection of even modest advantages of one treatment over another.

Adjuvant endocrine therapy and chemotherapy alone in women with operable breast cancer each reduce the annual risk of death by between 25 and 39% for at least 10 years. Benefits of adjuvant therapy add up to about 10 extra women alive at 10 years for every 100 women with stage 2 disease and five extra women alive at 10 years for every 100 women with stage 1 disease.

The relative reductions in mortality are the same in women with axillary negative or axillary positive nodes. This suggests that adjuvant therapy is equally active in both low- and high-risk groups. The absolute reduction in mortality depends on the chances of a woman dying of disease. A 30% reduction in the relative risk of the odds of dying reduces a 10% mortality at 10 years by 3% and a 60% mortality at 10 years by 18%. The shape of the disease-free and overall survival curves over time indicates that for most patients the benefit is that of a delay in the onset of recurrence rather than long-term cure.

Hormonal therapy

Premenopausal patients

Results from the Early Breast Cancer Trialists' overview show that in women under 50 years of age ovarian suppression as the sole adjuvant therapy is associated with a 28% reduction in the annual risk of death, and this effect lasts for at least 15 years (Table 5.2).[16] The benefits of oophorectomy seem greatest in patients with ER-positive tumours. The overview suggests that tamoxifen produces benefits in premenopausal women equal to those in postmenopausal women (**Tables 5.2 and 5.3**), with the benefits again being restricted to patients with ER-positive tumours. The evidence on duration of tamoxifen in premenopausal women suggests that it should be given for 5 years (Table 5.3). Combining tamoxifen and ovarian suppression may have benefits compared with LHRH or tamoxifen alone in premenopausal women.[43]

	% Proportional reduction in	
	Recurrence (SD)	Mortality (SD)
Polychemotherapy	35 (4)	27 (4)
Ovarian suppression	30 (9)	28 (9)
Tamoxifen for 5 years	45 (8)	32 (10)

Adapted from Early Breast Cancer Trialists Collaborative Group, reference 13.

Table 5.2 Direct estimates of proportional reduction in odds of recurrence and death among women aged less than 50 in trials of adjuvant therapy

Duration of tamoxifen treatment	% ER positive	% Proportional risk reduction in	
		Recurrence (SD)	Deaths (SD)
1 year	74	2 (7)	–2 (8)
2 years	79	14 (5)	10 (6)
5 years	92	45 (8)	32 (10)

Adapted from Early Breast Cancer Trialists Collaborative Group, reference 13. ER, Oestrogen receptor.

Table 5.3 Proportional risk reductions in women aged less than 50 treated with tamoxifen subdivided by duration

Postmenopausal patients

Tamoxifen produces between a 37 and 54% reduction in the annual odds of recurrence in women aged 50 or over with ER-positive breast cancers (**Table 5.4**). The optimum duration of tamoxifen seems to be 5 years (**Table 5.5**). The meta-analysis included five studies which compared 1, 2 and 5 years of tamoxifen treatment, and on the basis of these data the current recommendations are that patients should take adjuvant tamoxifen for 5 years. There seems to be a significant interaction between ER status of the tumour and the benefit obtained by tamoxifen, and patients with ER-poor tumours gain no significant benefit (**Table 5.5**).

Chemotherapy

The overview concluded that when using chemotherapy a combination of drugs produced better results than a single drug alone and that six courses produced similar benefits to more prolonged treatment schedules.[13]

Tamoxifen for 5 years		% Proportional reduction in	
Age	% ER positive	Annual odds of recurrence (SD)	Annual odds of death (SD)
Age <50	92%	45 (8)	32 (10)
50–59	93%	37 (6)	11 (8)
60–69	95%	54 (5)	33 (6)
≥70	94%	54 (13)	34 (13)
Overall	94%	47 (3)	26 (4)

Table 5.4 Proportional risk reductions subdivided into age groups after exclusion of patients with oestrogen receptor (ER) poor disease

	% Recurrence (SD)	% Death (SD)
Tamoxifen for 1 year		
ER poor (< 10 fmol/mg^{-1})	6 (8)	6 (8)
ER unknown	20 (4)	10 (4)
ER positive	21 (5)	14 (5)
Tamoxifen for 2 years		
ER poor	13 (5)	7 (5)
ER unknown	28 (4)	15 (4)
ER positive	28 (3)	18 (4)
Tamoxifen for 5 years		
ER poor	6 (11)	−3 (11)
ER unknown	37 (8)	21 (9)
ER positive	50 (4)	28 (5)

Adapted from Early Breast Cancer Trialists Collaborative Group, reference 13.

Table 5.5 Odds reduction of risk of recurrence and absolute survival benefits for postmenopausal patients given tamoxifen subdivided by oestrogen receptor (ER) status

Chemotherapy given at the time of, or just after, surgery has theoretical advantages. Drugs given at the time of surgery might theoretically kill any circulating tumour cells dislodged by surgery. Cumulative data suggest, however, that there is little added benefit from administering perioperative chemotherapy.

Premenopausal patients

Adjuvant chemotherapy seems to produce similar reductions in odds of death to that of oophorectomy (**Table 5.2**). Data from a Scottish trial suggest that the greatest benefit from chemotherapy is in patients with ER-negative tumours.[73] Adjuvant chemotherapy given for at least four cycles produces a highly significant 37% reduction in annual odds of recurrence in women aged under 40 and a 27% reduction in annual odds of death (**Table 5.6**).[13] Chemotherapy seems to be most effective in young patients (i.e. women under the age of 50). One third or more of recurrences and one quarter of the deaths in premenopausal women seem to be avoided or delayed at 10 years by chemotherapy. This effect is similar in patients who are node positive and node negative (**Table 5.7**). The effects of chemotherapy in reducing the risks of dying are prolonged beyond 5 years (**Table 5.7**).

Postmenopausal patients

Ten-year survival data do show a significant reduction in recurrence and improved survival in postmenopausal patients given adjuvant chemotherapy.

Age at randomisation	% Proportional risk reductions	
	Recurrence (SD)	Mortality (SD)
<40	37 (7)	27 (8)
40–49	34 (5)	27 (5)
50–59	22 (4)	14 (4)
60–69	18 (4)	8 (4)

Adapted from Early Breast Cancer Trialists Collaborative Group, (reference 13).

Table 5.6 Proportional risk reductions with polychemotherapy subdivided by age at randomisation

Age at randomisation	Nodal status	% Proportional risk reduction in mortality	
		0–4 years (SD)	≥5 years (SD)
<50	Negative	18 (11)	23 (14)
<50	Positive	24 (7)	39 (8)
50–69	Negative	23 (10)	17 (12)
50–69	Positive	10 (4)	9 (5)

Table 5.7 Proportional risk reductions in mortality with polychemotherapy during first 5 years of follow-up (years 0–4) and later years (≥5) subdivided by age at randomisation and nodal status

Overall, a 14% reduction in the proportional reduction in the odds of dying was observed in women aged 50–60 (Table 5.6). This reduction is about half that of younger patients. The benefits seem to be less pronounced in women aged 60–69 years than in younger, postmenopausal women. Too few women aged over 70 years of age were included in the overview to provide a valid estimate of the effects. Some of these differences between premenopausal and post-menopausal women have been attributed to the added endocrine effects of chemotherapy in premenopausal patients. Since publication of the overview, other data from recent trials have suggested that the benefits of chemotherapy are significant for older patients.[60]

Optimal regimen for adjuvant chemotherapy

The most commonly used treatment is six cycles of CMF over 6 months. Studies have shown that four cycles of AC (given over approximately 3 months) is as effective as six cycles of CMF.[74] In this direct comparison the days of nausea were fewer with the AC regimen, and many investigators have concluded that AC is the preferred regimen. Cardiac toxicity was not a major problem, but alopecia was worse with the AC regimen.

Direct comparisons of anthracyclines and other chemotherapeutic regimens have shown that anthracyclines produce a 12% (SD 4) proportional reduction in the odds of recurrence over other regimens and a marginally 11% (SD 5) proportional reduction in mortality. This suggests that there are potential benefits of anthracycline-containing combinations over the CMF regimen.

In a randomised trial from Milan of patients with four or more positive nodes the sequence of doxorubicin for four cycles followed by intravenous CMF for eight courses was compared with CMF for two cycles followed by doxorubicin for one cycle repeated to a total of 12 courses of chemotherapy, there was a highly significant improvement in disease-free and overall survival in the patients treated with adriamycin and then CMF.[74] The survival curve of patients having the sequential regimen flattens out a few years after the start of treatment suggesting that this regimen may be curing some patients. No CMF arm alone was included in this trial, but comparison with earlier results with CMF suggests that a sequence of four cycles of adriamycin and eight of CMF is a potent regimen for high-risk patients who are node positive.

A more recent study of over 3000 patients has suggested that after an anthracycline regimen the addition of paclitaxel produces additional benefits.[58] AC followed by paclitaxel produced a 40% reduction in the odds of relapse and a 25% reduction in the odds of death compared with AC alone. This relative gain at 30 months is similar to the benefit conferred by standard polychemotherapy (CMF) when compared with observation alone. At the last follow up the relative benefit in the paclitaxel-treated group had reduced, but it was still significant. Paclitaxel is now licensed for adjuvant chemotherapy in the USA.

Many physicians routinely use a doxorubicin or epirubicin regimen such as CAF or FEC for patients who are node positive and particularly for younger patients. Data of the superiority of anthracycline regimens over CMF are now consistent.[75,76]

Dose-intensive adjuvant chemotherapy

The issue of dose intensity first received attention in 1981 when the Milan group reported that only those patients who received at least 85% of the planned CMF dose benefited significantly from adjuvant chemotherapy, whereas those receiving less than 65% of the planned dose had the same disease-free and overall survival as the control group treated by surgery alone.[77] Later, in a retrospective analysis of published randomised trials, Hryniuk and Levine showed a direct correlation between survival and dose intensity.[78] One prospective study compared three doses of CAF, and after a median follow-up of 3.4 years, the higher and moderate dose-intensity regimens yielded superior disease-free and overall survivals than the low dose.[79] The 'low-dose' chemotherapy was well below the intensity most oncologists would accept. There may be a threshold rather than a dose–response effect, i.e. a minimum dose below which cytotoxics are not effective. In a second study where the dose of cyclophosphamide was intensified in the AC regimen there was no difference in outcome in the three groups given different doses of cyclophosphamide.[80]

Studies of dose intensity using extremely high–dose chemotherapy and autologous bone marrow transplant or peripheral stem cell rescue have now been completed and early data presented.[81–83] (The validity of the trial in reference 83 has not been confirmed.) Only one of the three studies, the smallest, showed a potential benefit for high-dose chemotherapy.[84] There are problems with all three trials, which have so far been reported in abstract form only. One neutral study was reported before the planned date due to political pressure, the second, which was in favour of the non-high dose arm, compared high-dose chemotherapy with a non-standard intensive chemotherapy arm that relied on granulocyte colony stimulating factor support. Results of large-scale European trials are awaited, and an overview analysis will almost certainly be needed before definitive comments can be made on the value of high–dose chemotherapy either as initial treatment or as consolidation therapy for patients at high risk. Until data from any meta–analysis show benefits, high-dose chemotherapy with stem cell rescue should not be used outside randomised trials.

Adjuvant therapy

The benefit of adjuvant therapy—possible treatment side effects, long-term toxicities and their impact on quality of life—need to be considered when selecting adjuvant therapy for individual patients. Absolute improvements in survival seem greatest in patients at high risk of recurrence and death. Patients in these categories may therefore be prepared to accept higher degrees of toxicity and side effects. The current philosophy in adjuvant therapy is to stratify patients in relation to their risk of recurrence and death and to tailor the adjuvant treatment to that risk. Patients can be stratified on the basis of number of involved nodes (**Table 5.8**) and tumour size and grade in patients who are node negative.[60] More recently, age has been identified as an important prognostic factor and has been suggested by the St Gallen group as a factor that should be considered when prescribing adjuvant chemotherapy. Alternatively, patients can be stratified on the basis of a single index such as the Nottingham Prognostic Index, which combines tumour size, histological tumour grade and node status.[85] Having identified risk groups, adjuvant treatment is tailored to that risk. An outline of the current recommendations for adjuvant treatment for patients with operable breast cancer is given in **Table 5.9**.

Combinations of hormonal and chemotherapy

The Early Breast Cancer Trialists' overview predicted that in postmenopausal women there were additional survival gains from addition of chemotherapy to tamoxifen.[13] These gains, although not significant in terms of survival, did make major differences in terms of recurrence, and these are expected eventually to translate into improvements in survival. Trials are currently underway to investi-

Risk group	Age	% Survival without relapse at 5 years
Node-negative patients		
Low risk	>35; tumour ≤1 cm in diameter	>90
Intermediate risk	≤35; tumour ≤1 cm in diameter	75–80
	>35; tumour >1 cm grade 1 or 2	
High risk	≤35; tumour >1 cm grade 1 or 2	50–60
	Any tumour >1 cm grade 3	
Node-positive patients		
Low or intermediate risk	>35; 1–3 positive nodes	40–50
High risk	≤35; 1–3 positive nodes	20–30
	>35; 4–9 positive nodes	
Very high risk	≤35; ≥4 nodes involved	10–15
	>35; ≥10 nodes involved	

Table 5.8 Definitions of risk groups and associated risk of relapse

gate combinations of hormonal therapy and chemotherapy in premenopausal and postmenopausal women.

Adjuvant immunotherapy

More than 20 randomised trials of adjuvant immunotherapy have been completed, and currently no evidence exists to support the use of this modality.[61] The latest consensus-report from the St Gallen group advocates a more aggressive policy of including lower risk groups for chemotherapy compared with earlier reports. This reflects an emphasis on aiming to achieve the gain in disease-free survival rather than overall survival.

Adjuvant use of bisphosphonates

Other drugs that are not strictly cytotoxic are being investigated in combination with standard adjuvant therapy strategies. Bisphosphonates inhibit the osteoclast over-activity in bone that results from metastatic tumour cells and reduces the incidence of bone metastases in experimental animal models. In one study, patients with primary breast cancer who had microscopic bone marrow involvement detected by sensitive assays received standard adjuvant therapy and were randomised either to receive clodronate for 2 years or placebo. At 3 years of follow-up, patients who received clodrinate not only had a reduction in the incidence of bone metastases but also had a reduced incidence of soft tissue and visceral metastases.[86] Preliminary results of a second trial also showed a signifi-

	ER status	Premenopausal patients	Postmenopausal patients
Node negative patients			
Low risk	Positive	Tamoxifen or nil	Tamoxifen or nil
	Negative	Nil	Nil
Intermediate risk	Positive	Tamoxifen	Tamoxifen
	Negative	Chemotherapy	Chemotherapy
High risk	Positive	Chemotherapy + tamoxifen	Tamoxifen ± chemotherapy
	Negative	Chemotherapy	Chemotherapy
Node positive patients			
Low + intermediate risk	Positive	Chemotherapy + tamoxifen ± LHRH	Chemotherapy + tamoxifen
	Negative	Chemotherapy	Chemotherapy
High + very high risk	Positive	More intensive chemotherapy + tamoxifen + LHRH	More intensive chemotherapy + tamoxifen if fit
	Negative		

ER, oestrogen receptor; LHRH, luteinising hormone releasing-hormone.

Table 5.9 Adjuvant treatment for patients with breast cancer

cant reduction in the development of bone metastases when the drug was used as an adjuvant to other treatment modalities.[87] A large trial is ongoing in the USA to further evaluate the role of bisphosphonates.

Locally advanced breast cancer

Locally advanced breast cancer is characterised clinically by features suggesting infiltration of the skin or chest wall by tumour or matted involved axillary nodes (**Table 5.10**).[88] Large operable cancers and tumours fixed to muscle should not be considered locally advanced. Depending on referral patterns and clinical definitions, between 1 in 12 and 1 in 4 patients present with locally advanced disease.[88] Differences in definition and the different forms of breast cancer explain why the reported 5-year survival rates for locally advanced disease vary between 1 and 30%. Overall median survival is about 2.5 years, which is not very different from the survival described for breast cancer in the late 19th and early 20th centuries.

Locally advanced breast cancer may arise because of its position in the breast (for example, if the lesion is peripheral), because of neglect or because the cancer is biologically aggressive (inflammatory cancers and most of those with peau d'orange). Inflammatory cancers are uncommon and are characterised by brawny, oedematous, indurated and erythematous skin changes; these cancers have the worst prognosis of all locally advanced breast cancers.

Treatment

Current treatments have had a significant impact on local control rates and have had some impact on overall survival.[89] Patients with hormone-sensitive disease have a much longer survival than those with hormone-insensitive disease. Local

Skin
Ulceration
Dermal infiltration
Erythema over tumour
Satellite nodules
Peau d'orange

Chest wall
Tumour fixation to
    Ribs
    Serratus anterior
    Intercostal muscles

Axillary nodes
Nodes fixed to one another or to other structures

Table 5.10 Clinical features of locally advanced breast cancer

and regional relapse remains a major problem in locally advanced disease and affects approximately half of all patients.

Surgery

Mastectomy is generally not indicated in the presence of features of locally advanced disease, but after treatment with a combination of cytotoxic drugs or initial hormonal treatment, surgery may become feasible weeks or months later.[90] It may be possible to perform a wide excision, although mastectomy is the most commonly performed procedure. Some cancers, principally those with direct skin involvement because of position or neglect, are suitable for primary surgical treatment.

Role of systemic and local treatments

The mainstay of local treatments has been radiotherapy because surgery is associated with high rates of local recurrence.[90-92] Radiotherapy can produce high rates of local remission in both the breast and axilla, but when radiotherapy is used alone only 30% of patients remain free of locoregional disease at death. By combining appropriate systemic therapy and radiotherapy, response rates of over 80% have been reported, and over two thirds of patients retain locoregional control at death. Radiotherapy should be given to patients managed initially by surgery, to those who have operations after a course of systemic therapy and to those whose cancer remains inoperable after primary systemic therapy.

Choice of systemic treatment

Systemic therapy should be given as part of a planned programme of combined systemic and local therapies.[89] Factors influencing the choice of systemic therapy for locally advanced breast cancer are outlined in **Table 5.11**. Standard chemotherapy, such as CMF, increases rates of local control but has little impact on survival. There are some data to suggest that infusional therapies based on 5-FU combined with doxorubicin (AF), sometimes with the addition of

Hormonal treatment
Slow-growing or indolent disease
Oestrogen receptor-positive tumour
Elderly or unfit patients

Chemotherapy
Inflammatory cancer
Oestrogen receptor-negative tumour
Rapidly progressive cancer

Table 5.11 Factors affecting choice of systemic therapy for locally advanced breast cancer

Figure 5.4
Locally advanced breast cancer before (a) and after (b) treatment with six months of tamoxifen. The mass in the supraclavicular region is a lipoma.

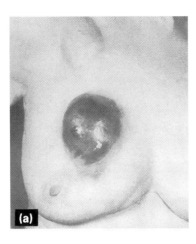 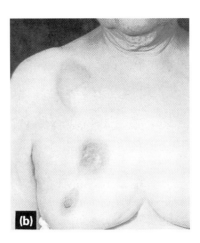

Hormonal treatment
Premenopausal patients Ovarian ablation (surgery, radiation or gonadotrophin releasing hormone antagonists)
Postmenopausal patients Tamoxifen or Aromatase inhibitor

Chemotherapy
Intravenous Infusion of 5-fluorouracil combined with an anthracycline (e.g. epirubicin, cyclophosphamide and 5-fluorouracil; or epirubicin, cisplatin and 5-fluorouracil)

Table 5.12 Choice of treatment for patients with locally advanced breast disease

cyclophosphamide (ACF) or 5-FU combined with epirubicin and cisplatin (ECF) or cyclophosphamide (ECF), do produce higher local response rates than the intermittent regimens used for adjuvant chemotherapy. Despite apparently high response rates these have not been associated with significant improvements in survival.[69]

Primary hormonal therapy can be given to patients with locally advanced breast cancer provided that their tumours are ER positive and appear to be relatively slow growing or indolent (**Fig. 5.4**). The choice of treatments in these patients is outlined in **Table 5.12**.

Metastatic breast cancer

The pattern of survival of patients with metastatic disease is variable. Some patients with hormone-sensitive disease survive many years after sequential hormone manipulation. Patients with disease that is not hormone sensitive have much shorter survivals.[29] The clinical pattern of relapse predicts future behaviour. Patients with a long disease-free interval (>2 years after primary diagnosis) and favourable sites of recurrence (such as local lymph nodes and chest wall) survive much longer than patients who have either a short disease-free interval

Figure 5.5
Median time of survival associated with sites of metastasis in patients with breast cancer.

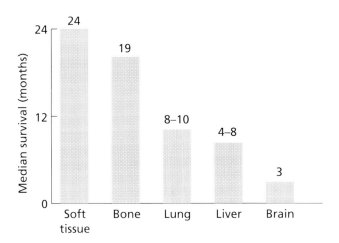

Median survival (months)

24 — 24
19
12 — 8–10
4–8
0 — Soft tissue, Bone, Lung, Liver, Brain, 3

or recurrence at other sites.[93,94] Patients with lung, liver and brain disease have the poorest outlook (**Fig. 5.5**).

Treatment should produce effective control of symptoms and at the same time prolong survival. The primary aim, however, is to improve quality of life. At the present time there is no evidence that treating asymptomatic metastases improves survival, and it is not appropriate to perform regular routine screening investigations looking for systemic disease during follow up.[10]

The choice of whether patients should have hormonal treatment or chemotherapy depends on the biology of the disease. Disease with a potentially good prognosis is best treated by hormonal treatment, whereas that with a poor prognosis usually requires chemotherapy (**Fig. 5.6**).[10,30]

Figure 5.6
Choices of treatment for metastatic or recurrent breast cancer.

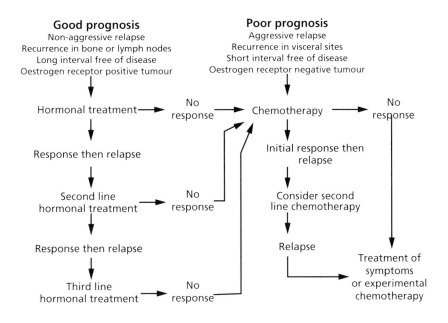

Good prognosis
Non-aggressive relapse
Recurrence in bone or lymph nodes
Long interval free of disease
Oestrogen receptor positive tumour

Poor prognosis
Aggressive relapse
Recurrence in visceral sites
Short interval free of disease
Oestrogen receptor negative tumour

Hormonal treatment → No response → Chemotherapy → No response

Response then relapse

Second line hormonal treatment → No response

Response then relapse

Third line hormonal treatment → No response

Initial response then relapse

Consider second line chemotherapy

Relapse

Treatment of symptoms or experimental chemotherapy

Hormonal treatment

Although generally regarded as causing few side effects, all hormonal therapies can cause distressing symptoms. Objective responses to hormonal agents are seen in 30% of all patients and in 50–60% of patients with ER–positive tumours, although when symptomatic response rates are included the final response rate is higher. Response rates of 25% are seen with second-line hormonal agents, although less than 15% of patients who get no response to first-line hormonal treatment will respond to second-line treatment.[30] Approximately 10–15% of patients respond to third-line treatment.

 In premenopausal women combinations of LHRH and tamoxifen seem superior to either agent alone.[95]

For second-line treatment after tamoxifen the choice would be LHRH agonists alone or LHRH agonists combined with an aromatase inhibitor. In post-menopausal women, if tamoxifen has not been used then this would be the first-line agent, although this may change as results of first-line studies with the aromatase inhibitors are becoming available.[10] If tamoxifen has already been used, one of the newer aromatase inhibitors such as anastrozole, letrozole or exemestrone is the hormonal treatment of choice. The next agent to be used is exemestrone if anastrozole or letrozole has been used previously, or faslodex when it becomes available. Progestogens, such as megestrol acetate or medroxy-progesterone acetate are now used much less frequently, but can be used following exemestrone failure (**Table 5.13**).[30]

Treatment	Premenopausal patients	Postmenopausal patients
First-line	LHRH agonists if not previously used. If patients had previous oophorectomy, LHRH agonists and tamoxifen	Tamoxifen if not previously used or an aromatase inhibitor such as anastrozole or letrozole
Second-line	LHRH agonists combined with in patients who have aromatase inhibitors in patients who have relapsed on LHRH agonists	After tamoxifen, anastrozole, letrozole or exemestrone. After anastrozole or letrozole, exemestrone or faslodex when it becomes available
Third-line		After anastrozole, or letrozole, exemestrone; After exemestrone progestogens

LHRH, luteinising hormone-releasing hormone.

Table 5.13 Hormonal treatment of metastatic breast cancer

Chemotherapy

With chemotherapy a balance has to be achieved between obtaining a high rate of response and limiting side effects. The best palliation and subsequent quality of life is obtained with regimens that produce the highest response rates. Studies that have compared different intensities of chemotherapy have shown that quality of life is better with more intensive regimens even with their associated side effects rather than with less intensive regimens that have lower response rates and fewer side effects.[96,97] Overall rates of response to chemotherapy are about 40–60%, with a median time to relapse of 6–10 months.[30] The current chemotherapy regimens of choice usually include an anthracycline, although elderly patients or those with significant comorbid (e.g. heart) disease are usually treated with alternative regimens. Combinations of anthracyclines and taxanes are currently being studied and seem to be superior than either agent alone. These may become the treatment of choice because of their high response rates.[98] Subsequent courses of chemotherapy have low rates of response (<25%).[10,30] The agents used for treating metastatic disease are similar to those used in the adjuvant or primary systemic therapy settings.

Short-term results from high-dose chemotherapy with bone marrow or stem cell rescue for metastatic breast cancer seem promising, with 15–20% of patients being disease free after 3–10 years.[99] One randomised study did show a significant survival benefit for patients having stem cell rescue, but this study has been criticised because the survival of patients given standard doses of chemotherapy was less than would have been expected and long-term tamoxifen was given only to the chemotherapy responders in a population of women that included a substantial number with ER-positive tumours. Larger, long-term controlled studies are currently underway.[84]

The emphasis on objective response rates in chemotherapy reports is to some extent a cultural inheritance reflecting the experimental nature of chemotherapy development over the years. Clinical experience tells us that the subjective benefit and improvement in quality of life is not always indicated by improvements in X-ray films or scans. Too few reports have looked at quality of life issues but those that have done so have tended to show that patients seem to derive a benefit even from toxic therapies in the absence of high rates of objective response.[85,100]

New agents

The erb-B2 targeting antibody trastuzamab or herceptin has anti-tumour activity in erb-B2 over-activity expression malignancies and phase 1 and phase 2 clinical trials have shown that multiple doses of antibody can be given safely. The results of a large randomised trial have demonstrated that herceptin is at least additive or perhaps synergistic with other chemotherapeutic agents. In combination with first-line doxorubicin and cyclophosphamide chemotherapy, herceptin moderately increased response rates and time to regression than did AC alone. In the second part of this same clinical trial, patients with metastatic breast cancer refractory to doxorubicin were randomly assigned to treatment with either trastuzamab and paclitaxel or paclitaxel alone. Patients treated with the combination had almost double the response rate and improvements in the time to progression and survival than did those treated with paclitaxel alone. The only worrisome effect was an increase in congestive cardiac failure rate.[98]

Specific problems

Soft tissue or local chest wall disease

Although local disease can be isolated, up to 50% of patients have associated systemic relapse. Local recurrence after mastectomy can be classified as single-spot relapse, multiple-spot relapse or field change.[101] Treatment and prognosis differ

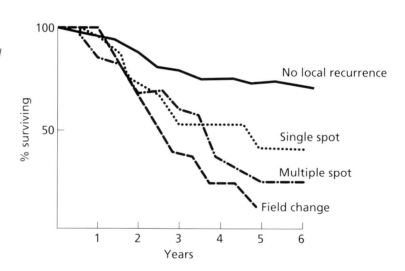

Figure 5.7 *Survival of patients with local recurrence separated into three groups; single spot, multiple spot and field change compared with patients without local recurrence. Modified from reference 101.*

Type of recurrence	Treatment
Single spot	Excise and consider radiotherapy if short disease-free interval If oestrogen receptor positive, change endocrine therapy
Multiple spot	Radiotherapy, unless already given, or more radical excision (possibly with coverage with myocutaneous flap) Change hormonal systemic therapy if ER positive
Widespread	Consider radiotherapy unless already given or disease too widespread. Appropriate systemic treatment (and/or local application of chemotherapy such as miltefosine applied daily

Table 5.14 Treatment of local recurrence in chest wall

for these three categories (**Fig. 5.7, Table 5.14**). If the recurrence is focal and occurs many years after the original, surgery alone can provide long-term control.[102] If the disease-free interval is short then surgery could be combined with radiotherapy and a change in hormonal therapy if the tumour is ER positive. If the recurrence is multiple spot but still localised the options are radiotherapy or more radical excision combined, if the tumour is ER positive, with a change in hormonal systemic therapy.[30] In widespread recurrence, standard treatments are often disappointing, although intra-arterial chemotherapy and infusional 5-FU is sometimes effective for chest wall and soft tissue disease (**Fig. 5.8**).[103] The topical agent miltefosine is active for small-volume multiple-skin nodules and has been tested in a randomised controlled clinical trial against placebo (about 30% of patients show response for up to 10 months). It does not yet, however, have a product licence in the UK. Failure to halt the progress of local disease can lead to carcinoma en cuirasse where the chest wall is encircled by tumour—a most unpleasant situation for the patient.[102]

The control of ulceration and focal malodorous infected tissue is a considerable problem for carers and patients. Excision of dead tissue and the use of topical and oral antibiotics with antianaerobic activity combined with charcoal dressings may help to control malodour.[30]

Recurrent axillary disease

If initial axillary therapy has been suboptimal, axillary disease can represent residual untreated disease rather than recurrence. Isolated mobile recurrences should be excised and combined with a level 3 dissection if this has not already been performed.[104,105] Patients with isolated inoperable recurrence may be given radiotherapy (if not previously given) or systemic therapy, or both; these are sometimes effective at palliation but rarely produce long-lasting control of the disease.[102] When, as is often the case, axillary recurrence occurs in

Figure 5.8
Patient with symptomatic skin and soft tissue disease in left supraclavicular fossa before (a) and after (b) a 12-week course of single agent continuous 5-fluorouracil.

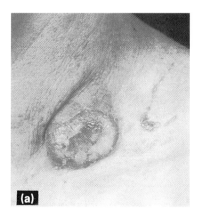
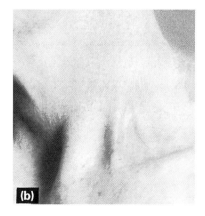

association with metastases at other sites, then appropriate systemic therapy with or without local treatments is required.[106,107]

Bone disease

Up to 75% of patients with recurrence will develop bone disease in the skeleton. Widespread bone disease alone often responds well to hormonal treatment (**Fig. 5.9**) but when associated with visceral disease or young patients, chemotherapy is usually required.[61] Assessing response to treatment is difficult and studies suggest that serological tumour markers may be of more use than repeated radiographs or bone scans.[108] Most clinicians use control of symptoms to determine response to therapy.

Bisphosphonates have had a major effect on the treatment of bone disease and hypercalcaemic bone disease associated with breast cancer. Bisphosphonates are small molecules based on organic phosphate, which bind to mineral calcium in the bone but also exert an inhibitory effect on the activity of osteoclasts and possibly on tumour cells directly. Given by mouth the absorption is unreliable and poor probably owing to calcium binding in the gut. Both oral and intravenous preparations have, however, been tested in clinical trials to treat hypercalcaemia and symptomatic bone disease. Pamidronate, the intravenous preparation given as a 4-weekly infusion, and oral clodronate have both shown important clinical benefits in symptomatic bony metastases regardless of whether the patient is receiving chemotherapy or endocrine therapy.[98]

Biphosphonates produce a substantial reduction in skeletal morbidity such as pain, incidence of fractures and the need for radiotherapy, with benefits lasting for up to 2 years in about 25% of patients.[109,110]

Figure 5.9
Radiograph showing metastatic lesions in humerus before (a) and after (b) course of hormonal treatment with consequent reduction in bone pain and increase in bone density. From Dixon JM. ABC of Breast Diseases, BMJ Publishing Group, 1995.

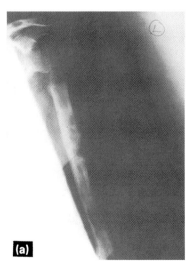

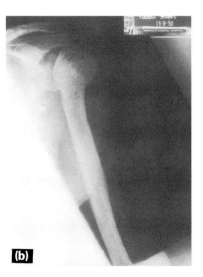

Localised bone pain can be treated by a single fraction of radiotherapy.[111] Widespread bone pain can be treated with radioactive strontium, with few side effects, or with sequential upper and lower body hemibody radiotherapy.[111,112] This latter treatment is associated with more toxicity. Bisphosphonates are useful for diffuse bone pain although their true role remains to be determined.[113]

When bone lysis threatens fracture, internal fixation followed by radiotherapy (low doses in a few fractions) improves quality of life and maintains mobility (**Fig. 5.10**). Such treatment is often associated with a reasonable survival. If a pathological fracture does occur, a combination of internal fixation and radiotherapy should be used, although the functional result is usually inferior to that of prophylactic treatment.[111]

Detection of bone metastases can be a problem. Some patients have infiltration of marrow causing the pain rather than bony destruction. Such disease is often best detected by MRI or CT rather than by bone scanning or plain radiography.[29]

Widespread marrow infiltration can cause a leucoerythroblastosis (immature cells in the peripheral blood). In such patients chemotherapy is generally required, although it has to be given initially at reduced doses with careful monitoring and adequate supportive therapy.[114]

Malignant hypercalcaemia

The onset of confusion, thirst and polyuria can be insidious and in patients with bone disease non-specific illness should always arouse suspicion of malignant hypercalcaemia. After diagnosis, patients should be treated with hydration with saline (about 3 l over 24 hours) and then intravenous bisphosphonates.

Figure 5.10
Radiograph showing lytic lesion in the neck of the right femur before (a) and after (b) prophylactic replacement. Patient was alive and well three years later. From Dixon JM. ABC of Breast Diseases, BMJ Publishing Group, 1995.

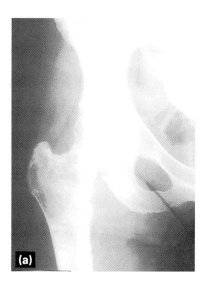
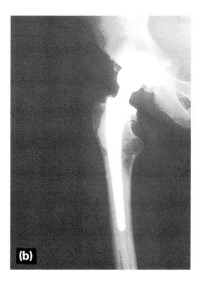

Effective anticancer treatment reduces the risk of recurrence, but patients who exhibit continuing hypercalcaemia can be treated with repeated intravenous bisphosphonates. Gastrointestinal absorption of oral bisphosphonates is poor and variable, and their role in recurrent hypercalcaemia is being investigated.[115]

Malignant pleural effusion

Up to 50% of patients with metastatic breast cancer develop a malignant pleural effusion, but only some will require specific treatment. Only 85% of patients have malignant cells in the effusion.[116] Although aspiration is effective at establishing a diagnosis, it is not an effective treatment. Tube drainage followed by new or changed systemic therapy controls effusions in just over one third of patients.[30] For the other two thirds installation of bleomycin, tetracycline or talc (the latter inserted under general anaesthesia) is required to control recurrence.[117–119] The effusion should be aspirated to complete dryness and then a small amount of local anaesthetic placed before adding bleomycin or tetracycline. This reduces the pain associated with the procedure. Talc seems to have the lowest rates of recurrence. Patients often get transient pyrexia after chemical pleurodesis.

Neurological complications

Although non-metastatic syndromes of the CNS can occur, any focal neurological symptom must be investigated. CT or MRI detects even small volumes of disease in the brain or spinal cord.[120–123]

Initial treatment of brain metastases is to reduce oedema with high-dose corticosteroids (dexamethasone 12–16 mg daily) pending local treatment with fractionated radiotherapy.[30] Radiotherapy produces most benefit in patients whose neurological symptoms improve after taking steroids. Radiotherapy is delivered in five daily fractions.[124] The long-term results of treating CNS disease are disappointing, with most patients, especially those with leptomeningeal disease, surviving only a few weeks or months. Long-term survival is seen quite often, however, especially in patients with isolated brain metastases after excision of metastasis and postoperative radiotherapy.[125]

Cord compression is not usually amenable to surgery and is seen most often in patients with thoracic spinal metastases.[118] Treatment is with steroids and fractionated radiotherapy. Treatment needs to be started as soon as possible and before any neurological deficits are severe. Occasionally patients do have isolated metastases causing cord compression and in these laminectomy can be effective.[30,126]

References

1. Vessey MP. The involvement of oestrogen in the development and progression of breast disease: epidemiological evidence. Proc R Soc Edinb 1989; 95B: 3.

2. Dupont WD, Page DL. Menopausal oestrogen replacement therapy and breast cancer. Arch Intern Med 1991; 51: 67–72.

3. Fuqua SAW. Estrogen and progestogen receptors in breast cancer. In: Harris IK, Lippman ME, Morrow M, Hellman S (eds). Diseases of the breast. Philadelphia: Lippincott-Raven, 1996: 261–71.

4. Bezwoda WR, Esser JD, Dansey R et al. The value of estrogen and progesterone receptor determination in advanced breast cancer. Cancer 1991; 68: 867–72.

5. Osborne CK, Yochmovit MG, Knight WA et al. The value of estrogen and progesterone receptors in the treatment of breast cancer. Cancer 1980; 46: 2884–8.

6. Hawkins RA, Tesdale I, Sangster K et al. The quantitative importance of oestrogen receptor (ER) assay in elderly patients with breast cancer treated with tamoxifen. Br J Surg 1996; 83 (suppl 1): 11.

7. Hawkins RA, White C, Bundred NJ et al. Prognostic significance of oestrogen and progestogen receptor activities in breast cancer. Br J Surg 1987; 74: 1009–13.

8. Wenger CR, Beardslee S, Owens MA et al. DNA ploidy, S-phase and steroid receptors in more than 127,000 breast cancer patients. Breast Cancer Res Treat 1993; 28: 9–20.

9. Beatson GT. On the treatment of inoperable cases of carcinoma of the mamma. Suggestions for a new method of treatment with illustrative cases. Lancet 1896; ii: 104–7, 162–5.

10. Honig SF. Hormonal therapy and chemotherapy. In: Harris JR, Lippman ME, Morrow M, Hellman S (eds). Diseases of the breast. Philadelphia: Lippincott-Raven, 1996: 669–73.

11. Muss HB. Endocrine therapy for advanced breast cancer: a review. Breast Cancer Res Treat 1992; 21: 15–26.

12. Hoogstraten B, Fletcher WAS, Gad-el-Mawla N et al. Tamoxifen and oophorectomy in the treatment of recurrent breast cancer. Cancer Res 1982; 42: 4788–91.

13. Early Breast Cancer Trialists Collaborative Group. Tamoxifen for early breast cancer: an overview of the randomised trials. Lancet 1998; 351: 1451–67.

14. Santen RJ, Manni A, Harvey H et al. Endocrine treatment of breast cancer in women. Endocr Rev 1990; 11: 221–65.

15. Harvey HA, Santen RJ, Osterman J et al. A comparative trial of transphenoidal hypophysectomy and estrogen suppression with aminoglutethimide in advanced breast cancer. Cancer 1979; 43: 2207.

16. Early Breast Cancer Trialists Collaborative Group. Ovarian ablation in early breast cancer: overview of the randomised trials. Lancet 1996; 348: 1189–96.

17. Harris AL, Carmichael J, Cantwell BMJ et al. Zoladex: endocrine and therapeutic effects in postmenopausal breast cancer. Br J Cancer 1989; 59: 97.

18. Miller WR, Scott WN, Morris R et al. Growth of human breast cancer cells inhibited by a leutinizing hormone-releasing hormone agonist. Nature 1985; 313: 231.

19. Nicholson RJ, Walker KJ, Davies P. Hormone agonists and antagonists in the treatment of hormone sensitive breast and prostate cancer. Cancer Surv 1986; 5: 463.

20. Furr JA, Jordan VC. The pharmacology and clinical uses of tamoxifen. Pharmacol Ther 1984; 25: 127.

21. Langan-Fahey SM, Tormey DC, Jordan VC. Tamoxifen metabolites in patients with longterm adjuvant therapy for breast cancer. Eur J Cancer 1990; 26: 883–8.

22. Wittliff JL. Steroid-hormone receptors in breast cancer. Cancer 1984; 53: 630.

23. Osborne CK, Coronado E, Allred DC et al. Acquired tamoxifen resistance: correlation with reduced breast tumour levels of tamoxifen and isomerization of trans-4-hydroxy-tamoxifen. J Natl Cancer Inst 1991; 83: 1477–82.

24. Turken S, Siris E, Seldin D et al. Effects of tamoxifen on spinal bone density in women with breast cancer. J Natl Cancer Inst 1989; 81: 1086.

25. Love RR, Mazess RB, Barden HS et al. Effect of tamoxifen on mineral density in postmenopausal women with breast cancer. N Engl J Med 1992; 326: 852–6.

26. Schapira DV, Kumar NB, Lyman GH. Serum cholesterol reduction with tamoxifen. Breast Cancer Res Treat 1990; 1: 3–7.

27. McDonald CC, Stewart HJ. Fatal myocardial infarction in the Scottish adjuvant tamoxifen trial. BMJ 1991; 303: 435–7.

28. Fisher B, Costantino J, Redmond C et al. A randomised clinical trial evaluating tamoxifen in the treatment of patients with node-negative breast cancer who had estrogen-receptor positive tumours. N Engl J Med 1989; 320: 479.

29. Loprinzi CL, Michalak IC, Quella SK. Megestrol acetate for the prevention of hot flashes. N Engl J Med 1994; 331: 347–52.

30. Leonard RCF, Rodger A, Dixon JM. Metastatic breast cancer. In: Dixon JM (ed). ABC of breast diseases. London: BMJ Publishing Group, 1995: 45–8.

31. Jaiyesimi IA, Buzdar AU, Decker DA et al. Use of tamoxifen for breast cancer: 28 years later. J Clin Oncol 1995; 13: 513–29.

32. Love CDB, Muir BB, Scrimgeour JB et al. An investigation of endometrial abnormalities in asymptomatic women on tamoxifen and an evaluation of the role of endometrial screening. J Clin Oncol 1999; 17(7): 2050–4.

33. Jordan VC, Fritz NF, Langan-Fahey S et al. Alteration of endocrine parameters in premenopausal women with breast cancer during long-term adjuvant therapy with tamoxifen as the single agent. J Natl Cancer Inst 1991; 83: 1488–91.

34. Ingle JN, Krook JE, Green SJ et al. Randomized trial of bilateral oophorectomy versus tamoxifen in premenopausal women with metastatic breast cancer. J Clin Oncol 1986; 4: 178.

35. Buchanan RB, Blamey RW, Durrant KR et al. A randomized comparison of tamoxifen with surgical oophorectomy in premenopausal patients with advanced breast cancer. J Clin Oncol 1986; 4: 1326.

36. Howell A, DeFriend DJ, Robertson JFR et al. Clinical studies with the specific 'pure' antioestrogen ICI 182780. Breast 1996; 5: 192–5.

37. Dowsett M. Biological background to aromatase inhibition. Breast 1996; 5: 196–201.

38. Lonning PE. Pharmacology of new aromatase inhibitors. Breast 1996; 5: 202–8.

39. Jonat W. Results of phase II and phase III trials with new aromatase inhibitors. Breast 1996; 5: 209–15.

40. Wiseman LR, McTavish D. Formestane: a review of its pharmacodynamic and pharmokinetic properties and therapeutic potential in the management of breast cancer and prostatic cancer. Drugs 1993; 45: 66–84.

41. Mattson W. Current status of high dose progestin treatment in advanced breast cancer. Breast Cancer Res Treat 1983; 3: 231.

42. Dombernowsky P, Smith I, Falkson G et al. Letrozole, a new oral aromatase inhibitor for advanced breast cancer: double-blind randomised trial showing a dose effect and improved efficacy and tolerability compared with megestrol acetate. J Clin Oncol 1998; 16: 453–61.

43. Davidson N, O'Neill A, Vukov A et al. Effect of chemohormonal therapy in premenopausal, node +, receptor + breast cancer: an Eastern co-operative Oncology Group phase III inter-group trial (E5188, INT-0101). Proc Am Soc Clin Oncol 1999; 18: 67a.

44. Ahmann DL, Bisel HF, Eagan RT et al. Controlled evaluation of adriamycin (NSC-123127) in patients with disseminated breast cancer. Cancer Chemother Rep 1974; 58: 877.

45. Hoogstraten B, George SL, Samal B et al. Combination chemotherapy and adriamycin in patients with advanced breast cancer. Cancer 1976; 83: 13.

46. Robert J. Epirubicin: clinical pharmacology and dose–effect relationship. Drugs 1993; 45: 20–30.

47. Brambilla C, Rossi A, Bonfante V et al. Phase II study of doxorubicin versus epirubicin in advanced breast cancer. Cancer Treat Rep 1986; 70: 261.

48. Myers CE, Chabner BA. Anthracyclines: In: Chabner B, Collins JM (eds) Cancer chemotherapy: principles and practice. Philadelphia: JB Lippincott, 1990: 356.

49. Engelsman E, Klijn JCM, Rubens RD et al. Classical CMF versus 3-weekly intravenous CMF schedule in postmenopausal patients with advanced breast cancer. Eur J Cancer 1991; 27: 966–70.

50. Diasio RB, Harris BE. Clinical pharmacology of 5-fluorouracil. Clin Pharmacokinet 1989; 16: 215.

51. Chang AYC, Most C, Pandya KJ. Continuous intravenous infusion of 5-fluorouracil in the treatment of refractory breast cancer. Am J Clin Oncol 1989; 12: 453.

52. Davidson K, Cameron DAC, Dillon P et al. Locally advanced breast cancer: the outcome of primary polychemotherapy based on infusional 5-fluorouracil. Breast 1999; 8: 110–5.

53. Reed E, Kohn KW. Platinum analogues. In: Chabner B, Collins JM (eds). Cancer chemotherapy: principles and practice. Philadelphia: JB Lippincott, 1990: 465.

54. Verweij J, Den Hartigh J, Pinedo HM. Antitumour antibiotics. In: Chabner B, Collins IM (eds).

Cancer chemotherapy: principles and practice. Philadelphia: JB Lippincott, 1990: 382.

55. Jodrell DI, Smith IE, Mansi JL *et al.* A randomised comparative trial of mitoozantrone/methotrexate/ mitomycin C (MMM) and cyclophosphamide/ methotrexate/5 FU (CMF) in the treatment of advanced breast cancer. Br J Cancer 1991; 63: 794–8.

56. Rowinsky EK, Cazenave LA, Donehower RC. Taxol: a novel investigational antimicrobule agent. J Natl Cancer Inst 1990; 82: 1247–59.

57. Buzdar AU, Hortobagyi GN, Frye D *et al.* Second-line chemotherapy for metastatic breast cancer including quality of life issues. Breast 1996; 5: 312–7.

58. Henderson IC, Berry D, Demetri G *et al.* Improved disease-free and overall survival from the addition of sequential paclitaxel but not from the escalation of doxorubicin dose level in the adjuvant chemotherapy of patients with node-positive primary breast cancer. Proc Am Soc Clin Oncol 1998; 17: 101a.

59. Yarnold J. Breast cancer. In: Price P, Sikora K (eds). Treatment of breast cancer. London: Chapman and Hall, 1995: 413–36.

60. Richards MA, Smith IE. Role of systemic treatment for primary operable breast cancer. In: Dixon JM (ed). ABC of breast diseases. London: BMJ Publishing Group, 1995: 38–41.

61. Osborne CK, Clarke GM, Ravdin PM. Adjuvant systemic therapy of primary breast cancer. In: Harris JR, Lippman ME, Morrow M, Hellman S (eds). Diseases of the breast. Philadelphia: JB Lippincott-Raven, 1996: 548–78.

62. Bonadonna G, Valgussa P, Brambilla C *et al.* Adjuvant and neoadjuvant treatment of breast cancer with chemotherapy and/or endocrine therapy. Semin Oncol 1991; 15: 515–24.

63. Veronesi U, Bonadonna G, Zurrida S *et al.* Conservation surgery after primary chemotherapy in large carcinomas of the breast. Ann Surg 1995; 222: 612–8.

64. Mauriac L, Durand M, Avril A *et al.* Effect of primary chemotherapy in conservative treatment of breast cancer patients with operable tumours larger than 3cm: results of a randomised trial in a single center. Ann Oncol 1991; 2: 347–54.

65. Fisher B, Bryant J, Wolmark N *et al.* Effect of preoperative chemotherapy on the outcome of women with operable breast cancer. J Clin Oncol 1998; 1: 2672.

66. Veronesi U, Bonadonna G, Zurrida S *et al.* Conservation surgery after primary chemotherapy

in large carcinomas of the breast. Ann Surg 1995; 222: 612–8.

67. Smith IE. Primary (neoadjuvant) medical therapy: introduction. In: Powles T, Smith IE (eds) Medical management of breast cancer. London: Martin-Dunitz, 1991: 259–65.

68. Forouhi P, Walsh JS, Anderson TJ *et al.* Ultrasonography as a method of measuring breast tumour size and monitoring response to primary systemic treatment. Br J Surg 1994; 81: 223–5.

69. Smith IE, Walsh G, Jones A *et al.* High complete remission rates with primary neoadjuvant infusional chemotherapy for large early breast cancer. J Clin Oncol 1995; 13: 424–9.

70. Anderson EDC, Forrest APM, Levack PA *et al.* Response to endocrine manipulation and oestrogen receptor concentration in large, operable breast cancer. Br J Cancer 1989; 60: 223–6.

71. Dixon JM, Love CDB, Renshaw L *et al.* Lessons from the use of aromatase inhibitors in the neoadjuvant setting. Endocr Rel Cancer 1999; 6: 227–30.

72. Early Breast Cancer Trialists Collaborative Group. Polychemotherapy for early breast cancer: an overview of the randomised trials. Lancet 1998; 352: 930 42.

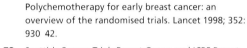
73. Scottish Cancer Trials Breast Group and ICRF Breast Unit, Guy's Hospital. Adjuvant ablation versus CMF chemotherapy in premenopausal women with pathological stage II breast carcinoma: the Scottish trial. Lancet 1993; 341: 1293–8.

74. Fisher B, Brown AM, Dimitrov NV *et al.* Two months of doxorubicin–cyclophosphamide with and without interval reinduction therapy compared with 6 months of cyclophosphamide, methotrexate and fluorouracil in positive-node breast cancer patients with tamoxifen-nonresponsive tumours: results from the National Surgical Adjuvant Breast and Bowel Project B-15. Clin Oncol 1990; 8: 1483–96.

75. Lavine MN, Bramwell VH, Pritchard K. Randomised trial of intensive cyclophosphamide, epirubicin and fluorouracil chemotherapy compared with cyclophosphamide, methotrexate and fluorouracil in premenopausal women with node positive breast cancer. J Clin Oncol 1998; 16: 2651–8.

76. Coombes RC, Bliss JM, Wills J *et al.* Adjuvant cyclophosphamide, methotrexate and fluorouracil, epirubicin and cyclophosphamide chemotherapy in premenopausal women with axillary node positive operable breast cancer: results of a randomised trial. J Clin Oncol 1996; 14: 35–45.

77. Bonadonna G, Valaguss P. Dose-response effect of adjuvant chemotherapy in breast cancer. N Engl J Med 1981; 304: 10.

78. Hryniuk W, Levine MN. Analysis of dose intensity for adjuvant chemotherapy trials in stage II breast cancer. J Clin Oncol 1986; 4: 1162.

79. Wood WC, Budman DR, Korzun AH et al. Dose and dose intensity of adjuvant chemotherapy for stage II, node-positive breast carcinoma. N Engl J Med 1994; 330: 1253–9.

80. Dimitrov N, Anderson S, Fisher B et al. Dose intensification and increased total dose of adjuvant chemotherapy for breast cancer (BC): findings from NSABP B22. Proc Am Soc Clin Oncol 1994; 13: 64.

81. Peters W, Rosner G, Vredenburgh J et al. A prospective, randomised comparison of two doses of combination alkyating agents as consolidation after CAF in high-risk primary breast cancer involving ten or more axillary lymph nodes: preliminary results of CALGB 9082/SWOG 9114/NCIC MA-13. Proc Am Soc Clin Oncol 1999; 18: 1a.

82. Scandinavian Breast Cancer Study Group 9401. Results from a randomised adjuvant breast cancer study with high dose chemotherapy with CTCb supported by autologous bone marrow stem cells versus dose escalated and tailored FEC therapy. Proc Am Soc Clin Oncol 1999; 18: 2a.

83. Bezwoda WR. Randomised, controlled trial of high dose chemotherapy (HD-CNVp) versus standard dose (CAF) chemotherapy for high risk, surgically treated primary breast cancer. Proc Am Soc Clin Oncol 1999; 18: 2a.

84. Bezwoda WR, Seymour L, Dansey RD. High-dose chemotherapy with hematopoietic rescue as primary treatment for metastatic breast cancer: a randomized trial. J Clin Oncol 1995; 13: 2483–9.

85. Galea MH, Blamey RW, Elston CE et al. The Nottingham prognostic index in primary breast cancer. Breast Cancer Res Treat 1992; 22: 207–19.

86. Diel IJ, Solomayer EF, Costa SD et al. Reduction in new metastases in breast cancer with adjuvant clodronate treatment. N Engl J Med 1998; 339: 357.

87. Powles TJ, Paterson AHG, Nevantaus A et al. Adjuvant clodronate reduces the incidence of bone metastases in patients with primary operable breast cancer. Proc Am Soc Clin Oncol 1998; 17: 123a (abstract 468).

88. Rodger A, Leonard RCF, Dixon JM. Locally advanced breast cancer. In: Dixon JM (ed). ABC of breast diseases. London: BMJ Publishing Group, 1995: 42–4.

89. Hortobagyi GN, Singletary SE, McNeese MD. Treatment of locally advanced and inflammatory breast cancer. In: Harris JR, Lippman ME, Morrow M, Hellman S (eds). Diseases of the breast. Philadelphia: Lippincott-Raven, 1996: 585–99.

90. Haagensen CD, Stout AP. Carcinoma of the breast: criteria of inoperability. Ann Surg 1943; 118: 859.

91. Zucali R, Islenghi C, Kenda R et al. Natural history and survival of inoperable breast cancer treated with radiotherapy and radiotherapy followed by radical mastectomy. Cancer 1976; 37: 1422.

92. Harris JR, Sawicka J, Gleman R et al. Management of locally advanced carcinoma of the breast by primary radiation therapy. Int J Radiat Oncol Biol Phys 1983; 9: 345.

93. Valagussa P, Bonadonna G, Veronesi U. Patterns of relapse and survival following radical mastectomy. Cancer 1978; 41: 1170.

94. Perez JE, Machiavelli M, Leone BA et al. Bone-only versus visceral-only metastatic pattern in breast cancer: analysis of 150 patients. Am J Clin Oncol 1990; 13: 294–8.

95. Jonat W, Klijn JGM, Blamey RW et al. Combination LHRH-agonist plys tamoxifen treatment is superior to medical castration alone in premenopausal metastatic breast cancer: a subgroup and meta-analysis of the combined hormonal agent trialists group (CHAT). Breast 1999; 8: 214 (abstract 005).

96. Carmo-Pereira J, Oliveira Costa F, Henriques E et al. A comparison of two doses of adriamycin in the primary chemotherapy of disseminated breast carcinoma. Br J Cancer 1987; 56: 471.

97. Tannock IF, Bovd NF, DeBoer C et al. A randomized trial of two dose levels of cyclophosphamide, methotrexate and fluorouracil chemotherapy for patients with metastatic breast cancer. J Clin Oncol 1988; 6: 137.

98. Ellis MJ, Hayes FD, Lippman ME. Treatment of metastatic breast cancer. In: Harris JR, Lippman ME, Morrow M, Osborne CK (eds). Diseases of the breast, 2nd edn. Philadelphia: Lippincott Williams & Wilkins, Philadelphia, 1999: 749–97.

99. Myers SE, Williams SF. Role of high-dose chemotherapy and autologous stem cell support in treatment of breast cancer. Hematol Oncol Clin North Am 1993; 7: 631–45.

100. McLachlan S-A, Pintilie M, Tannock IF. Third chemotherapy in patients with metastatic breast cancer: an evaluation of quality of life and cost. Breast Cancer Res Treat 1999; 54: 213–23.

101. Blacklay PF, Campbell FS, Hinton SP *et al.* Patterns of flap recurrence following mastectomy. Br J Surg 1995; 72: 719–20.

102. Recht A, Hayes DF, Eberlein TJ *et al.* Local-regional recurrence after mastectomy or breast-conserving therapy. In: Harris JR, Lippman ME, Morrow M, Hellman S (eds). Disease of the breast. Philadelphia: Lippincott-Raven, 1996: 649–67.

103. Ng JSY, Cameron DA, Lee L *et al.* Infusional 5-fluorouracil given as a single agent in relapsed breast cancer: its activity and toxicity. Breast 1994; 3: 87–9.

104. Halversoll KJ, Perez CA, Kuske RR *et al.* Isolated local-regional recurrence of breast cancer following mastectomy: radiotherapeutic management. Int J Radiat Oncol Biol Phys 1990; 19: 851–8.

105. Bundred NJ, Moragan DAL, Dixon JM. Management of regional nodes in breast cancer. In: Dixon JM (ed). ABC of breast diseases. London: BMJ Publishing Group, 1995: 30–3.

106. Recht A, Pierce SM, Abner A *et al.* Regional nodal failure after conservative surgery and radiotherapy for early-stage breast carcinoma. J Clin Oncol 1991; 9: 988–96.

107. Gateley CA, Mansel RE, Owen A *et al.* Treatment of the axilla in operable breast cancer (abstract). Br J Surg 1991; 78: 750.

108. Coleman RE. Evaluation of bone disease in breast cancer. Breast 1994; 2: 73–8.

109. Theriault R, Lipton A, Hortobagyi G *et al.* Pamidronate reduces skeletal morbidity in women with advanced breast cancer and lytic bone lesions: a randomised placebo controlled trial. J Clin Oncol 1999; 17: 846–54.

110. Hortobagyi G, Theriault R, Porter L *et al.* Efficacy of pamidronate in reducing skeletal complications in patients with breast cancer and lytic bone lesions. N Engl J Med 1996; 335: 1785–91.

111. Aaron AD, Jennings LC, Springfield DS. Local treatment of bone metastases. In: Harris JR, Lippman ME, Morrow M, Hellman S (eds). Diseases of the breast. Philadelphia: Lippincott-Raven, 1996: 811–9.

112. Robinson RG, Blake GM, Preston DF *et al.* Strontium-89: treatment results and kinetics in patients with painful metastatic prostate and breast cancer in bone. Radiography 1989; 9: 271.

113. Theriault RL. Medical treatment of bone metastases. In: Harris JR, Lippman ME, Morrow

M, Hellman S (eds). Diseases of the breast. Philadelphia: Lippincott-Raven, 1996: 819–26.

114. Come SE, Schnipper LE. Bone marrow metastases. In: Harris JR, Lippman ME, Morrow M, Hellman S (eds). Diseases of the breast. Philadelphia: Lippincott-Raven, 1996: 847–53.

115. Warrell RP Jr. Hypercalcemia. In: Harris JR, Lippman ME, Morrow M, Hellman S (eds). Diseases of the breast. Philadelphia: Lippincott-Raven, 1996: 840–7.

116. Prakash UBS, Reiman HM. Comparison of needle biopsy with cytologic analysis for the evaluation of pleural effusion: analysis of 414 cases. Mayo Clin Proc 1985; 60: 158.

117. Hausheer FH, Yarbro JW. Diagnosis and treatment of malignant pleural effusion. Semin Oncol 1985; 12: 54.

118. Pearson FG, Macgregor DC. Talc poudrage for malignant pleural effusion. J Thorac Cardiovasc Surg 1966; 51: 732.

119. Ruckdeschel JC, Moores D, Lee JY *et al.* Intrapleural therapy for malignant pleural effusions: a randomised comparison of bleomycin and tetracycline. Chest 1991; 100: 1528–35.

120. Shi M-L, Wallace S, Libshitz HI *et al.* Cranial computed tomography of breast carcinoma. J Comput Assist Tomogr 1982; 6: 77.

121. Hayman LA, Evans RA, Henck VC. Delayed high iodine dose contrast computed tomography. Radiology 1980; 136: 677.

122. Shalen PR, Hayman LA, Wallace S. Protocol for delayed contrast enhancement in computed tomography of cerebral neoplasia. Radiology 1981; 139: 397.

123. Kent DL, Larson FB. Magnetic resonance imaging of the brain and spine. Ann Intern Med 1988; 108: 402.

124. Borgelt B, Gelber R, Kramer S *et al.* The palliation of brain metastases: final results of the first of two studies by the Radiation Therapy Oncology Group. Int J Radiat Oncol Biol Phys 1980; 6: 1.

125. Posner JB. Surgery for metastases to the brain. (Editorial.) N Engl J Med 1990; 322: 544–5.

126. Freilich RJ, Foley KM. Epidural metastasis. In: Harris JR, Lippman ME, Morrow M, Hellman S (eds). Diseases of the breast. Philadelphia: Lippincott-Raven, 1996: 779–89.

6 Palliative care in breast cancer

Janet Hardy

As metastatic breast cancer is an incurable malignancy, the ability to palliate advanced disease is of major importance, particularly as around 14 000 women in the UK die of the disease each year. Palliative care is important not just in the terminal phase of disease but throughout the patient's illness. Chemotherapy, hormone therapy and radiotherapy (see Chapter 5) are probably the most effective means of palliation in breast cancer, but it is not always possible or appropriate to deliver these treatment modalities. The common symptoms of breast cancer relate directly to the pattern of metastatic disease spread, and any treatment should always be delivered in conjunction with measures to control symptoms.

Pain

Pain is the most common and certainly the most feared symptom in patients with cancer. Chronic pain is said to be controlled, however, in about 80% of patients by adhering to the analgesic guidelines from the World Health Organisation (WHO). These are based on a three-step ladder approach whereby increasing severity of pain is matched by increasing strengths of analgesia (**Fig. 6.1**).

A systematic review has challenged the validity of those studies that have claimed to show the effectiveness of the WHO ladder, mainly on methodological grounds.[1] The weight of anecdotal evidence, however, supports the conclusion that this method provides a simple, effective means of controlling cancer pain in most patients.

Physicians need to become familiar with the use of a relatively small number of drugs to adhere to these guidelines. Analgesia at each step can be supplemented by the use of additive drugs or co-analgesics (see below). Drugs at each

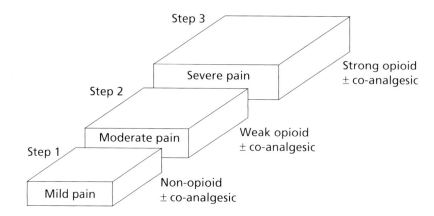

Figure 6.1
WHO analgesic ladder.

step of the ladder should be used up to the maximum dose and frequency prior to progression to the next step. The system is based on regular oral drug dosing rather than 'as required' medication. It is illogical to use an alternate drug of the same strength if the previous drug on the same step has failed to control pain. Recommended drugs at each step are shown in **Figure 6.2**. At step 1, paracetamol is used in preference to aspirin because of its relative lack of gastrointestinal toxicity.

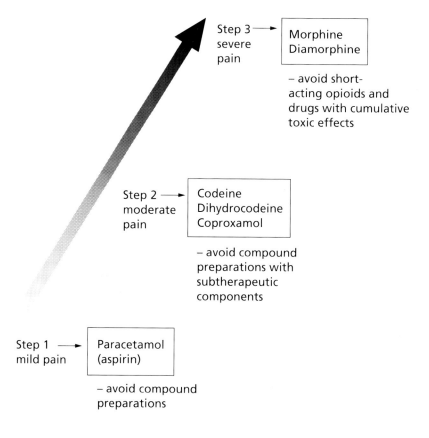

Figure 6.2
Recommended analgesics at each step of the WHO analgesic ladder.

Non-steroidal anti-inflammatory drugs (NSAIDs) are now also classed as step 1 analgesics rather than co-analgesics. They have proven efficacy in cancer pain[2] and, anecdotally, are particularly useful in bone pain. There are many of these agents available. Apart from differences in cost and some differences in side effect profile, there is little advantage of one NSAID drug over another. Their analgesic effect tends to be dose dependent up to a ceiling. The incidence of side effects (predominately gastric and renal toxicity) increases with dose and chronic use.[2] Meta-analysis has shown NSAIDs to be as effective as, if not better than, paracetamol and to be more effective than several of the opioids traditionally used either alone or in combination at step 2 of the analgesic ladder.[2,3] Many are now available in slow-release preparations (which are valuable for patients who are on a large number of drugs) as well as suppository and elixir form (**Table 6.1**). It is important to remember that the prescription of a NSAID 'per rectum' does not protect from gastrointestinal toxicity as this is a systemic effect. Other side effects include fluid retention and a reversible inhibition of platelet aggregation. All NSAIDs should be used with caution in elderly patients and in those with cardiac or renal impairment, and they should not be used in patients with low platelet counts.

The development of selective NSAIDs that inhibit only those prostaglandins that contribute to the pain and swelling of inflammation and not those that are protective to the gut and kidneys hold promise for the future development of NSAIDs with much improved side effect profiles.[4]

Drug	Usual oral dose	Comments
Naproxen[S,E]	500 mg b.i.d.	Available as enteric-coated preparation
Diclofenac[S,E,I]	50 mg t.i.d.	75 and 100 mg slow-release preparations available
Ibuprofen[E]	400 tds–600 mg q.i.d.	Fewer side effects than other non-steroidal anti-inflammatory drugs but weaker anti-inflammatory properties
Ketoprofen[S]	100–200 mg d^{-1}	Available as once daily slow-release preparation
Sulindac	200 mg b.i.d.	Similar tolerance to naproxen
Indomethacin[S,E]	50 mg t.i.d.	Intermediate risk of gastrointestinal toxicity
Ketorolac[I]	40 mg d^{-1}	Higher analgesic/anti-inflammatory ratio, can be given subcutaneously
Meloxicam[S]	7.5–10 mg d^{-1}	
Rofecoxib[E]	12.5–25 mg d^{-1}	Preferential COX-2 inhibitors

[S] Available as suppository.
[E] Available as elixir/dispersable tablet.
[I] Can be given subcutaneously (unlicensed route of delivery).

Table 6.1 Non-steroidal and anti-inflammatory agents

It has become clear that the previous ladder terminology of 'weak' and 'strong' opioids is misleading in that low-dose morphine produces effects that are indistinguishable from that of the opioids commonly used at step 2. All opioids are now classed together and separated only on the basis of those that are commonly used for mild to moderate pain at step 2 and those that are commonly used for moderate to severe pain at step 3.[5]

Many of the opioids used at step 2 are available in combination preparations, e.g. coproxamol (which is comprised of paracetamol and dextroproxyphene) and co-codamol (paracetamol and codeine). A common mistake at step 2 is to use combination analgesics that comprise low doses of opioid that are in fact subtherapeutic, e.g. co-codaprin and co-codamol 8/500, which both contain only 8 mg codeine in combination with aspirin and paracetamol, respectively. Dihydrocodeine is a semi-synthetic analogue of codeine and has the advantage of being available as an oral solution as well as a delayed-release preparation that can be given twice daily rather than 4-hourly as with coproxamol.

Although there are now a large number of alternate strong opioids available on the market, morphine remains the opioid of choice at step 3.[6] There are a large number of preparations and strengths of morphine available (**Table 6.2**).

When starting morphine, patients should ideally be prescribed one of the immediate-release preparations, e.g. Sevredol or Oramorph, that are given every

---

Immediate-release oral preparations

Duration of action 4 hours

• Morphine sulphate oral solution, e.g. (Oramorph)®	10 mg 5 ml^{-1} + taste mask suitable for dose titration
• Concentrated oral morphine sulphate solution	100 mg 5 ml^{-1} (no taste mask)
• Morphine sulphate unit dose vials	10 mg 5 ml^{-1}, 30 mg 5 ml^{-1}, 100 mg 5 ml^{-1}
• Morphine tablets (Sevredol®)	10 mg, 20 mg and 50 mg tablets suitable for those patients who prefer tablets
• Morphine suppositories	10, 15, 20, 30, 50 and 100 mg, similar bioavailability to oral morphine

Delayed release oral preparations

Duration of action 12 hours

• Morphine sulphate controlled release tablets, e.g. MST—Continus® Oramorph® SR	Available in 5, 10, 30, 60, 100 and 200 mg strengths Suitable for patients with good pain control on a stable dose of morphine
• Morphine sulphate slow release suspension	Sachet of granules to mix with water: 20, 30, 60, 100 and 200 mg

Duration of action 24 hours

• Morphine sulphate controlled-release tablets, e.g. MXL capsules®	Available in 30, 60, 90, 120, 150 and 200 mg capsules
• Morphine sulphate injection	Diamorphine is usually used in preference because of its greater solubility

Table 6.2 Morphine formulations commercially available for routine use

4 hours at a dose of 5–10 mg. The dose can then be increased every 24 hours or so until pain control is achieved. The total daily dose can then be given as a delayed-release preparation, either once or twice a day, e.g. 4-hourly 10 mg immediate-release morphine can be given as MST Continus 30 mg b.i.d. or as MXL capsules 60 mg once a day. A 'breakthrough dose,' which is equivalent to the 4-hourly dose (or one sixth the total 24 hours dose), can be given at any time in between planned doses for uncontrolled or 'breakthrough' pain. A patient should never be expected to wait the standard 4 hours for the next dose of morphine if they are in pain. The necessity for many breakthrough doses would suggest, however, that the baseline dose should be increased. It is unusual for patients to have to take delayed-release morphine more often than recommended. Very rarely, a patient may have to take MST Continus 8-hourly rather than 12-hourly, but this usually indicates that the baseline 12-hourly dose needs to be increased. There is no ceiling dose of morphine; the correct dose for any patient is the dose that controls the pain. Most patients can be controlled on <30 mg 4-hourly, but the dose range is huge (5–500 mg 4-hourly). Guidelines for the prescription of morphine are shown in **Table 6.3** and in the document produced by the Expert Working Group of the European Association for Palliative Care.[7] Patients are advised to take morphine regularly rather than 'as required', as morphine is a relatively poor analgesic when given orally in single doses. Morphine-6-glucuronide (M6G), an active morphine metabolite, is a potent analgesic but is produced in very small quantities after single doses of morphine. It is thought that repeated dosing is necessary to allow accumulation of M6G to sufficient concentrations to provide analgesia and specifically to cross into the cerebral spinal fluid to reach central opioid receptors.[8]

Patients should always be prescribed laxatives along with morphine as constipation is an inevitable side effect of the drug. Other side effects include nausea, vomiting and drowsiness, which usually resolve after a couple of days.

1. Start with a low dose of immediate-release morphine
2. Prescribe a regular 4-hourly dose (with a double dose at night to avoid the middle-of-the night dose)
3. Prescribe the same dose to be given 'as required' for 'breakthrough pain'
4. Review after 24–36 hours and, if pain not controlled, increase 4-hourly dose by one third, e.g. 10 → 15 → 20 → 30 → 40 mg
5. Once the pain is controlled, convert to once or twice daily slow-release morphine preparations
6. Continue to supply appropriate 'breakthrough' doses equivalent to the 4-hourly dose in an immediate-release preparation
7. If pain control is lost, recalculate total daily dose required according to 'breakthrough' requirements
8. Always prescribe a laxative to be taken concurrently
9. Ensure that out-patients have a supply of anti-emetics in case of opioid-induced nausea
10. Reassure that most of the initial side effects, e.g. drowsiness, light headedness and nausea, will pass
11. Ensure appropriate patient review

Table 6.3 Guidelines for the prescription of morphine

Respiratory depression can be used to advantage to palliate breathlessness in a patient without pain, but in patients with pain, this is not usually a problem. Pain does seem to provide physiological antagonism to the respiratory depressant effects of opioid analgesia. One explanation is that the respiratory centre receives nociceptive input, which counterbalances the respiratory depressant potential of the opioid.[9] Dry mouth is unfortunately a common side effect that does not tend to resolve. Itch and hallucinations are rarer side effects, which are generally a contraindication to the continued use of the drug.

Morphine toxicity is reflected by increasing drowsiness, miosis, myoclonic jerks and respiratory depression. This often reflects deteriorating renal function as M6G accumulates in renal failure. This situation can usually be managed by stopping the drug for a while and restarting at a lower dose given less frequently than 4-hourly. In severe toxicity the morphine effect may be reversed with naloxone, a synthetic opioid agonist that competitively antagonises the effects of opioids.

Unfortunately, many patients equate morphine with the 'end of the road,' and feel that if they agree to take morphine they are somehow 'giving up'. It is crucial, therefore, to explain that this is not the case and that morphine may in fact allow people to live longer by allowing them greater activity and relieving stress. Another common concern is a fear of addiction. Although patients can develop a physical dependence to morphine (as detected by a withdrawal syndrome when the drug is stopped suddenly), addiction encompasses psychological and behavioural factors that do not apply when morphine is taken for pain. There is no reason why a woman taking morphine cannot continue to undertake normal daily activities (including driving[10]), assuming her pain is under control.

When the oral route is not available, diamorphine is the agent of choice to be used parenterally at step 3 (see below). Fentanyl is a synthetic opioid that is available in a transdermal delivery system. Skin patches are applied every 72 hours and a 'fentanyl depot' concentrates in the upper skin layers from which the drug diffuses to the systemic circulation. The full clinical effects are not noted for 8–16 hours after application of the patch and persist for about 17 hours after patch removal. Fentanyl patches are, therefore, not suitable for patients with acute or changing pain as dose titration is difficult but offer an alternate non-invasive parenteral approach for patients with chronic stable pain.[11]

Some of the alternative opioids available and their respective advantages and disadvantages are listed in **Table 6.4**. There has been recent interest in the concept of opioid rotation, whereby improved pain relief with fewer side effects can sometimes be achieved by changing a patient from one strong opioid to another. The exact mechanism underlying this phenomenon is not clear.[6,12] The most simplistic explanation is that changing to a new drug allows toxic metabo-

Drug	Indication	Comments
Diamorphine	Nil by mouth Inability to take oral medications	Greater solubility than morphine allows injection of smaller volumes Drug of choice for subcutaneous strong opioid infusion
Phenazocine	Intolerance to morphine	Often better tolerated in elderly patients, can be given sublingually; dose limited by number of tablets (5 mg tablets only available)
Fentanyl transdermal patch	When oral route not available or gut absorption poor	Skin patch changed every 3 days Less constipating than morphine Not suitable for dose titration in unstable pain
Methadone	Opioid rotation Neuropathic pain	Long half-life Unique dosing schedule Toxic metabolites can accumulate with prolonged use
Oxycodone	Intolerance to morphine Morphine 'phobia'	Synthetic analogue of morphine available in both oral and per rectum formulations
Hydromorphone	Opioid rotation	Analogue of morphine, with similar pharmatokinetic properties Widely used in USA
Tramadol	WHO step 2 and 3 analgesic	Opioid and non-opioid analgesia by enhancement of serotoninergic and adrenergic pathways; therefore fewer opioid side effects
Pethidine	*Not* indicated in chronic pain because of short half-life	Less intense action at smooth muscle compared with morphine plus additional anticholinergic effects; toxic metabolites accumulate with prolonged use
Dextramoramide	Incident pain	Short half-life, duration of action 1–2 hours, unsuitable for regular analgesia in chronic pain

Table 6.4 'Alternative' strong opioids

lites of the previous drug to dispel, with the result that the new drug is better tolerated.[13]

Co-analgesics are drugs that often have little intrinsic analgesic effect but, when taken with standard analgesia, can confer an additive benefit with respect to pain control at any step of the WHO ladder. Examples include the use of antidepressants and anticonvulsants for neuropathic pain (see below; **Table 6.5**). Corticosteroids are valuable co-analgesics in several pain situations. As well as their non-specific benefit in mood elevation and general wellbeing, they can often provide added analgesia for bone pain, neuropathic pain and inflammatory tumours. Side effects after long-term use are significant, however, and include proximal myopathy, Cushing's syndrome, oral candida, glucose intolerance, sleep disturbance and even psychosis. Patients taking steroids should always be monitored so that the drug can be discontinued if the desired symptomatic benefit is not achieved. If effective, maintenance doses should be kept as low as possible.[14]

Indication	Appropriate agents	Comments
Bone pain	Non-steroidal anti-inflammatory drugs*	Anti-inflammatory action via inhibition of prostaglandin synthesis
	Bisphosphonates	Potent inhibitors of osteoclast-mediated bone resorption
Neuropathic pain	Antidepressants, e.g. amitriptyline, dosulepin	Analgesic effect via increased concentrations of serotonin in spinal cord
		Indicated for dysaesthetic, aching neuropathic pain
	Anticonvulsants, e.g. sodium valproate, carbamazepine, gabapentin	Analgesic effect via stabilisation of neuronal membrane
		Indicated for shooting, lancinating pain
	Antiarrhythmics, e.g. flecainide, mexiletine	Membrane stabilisers, usually used 'third line'
	Corticosteroids	Reduce perineuronal oedema
Soft tissue inflammation	Non-steroidal anti-inflammatory drugs	Useful for inflammatory breast tumours
	Corticosteroids	
	Antibiotics	
Muscle spasm	Benzodiazepines	Added anxiolytic effect
	Baclofen	Can be sedative

*WHO step 1 analgesic.

Table 6.5 Co-analgesics

Non-pharmacological means of pain control should also be considered. Acupuncture, transcutaneous electrical nerve stimulator (TENS), relaxation therapy, massage and distraction therapy can all be of great benefit to some patients. Similarly, anaesthetic techniques for pain control, e.g. spinal opioid administration and neurolytic blocks, are sometimes indicated for the control of particularly difficult pain or where standard analgesia cannot be tolerated because of unacceptable side effects.

Factors that predict for difficult or poor pain control are neuropathic pain, incident pain (pain only on movement), high previous narcotic exposure, major psychological distress, high tolerance (necessitating rapid increase in dose) and a history of alcoholism or drug addiction.

Special pain circumstances common in metastatic breast cancer

Pain secondary to metastatic bone metastases (Fig. 6.3)

Radiotherapy remains the treatment of choice for the palliation of bone disease. Single fractions have been shown to be as effective as multiple fractions in the achievement of pain control,[15] and this is obviously more acceptable to patients, especially those with a poor performance status.

Figure 6.3
Bone scan showing widespread metastases from breast carcinoma.

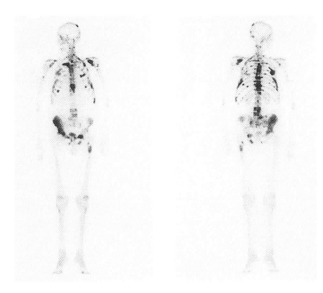

NSAIDs are specifically indicated in this situation and should be used as analgesics in their own right than as adjuncts to the basic analgesia as described above.

Bisphosphonates are now considered as part of the systemic treatment regimen of breast cancer rather than as just a treatment of hypercalcaemia.[16] Their mechanism of action is complex and not fully understood, but they are known to be potent inhibitors of normal and pathological bone resorption. Current evidence suggests that bisphosphonates, especially pamidronate, have an analgesic effect as well as a positive effect on the reduction of skeletal complications.[17] There is little evidence that oral bisphosphonates have a role in the control of bone pain, but pooled data of phase 2 studies of pamidronate infusions show relief of pain in more than one half of patients. Placebo controlled trials of both pamidronate and clodronate have confirmed this analgesic effect.[16] Responding patients also showed in improvement in quality of life.

Optimal doses and schedules are still to be determined, but 60–90 mg pamidronate every 3–4 times weeks and 1500 mg of clodronate every two weeks can now be recommended for the palliation of bone pain.

Several studies have shown that both oral and intravenous bisphosphonates can reduce the morbidity from bone metastases by significantly reducing skeletal 'events' (i.e. pathological fractures, bone pain requiring radiotherapy and hypercalcaemia).[16] Infusional therapy is probably more effective both for analgesia and for the prevention of complications, but it is difficult for some patients to attend regularly for intravenous therapy. Oral therapy is more convenient for many patients despite the low oral availability of the tablets and the dietary restrictions (patients are advised to take the tablets on an empty stomach at least 1 hour before eating). The drugs are generally well tolerated, apart from occasional gastrointestinal side effects. They are even said to be cost effective if the reduction in admission to hospital secondary to reduced skeletal complications is taken into account.[18]

The exact details of route, dose, scheduling and duration of therapy is still unclear. One approach is to start with intravenous therapy to assess effectiveness and then to convert to oral therapy, but this practice is not based on any scientific evidence.

Incident pain

Incident pain is a descriptive term for pain that occurs only on movement, e.g. on mobilising. It is difficult to control especially when pain control at rest is satisfactory. Short-acting analgesics are recommended such as immediate-release morphine or short-acting opioids (e.g. palfium), preferably given just prior to an anticipated activity. A short-acting oral preparation of fentanyl is under development.[19] If tolerated, entonox can be useful for situations such as painful wound care, e.g. when changing dressings.

The most common cause of incident pain in breast cancer is a lytic bone metastasis or pathological fracture. Orthopaedic procedures, such as pinning of a femur or a total hip joint replacement should be undertaken prophylactically

Figure 6.4
Pathological fracture of a humerus that may have been prevented by prophylactic pinning.

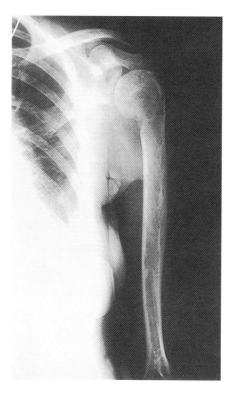

where there is loss of integrity of bone cortex or as a palliative procedure after pathological fracture (**Fig. 6.4**). Pain control will be difficult without stabilisation.[20]

Neuropathic pain

Neuropathic pain results from damage or compression to a peripheral nerve. The most common example of this in breast cancer is brachial plexopathy after treatment of the axilla or recurrent disease in the axilla. Neuropathic pain is classically resistant to standard analgesia, and it is often necessary to use co-analgesics at an early stage. Agents that are widely used in this situation include antidepressants and anticonvulsants. Although there are few studies in cancer pain, both antidepressants and anticonvulsants have proven effectiveness in non-cancer related neuropathic pain. It is still unclear which drug class should be first choice.[21] All of these drugs have their own inherent side effects (sedation being the most common) and should be used with care. The doses required to achieve an analgesic effect are often well below the doses required to achieve the usual effect, e.g. the analgesic effect of amitriptyline is seen well below its antidepressant effect. Second-line management of neuropathic pain with anti-arrythmics (e.g. flecainide) or N-methyl-D-aspartate antagonists such as keta-mine or methadone is potentially hazardous and usually requires specialist pain input or palliative care input. Neurolytic blocks, such as intercostal or brachial plexus blocks should be considered for neuropathic pain that does not respond to the measures described above.

Liver capsular pain

Pain in the right upper quadrant is common in patients with liver metastases. This follows not only swelling of the liver capsule but may also be particularly severe after a bleed into a liver metastasis. NSAIDs can provide excellent analgesia in this situation and are often used in conjunction with opioids. Similarly, corticosteroids can reduce swelling, inflammation and pain in an enlarged liver. Dexamethasone should be started at an oral dose of about 8 mg day^{-1} and then reduced to the lowest effective dose to avoid side effects. A maintenance dose of 2–4 mg is often necessary to maintain control.

Headache

In the scenario of metastatic breast cancer, especially if associated with vomiting, headache is often a sign of cerebral metastases. It is often taught that codeine and strong opioids should be avoided in this situation because of the possibility of respiratory depression associated with hypercapnia leading to reflex cerebral vasodilation, a further increase in intracranial pressure and increased headache. This does not occur in everyday practice, especially if these agents are used in conjunction with dexamethasone and should not be cited as a contraindication to opioids. The prompt use of opioid analgesia can avoid dependence on corticosteroid therapy and reduce side effects.

Spiritual pain

Pain is multifactorial and is often exacerbated by added burdens such as fear, anxiety, anger, depression, sleep disturbance, uncertainty and other uncontrolled symptoms. These factors are often overlooked with the main focus of pain control being on the physical aspects. It is crucially important, therefore, to make every attempt to relieve these aspects if 'complete pain control' is to be achieved. Simple measures such as explanation, reassurance, understanding and empathy can have profound pain-relieving effects.

Depression has been shown to have a significantly detrimental effect on survival in breast cancer.[22] Clinical depression must be actively looked for and appropriately treated in all women with breast cancer. Similarly, anxiety may require specific treatment with anxiolytics (e.g. buspirone, diazepam, lorazepam). Buspirone hydrochloride may have less addictive potential and should therefore be used in preference to diazepam for long-term use.

Dyspnoea

It is not always the malignancy that causes shortness of breath in a patient with metastatic breast cancer and it is important to look for and treat any other contributing causes such as infection, pulmonary embolism or anaemia. Specific causes include malignant pleural effusions, lymphangitis carcinomatosis, intrapulmonary metastases, pericardial effusions and constricting chest wall disease.

Aspiration of a pleural effusion often results in significant improvement of a patient's dyspnoea. Chemical pleurodesis with sclerosing agents such as bleomycin, tetracycline and doxycycline is reportedly effective in about two thirds of patients.[23] When factors such as length of response, patient comfort, adverse effects and length of stay in hospital are considered, bleomycin is recommended as the agent of choice (Royal Marsden Trust Drug Information Service). Talc pleurodesis via thoracoscopy is probably the most effective way of preventing reaccumulation of the fluid in selected patients.[24] A pleuroperitoneal shunt should be considered in a fit patient whose major problem is recurrent effusions. Lymphangitis carcinomatosis is a common complication of metastatic disease, and patients present with gradually progressive shortness of breath and a dry cough. Auscultation of the chest is often non-contributory but a chest radiograph will show fine septal lines reflecting interstitial oedema. This is best palliated with corticosteroids, given at the lowest possible dose that controls symptoms. Corticosteroids can also help dyspnoea associated with intrapulmonary disease almost certainly by reducing inflammation around a tumour.

The respiratory depressive effect of opioids can often be used to great advantage in patients who are dyspnoeic, especially those without pain. There is now some evidence to support the use of oral opioids for the palliation of dyspnoea, whereas systemic review has failed to define a role for nebulised morphine.[25] Regular morphine used in conjunction with anxiolytics such as diazepam can calm both the patient and the respiratory drive. Opioids are also effective cough suppressants. Small doses of methadone given at night can successfully control a troublesome nocturnal cough without leading to unbearable drowsiness. Lignocaine or bupivacaine nebulisers are rarely required. A short course of palliative radiotherapy to an obstructed bronchus, especially if this is associated with haemoptysis, is often worthwhile.

Nausea and vomiting

The commonest causes of nausea and vomiting in metastatic breast disease are therapy, specifically chemotherapy and radiotherapy. Other common causes are hypercalcaemia, liver metastases and constipation.

Nausea and vomiting is often multifactorial in origin, however, and a specific treatable cause may not be identified. There are a large number of anti-emetics available, which act at different sites or via different mechanisms. The appropriateness of each in specific situations is shown in **Table 6.6**. Levomepromazine is a 'broad-spectrum' anti-emetic acting at $5-HT_2$, dopaminergic, cholinergic and histamine receptor sites.[26] It is therefore the most logical anti-emetic to use when no specific cause can be identified. There is little evidence to support the use of the $5-HT_3$-receptor blockers other than for chemo- or radiotherapy-induced vomiting. Corticosteroids can often achieve control when all other anti-emetics have failed, especially in the case of metastatic liver disease. A cycle of protracted vomiting can be broken by giving antiemetics via a continuous subcutaneous infusion. Those drugs suitable for delivery by this route are shown in Table 6.6.

Anorexia and weight loss

Anorexia and weight loss is not as common in breast cancer as it is in many other advanced malignancies, e.g. carcinoma of the pancreas or lung. Corticosteroids improve appetite and general wellbeing, and there is some evidence that they result in non-fluid weight gain.[27] Progestogens are commonly used as

Drug	Specific indication	Comments
Metoclopramide*	Treatment-related nausea and vomiting Gastric stasis	Dopamine antagonist ($5-HT_3$ antagonist at high dose) Gastrokinetic, may induce acute dystonic reaction
Domperidone	Speeds gastric emptying and gut transit time	Available as suppository Gastrokinetic
Haloperidol*	Drug of choice for opioid-induced nausea and vomiting	Sedative at dose >3 mg d^{-1} Long half-life, can be given once or twice daily
Cyclizine*	Nausea and vomiting associated with bowel obstruction	Antihistamine; can cause dry mouth Will not exacerbate bowel colic
Levomepromazine*	If sedation is desirable	Powerful, broad-spectrum anti-emetic, with activity at several different receptors
Prochlorperazine	Motion sickness	Phenothiazine derivative
Ondansetron* and granisetron	Chemo- and radiotherapy-induced vomiting; also postoperative vomiting	Potent $5-HT_3$-receptor antagonists
Corticosteroids*	Vomiting, secondary to raised intracranial pressure or liver metastases	Broad-spectrum anti-emetic

* Can be given subcutaneously (unlicensed route).

Table 6.6 Anti-emetics

third-line hormonal therapy in breast cancer. Increased appetite and weight gain is a well documented side effect of these agents that can be used to advantage in metastatic disease.[28]

Sore mouth

One of the commonest causes of a sore mouth is a dry mouth, developing as a consequence of drugs, anticancer treatment or general debility. This in turn can lead to the development of oral infections with *Candida albicans*. Nystatin gives local control of oral thrush but is unlikely to eradicate the infection. A 5-day course of fluconazole is therefore usually indicated, care being taken in those patients with renal impairment. Most patients find amphotericin lozenges unpalatable as they are large and sticky. The underlying xerostomia must be corrected to avoid reinfection. Artificial saliva is the treatment of choice but must be used frequently. Fluoride may stimulate saliva in some patients, and fluoride mouth washes and toothpaste are recommended. Regular tooth brushing and mouth care should be encouraged to avoid infection. Many mouth washes (e.g. chlorhexidine gluconate) may exacerbate mouth dryness. Saliva stimulants, e.g. chewing gum, pilocarpine and parasympathomimetic agents (e.g. bethane-chol) are under investigation.[29]

Abdominal distension

The commonest cause of abdominal distension in metastatic breast cancer is ascites, usually associated with liver metastases or intraperitoneal disease. Abdominal paracentesis can lead to considerable relief and should be relatively painless when performed with a narrow-bore tube, e.g. a suprapubic catheter. Leaving a tube 'in situ' provides a route of infection, and therefore, the proce-dure should be repeated on an 'as required' basis. The use of diuretics in this situation may serve only to dehydrate the patient and rarely results in satisfac-tory control of ascites.

Lymphoedema

Lymphoedema of the upper limb develops after recurrence in the axilla and as a complication of treatment (surgery and radiotherapy). It is associated with pain and often loss of mobility and function of the arm. This is a specialist treatment area requiring the input of specialised lymphoedema teams.

Diuretics may help, but meticulous skin care, massage, elevation of the limb, bandaging and use of support sleeves to prevent recurrence are other practical measures.[30] Oedematous limbs are prone to infection, and antibiotics should be prescribed at the earliest suggestion of cellulitis.

Swelling of the ankle often causes the patient great alarm even in the face of widespread metastatic disease. Hypoalbuminaemia, immobility and concurrent drugs as well as mechanical blockage by tumour can all exacerbate this condi-tion. Diuretics, appropriate mobilisation and a support hose remain the mainstay of treatment. Intravenous albumin supplementation provides short-lasting benefit and is not generally recommended.

Wounds

Many women live with an extensive locally recurrent malignancy for many months before they die. Chest wall disease can be most distressing, particularly because of its detrimental effect on body image. Poor nutritional state, infec-tion and oedema all have an adverse effect on a malignant wound. There are a large number of dressings available with different properties appropriate for different types of wound (**Table 6.7**). The aim is not to heal but to keep wounds clean and free of infection, to control pain and to provide maximum comfort. Dressings must be cosmetically acceptable. Antibiotics effective against

Type of wound	Management
Necrotic Brown/black hard dead tissue must be removed to allow granulation	Requires debridement by surgery, hydrocolloid gels, hydrogels and/or enzymes
Sloughy Yellow dead tissue must be removed to allow granulation	Hydrogels, hydrocolloid gel sheets and paste Alginate/hydrofibre dressings for high exudate
Infected Identified by clinical signs: pain, heat, swelling, redness	Hydrocolloid gel/hydrogels Alginates/hydrofibre or foam cavity dressing for high exudate Change dressings daily Consider systematic (*not* topical) antibiotics Irrigate with 0.9% saline, avoid topical antiseptic agents
Malodorous	Consider systemic antibiotics if malodour is related to infection Metronidazole gel and primary and secondary dressings of choice Charcoal dressing can absorb odour
Granulating Pink/red appearance, bleeds easily, requires protection	Avoid frequent changes of dressings Hydrocolloid gel/hydrogels plus hydrofibre/alginates or foam cavity dressing for high exudate Hydrocolloid sheets Hydrogel sheets
Bleeding wounds	Initial management with pressure dressings Then consider adrenalin soaks, tranexamic acid (systemically and topically) and/or haemostatic swabs

Table 6.7 Wound management

anaerobes, e.g. metronidazole, given either systemically or topically, can relieve malodour. Tranexamic acid can be applied topically to prevent bleeding. Superficial radiotherapy prevents ulceration of a subcutaneous lesion and can provide local control over limited areas.

Constipation

Constipation is a common and most distressing symptom to those with advanced breast cancer and, as with pain, treatment should be continuous and anticipatory. Constipation can lead to considerable abdominal discomfort and is a common cause of nausea and vomiting. Unfortunately, almost all strong analgesics cause constipation, and the situation is often exacerbated by inactivity, poor diet, dehydration and hypercalcaemia. This condition should be taken seriously and treated aggressively with regular oral laxatives along with enemas and suppositories as indicated (**Table 6.8**). Opioid-induced constipation is best treated with compound preparations such as co-danthramer, which contains both a faecal softener (poloxamer) and a stimulant (danthron) or co-danthrusate (danthron 50 mg, docusate 60 mg). Care must be taken in those patients who

Drug	Indication/mechanism of action	Comments
	Bulking agents	
Bran	Increase stool by absorbing water	Avoid in patients with bowel obstruction
Isphaghula husk (Fybogel®)		Maintain adequate fluid intake
Stercula (normacol®)		
	Faecal softeners	
Liquid paraffin	Lubricates and softens impacted faeces	Should not be used in patients with swallowing difficulties (danger of aspiration lipoid pneumonia)
Docusate sodium		Added stimulant properties
Arachis oil enema	For 'per rectum' intervention'	
	Osmotic laxatives	
Magnesium sulphate	Retain fluid in bowel	Useful when rapid bowel evacuation is required; use with caution in elderly and debilitated patients
Lactulose		Semisynthetic disaccharide, not absorbed from bowel, added antimicrobial effect may take up to 48 hours to act
Phosphate suppositories	For clearance of rectal impaction	
	Bowel stimulants	
Senna	Increase colonic motility	May increase colicky pain
Bisacodyl		Avoid in bowel obstruction
Danthron		Colours urine red, skin contact can cause irritation and excoriation
Glycerol suppositories	Rectal stimulant because of irritant action of glycerol	

Table 6.8 Aperients

are incontinent or catheterised as the danthron can cause skin staining, irritation and occasionally excoriation. The combination of bisacodyl and docusate is a logical alternative in this situation. There is increasing interest in the use of opioid antagonists for the treatment of morphine-induced constipation. Initial studies suggest that oral naloxone may counteract the gut-slowing effect of morphine without effecting its analgesic activity.[31]

Confusion

Common causes of confusion are drug toxicity, infection, hypoxia, hypercalcaemia and direct cancer involvement of the CNS. The cause should be actively sought and treated accordingly.

Hypercalcaemia presents with polyuria, polydypsia, dehydration, nausea and vomiting, confusion and somnolence that can progress to coma and death if not treated. Tumour-induced hypercalcaemia (TIH) is a particularly common complication of advanced metastatic bone disease. Intravenous bisphosphonates remain the treatment of choice for TIH.[16] They are easy to deliver and relatively devoid of side effects. Patients should be rehydrated with at least 2 litres of normal saline prior to treatment with intravenous bisphosphonates (either pamidronate 90 mg or sodium clodronate 1500 mg in 500 ml normal saline over 3–4 hours). The serum calcium concentration should return to normal within 3 to 4 days with an improvement in symptoms. The hypercalcaemia will almost certainly recur after 2 to 4 weeks if no further specific systemic anticancer therapy is available. It can be retreated but will eventually become resistant. TIH is a preterminal event, and the median survival after an initial episode of TIH is 2 months, except in those patients in whom further systemic anticancer therapy is available.[32] Although the symptoms associated with hypercalcaemia are distressing and should be treated, the benefit of treating TIH in a patient in whom no further anticancer therapy is possible and who presents with no symptoms must be questioned.

The brain is a common site of metastases, and patients may present with localised weakness, convulsions or personality change as well as confusion. If cerebral secondaries are suspected, the patient should be started on high-dose steroids (e.g. dexamethasone 8 mg b.i.d.) while awaiting confirmation of the diagnosis. An improvement while taking steroids bodes well for subsequent response to radiotherapy. Short courses of radiotherapy (up to 5 fractions) are as effective as prolonged courses. In one series, the median survival after radiotherapy for cerebral metastases was about 6 months, compared with 1 month for those patients who received symptomatic (corticosteroid) therapy only.[33]

Weakness

Weakness, lethargy and fatigue are common but rarely reported symptoms of advanced breast cancer. A 41% incidence of asthenia (defined as physical or mental fatigue/weakness) has been reported in a controlled study of women with advanced breast cancer.[34] Physical (cachexia and weight loss, muscle abnormalities), biochemical, haematological, endocrine and psychological factors (depression, personality, stress) can all contribute. Corticosteroids, progestogens, anabolic steroids and psychostimulants have all been tried, but to date no pharmacological treatment has a proven role in this condition.[35]

If a patient suddenly 'goes off her legs,' especially if this is associated with bowel or bladder disturbance and sensory loss, malignant cord compression should be considered and investigated immediately. Vertebral bone disease is common in metastatic breast cancer and is often unsuspected until imaged by magnetic resonance[36] (**Fig. 6.5**). Cord compression is not uncommon and must be treated with urgency. The success of treatment often depends on early detection. High-dose steroids should be started at first suspicion and continued until treatment is complete. Surgical decompression may be appropriate for single

Figure 6.5
Malignant cord compression as demonstrated by MRI.

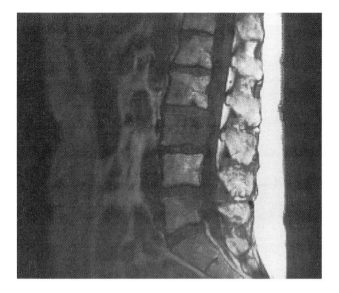

lesions or early on in the disease course, but as this condition is often associated with widespread metastatic disease, radiotherapy is normally the treatment of choice. The success of treatment is limited, and although the prognosis of these patients is generally poor, several patients will survive for a considerable period, which has significant implications for continuing care and local palliative care services.[37]

The dying

The ability to deliver drugs subcutaneously has in some ways revolutionised the dying process, although some believe that this has resulted in the institutionalisation of death and a further loss of the ability of a patient to die naturally.[38] Drugs that can be delivered subcutaneously via a syringe driver in this situation are listed in **Table 6.9**. Recommended sites for the placement of subcutaneous needles are shown in **Figure 6.6**, and some guidelines for the use of a syringe driver are given in **Table 6.10**.

It is crucial to continue to deliver analgesia to dying patients. Those women who can no longer take oral medications can be given drugs per rectum, transdermally or via a subcutaneous infusion. Diamorphine is the strong opioid of choice when delivered subcutaneously. It is much more soluble than morphine, allowing for larger doses to be delivered in a smaller volume. The appropriate dose of subcutaneous diamorphine is one third the total daily dose of oral morphine, although this often needs to be increased during the terminal phase.

Drug	Indication	Comments
Diamorphine	Analgesia	The 24-hour dose of diamorphine is one third the 24-hour oral morphine dose
Midazolam	Terminal restlessness and agitation, control of convulsions	Can be mixed with diamorphine in syringe driver Usual dose 20 to 60 mg 24-hourly
Levomepromazine	Terminal restlessness plus vomiting	Antipsychotic effect can help terminal confusion, usual starting dose 25 mg 24-hourly
Dexamethasone	Chronic steroid use	Sudden discontinuation can exacerbate terminal distress
Haloperidol	Nausea and vomiting	Commonly used with diamorphine to combat opioid-induced vomiting Sedative at doses >3 mg d^{-1}
Cyclizine	Nausea secondary to bowel obstruction	Does not exacerbate colicky pain, may precipitate at concentrations > 10 mg ml^{-1}
Glycopyrronium	Retained bronchial secretions	No CNS effects, can be used at an earlier stage than hyoscine
Hyoscine hydrobromide	Retained bronchial secretions 'death rattle'	Can result in profound dryness Maximum 24 hour dose 2.4 mg s.c.

Table 6.9 Drugs suitable for subcutaneous administration of the dying patient

A common problem encountered when managing the dying patient is terminal restlessness. This state of agitation may be exacerbated by several factors, e.g. infection, pain, drug toxicity or withdrawal, the treatment of which are often inappropriate or impossible. Midazolam, a benzodiazepine derivative, is the drug most commonly used to combat terminal restlessness. When nausea and vomiting has been a major problem, a more appropriate agent to use in this situation

1. Use of a simple battery-operated portable syringe driver with a butterfly infusion set to deliver drugs at a predetermined site
2. Place the subcutaneous needle over the shoulder area, abdomen or upper outer thigh (Fig. 6.6)
3. Provided there is evidence of compatibility, selected injections can be mixed in syringe drivers e.g: the following can be used with diamorphine: midazolam, methotrimeprazine, hyoscine, haloperidol, cyclizine* and dexamethasone*—avoid more than three drugs in one combination
4. Some medications are *not* suitable for subcutaneous infusion, e.g. chlorpromazine, prochlorperazine and diazepam, all of which cause skin reactions at the injection site
5. Small volumes of water for injection are usually used to dissolve drugs, as normal saline increases the likelihood of precipitation when more than one drug is used
6. The infusion site should be checked regularly—swelling at the site of injection is not an indication for site change whereas pain or obvious inflammation is
7. Cover the infusion site with a semi-occlusive dressing, e.g. Tegaderm®, to allow observation of needle site
8. The infusion can be programmed to run over 6, 12 and 24 hours, and drug doses should be reviewed regularly
9. Check syringe driver often to ensure correct administration rate

* May precipitate at higher doses.

Table 6.10 Guidelines for the use of subcutaneous infusions in palliative care

Figure 6.6
Recommended sites for the placement of subcutaneous needles.

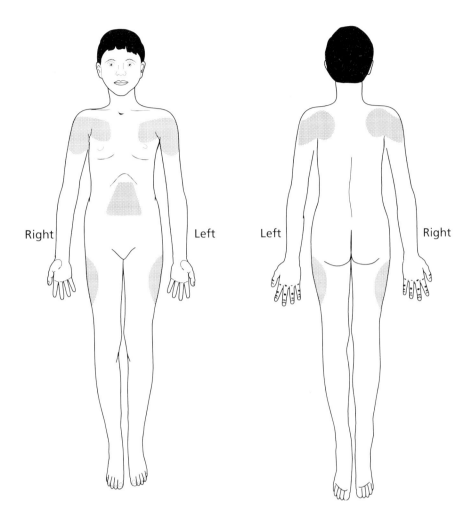

Right   Left   Left   Right

may be levomepromazine, which has both antipsychotic, sedative and antiemetic properties.[39] Both drugs can be delivered subcutaneously. Rectal diazepam provides an alternative choice if the subcutaneous route is not being used.

In terminal dyspnoea the primary aim is to depress respiratory drive, control anxiety and calm the patient. This can be achieved pharmacologically, with small doses of morphine or diamorphine given regularly in conjunction with benzodiazepines. Retained bronchial secretions can result in alarming sounds of laboured breathing in the dying patient. This can be distressing to relatives and carers but can be lessened with the judicious use of antimuscarinic agents, e.g. hyoscine hydrobromide or glycopyrronium bromide, to dry secretions in large airways.

Many relatives and carers find it difficult to cope with the fact that their loved ones are dying and yet not receiving fluid or nourishment when intravenous lines are taken down or removed. Up to 2 litres day^{-1} normal saline can be delivered via the subcutaneous route, but in a patient who is obviously dying of an incurable disease, a death without lines or tubes seems more dignified and can break down barriers between carers and a dying patient.

Conclusion

Although metastatic breast cancer is an incurable malignancy, it is possible to live with advanced disease for many years. With the provision of good palliative measures it is possible to achieve good quality of life for many women. This care encompasses not only the patient but their relatives and carers. Palliative care should be considered early in the course of the disease and should continue throughout the illness trajectory.

Many thousands of women die of breast cancer each year. In the UK, women can usually have the choice of place of death (hospice, hospital or home), because of the well developed hospice and palliative care services.[40] Similarly there is a large number of support services available in the community for patients with breast cancer (e.g. Macmillan nurses, Marie Curie Cancer Care, the Sue Ryder Foundation and the British Association of Cancer United Patients) to provide counselling and general support to women with breast cancer and their friends and carers.

References

1. Jadad AR, Browman GP. The WHO analgesic ladder for cancer pain management. JAMA 1995; 274: 1870–3.

 2. Eisenberg E, Berkey CS, Carr DB et al. Efficacy and safety of nonsteroidal anti-inflammatory drugs for cancer pain: a meta-analysis. J Clin Oncol 1994; 12: 2756–65.

3. McQuay H, Moore A. An evidence-based resource for pain relief, 1998. Oxford: Oxford University Press, 1998.

4. Hawkey CJ. COX-2 inhibitors. Lancet 1999; 353: 307–14.

5. World Health Organisation. Cancer pain relief, with a guide to opioid availability, 2nd edn, Geneva: WHO, 1996.

6. McQuay H. Opioids in pain management. Lancet 1999; 353: 2229–32.

7. European Association of Palliative Care. Morphine in cancer pain: modes of administration. BMJ 1996; 312: 823–6.

 8. Faura CC, Collins SL, Moore RA et al. Systematic review of factors affecting the ratios of morphine and its major metabolites. Pain 1998; 74: 43–53.

9. Borgbjerg FM, Nielsen K, Franks J. Experimental pain stimulates respiration and attenuates morphine-induced respiratory depression: a controlled study in human volunteers. Pain 1996; 64: 123–8.

10. Vainio A, Ollila J, Matikainen E et al. Driving ability in cancer patients receiving long term morphine analgesia. Lancet 1995; 346: 667–70.

11. Zech DFJ, Lehmann KA, Grond S. A new treatment option for chronic cancer pain. Eur J Palliat Care 1995; 1: 26–30.

12. Fallon M. Opioid rotation: does it have a role? Palliat Med 1997; 1: 177–8.

13. de Stoutz ND, Bruera E, Suarez-Almazor M. Opioid rotation for toxicity reduction in terminal care patients. J Pain Sym Man 1995; 10: 378–84.

14. Hardy JR. The use of corticosteroids in palliative care. Eur J Palliat Care 1998; 5: 46–50.

 15. Bone Pain Trial Working Party. 8Gy single fraction radiotherapy for the treatment of metastatic skeletal pain: randomised comparison with a multifraction schedule over 12 months of patient follow-up. Radiother Oncol 1999; 52: 111–21.

16. Body JJ, Bartl R, Burckhardt PD et al. Current use of bisphosphonates in oncology. International bone and cancer study group. J Clin Oncol 1998; 12: 3890–9.

17. Fulfaro F, Casuccio A, Ticozzi C et al. Role of bisphosphonates in treatment of painful metastatic bone disease: a review of phase III trials. Pain 1998; 78: 157–69.

18. Bierman WA, Cantor RI, Fellin FM et al. An evaluation of the potential cost reductions resulting from the use of clodronate in the treatment of metastatic carcinoma of the breast to bone. Bone 1991; 12 (suppl 1): 37–42S.

19. Christie JM, Simmonds M, Patl R et al. Dose titration, multicenter study of oral transmucosal fentanyl citrate for the treatment of breakthrough pain in cancer patients using transdermal fentanyl for persistent pain. J Clin Oncol 1998; 16: 3238–45.

20. British Association of Surgical Oncology. The management of metastatic bone disease in the UK. Eur J Surg Oncol 1999; 25: 3–23.

21. McQuay H, Moore A. Antidepressants in neuropathic pain. In: An evidence-based resource for pain relief. Oxford: Oxford Medical, 1998: 231–41.

22. Watson M, Haviland JS, Greer S et al. Influence of psychological response on survival in breast cancer: a population based cohort study. Lancet 1999; 354: 1331–6.

23. Walker-Renard PB, Vaughan LM, Sahn SA. Chemical pleurodesis for malignant pleural effusions. Ann Intern Med 1994; 120: 56–64.

24. Miles DW, Knight RK. Diagnosis and management of malignant pleural effusion. Cancer Treat Rev 1993; 19: 151–68.

25. Jennings A-L, Broadley KE. Systematic review of the palliative use of opioids in dyspnoea. (Abstract) 6th Congress of the European Association for Palliative Care, Geneva, Sept 1999.

26. Twycross RG, Barkby GD, Hallwood PM. The use of low dose levomepromazine (methotrimeprazine) in the management of nausea and vomiting. Progress in Palliat Care 1997; 5: 49–53.

27. Loprinzi CL, Kugler JW, Sloan JA et al. Randomised comparison of megestrol acetate versus dexamethasone versus fluoxymesterone for the treatment of cancer anorexia/cachexia. J Clin Oncol 1999; 17: 3299–306.

28. Tchekmedvian NS, Hickman M, Sian J et al. Megesterol acetate in cancer anorexia and weight loss. Cancer 1992; 69: 1268–74.

29. Davies AN. The management of xerostomia: a review. Eur J Cancer Care 1997; 6: 209–14.

30. Foldi E. The treatment of lymphedema. Cancer 1998; 83: 2833–4.

31. Sykes N. The treatment of morphine-induced constipation. Eur J Palliat Care 1998; 5: 12–5.

32. Ling PJ, A'Hern RP, Hardy JR. Analysis of survival following treatment of tumour-induced hypercalcaemia with intravenous pamidronate (APD). Br J Cancer 1995; 72: 206–9.

33. Lentzsch S, Reichardt P, Weber F et al. Brain metastases in breast cancer: prognostic factors and management. Eur J Cancer 1999; 35: 580–5.

34. Bruera E, Brenneis C, Michaud M et al. Association between asthenia and nutritional status, lean body mass, anaemia, psychological status, and tumor mass in patients with advanced breast cancer. J Pain Sym Man 1989; 4: 59–63.

35. Stone P, Richards M, Hardy J. Review article: fatigue in patients with cancer. Eur J Cancer 1998; 34: 1670–6.

36. Jones AL, Williams MP, Powles TJ et al. Magnetic resonance imaging in the detection of skeletal metastases in patients with breast cancer. Br J Cancer 1990; 62: 296–8.

37. Cowap J, Hardy J, A'Hern R. Outcome of spinal cord compression at a cancer centre—implications for palliative care services. J Pain Sympton Manag 2000; 19: 257–64.

38. O'Neil WM. Subcutaneous infusions—a medical last rite. Palliat Med 1994; 8: 91–3.

39. O'Neill J, Fountain A. Levomepromazine (methotrimeprazine) and the last 48 hours. Hosp Med 1999; 60: 564–7.

40. Higginson IJ, Astin P, Dolan S. Where do cancer patients die? Ten year trend in the place of death of cancer patients in England. Palliat Med 1998; 12: 353–63.

7 Breast cancer in men

Anthony R. Hyett
Nigel P.M. Sacks

Carcinoma in the vestigial breast of men is an uncommon disease accounting for only 0.87% of all breast cancers.[1] Initial investigation is in exactly the same way as breast cancer in women, where the triple assessment of breast examination, breast imaging with mammography and/or ultrasonography and fine needle aspiration cytology (FNAC) provide the means of diagnostic assessment.[1] As in breast cancer in women, a selective investigation policy for symptoms suggestive of metastatic breast disease in men should be adopted rather than screening for asymptomatic metastases.[1] Unlike women, breast conservation surgery is not appropriate for men, and a modified radical mastectomy with concomitant ipsilateral axillary node clearance is the standard surgical operation. Up until now decisions regarding surgery, endocrine therapies, cytotoxic chemotherapy and radiotherapy were extrapolated from the literature of the treatment of women.[2,3] Prospective double-blind randomised trials of different surgical therapies and different adjuvant therapies are non-existent in this condition[1] because of the rarity of the disease and the failure to consolidate treatment and outcome experiences across institutions. Postoperative adjuvant radiotherapy to the chest wall and the supraclavicular fossa is being used increasingly, as is cytotoxic chemotherapy.

Tamoxifen as an adjuvant endocrine therapy is beneficial, given the 85% rates for oestrogen receptor (ER)-positivity in men with breast cancer[1,2], but there are no data showing that tamoxifen has no role in those with ER-negative breast tumours. Other historically important surgical endocrine therapies including bilateral orchidectomy, adrenalectomy and hypophysectomy are now used very infrequently.

There is a greater trend in using adjuvant cytotoxic chemotherapy, non-surgical endocrine therapy and radiotherapy, and these are critical to improving effective disease-free intervals and survival rates.[1,4] The overall prognosis for male breast cancer compared with that in women is worse.[1,2,4] The reasons for this are related to delayed diagnosis, inappropriate staging, anatomical factors and more advanced diseases at presentation due to inappropriately low index of suspicion. There is a higher rate of histologically proven nodal positivity at the first diagnosis in men (65% node positive) compared with women with symptomatic and screen-detected cancers (30–50% node positive).[1]

There is an older average age at diagnosis and higher death rates for men from non-breast cancer reasons. Up to one third of deaths in men with breast cancer are due to other causes.[1,5] It is now clear that the cure rates in men and women are similar when they are accurately matched for stage and age.[1,5] An improved understanding of the incidence, prevalence, aetiology, genetics, tumour characteristics and anatomical and hormonal receptor differences between men and women with breast cancer will allow more appropriate and effective therapeutic strategies in the future.

Epidemiology

When reliable population statistics are considered there has been a relatively stable incidence of breast cancer in men over the past 40 years[6] in contrast to that in women, which continues to increase gradually.[2]

Breast cancer in men now accounts for 0.87% of all new incident breast cancers in men and women but only accounts for 0.2% of all cancers in men and is consequently a rare cause of death in men.[1] In the USA the 1998 estimates showed that there were 1600 new cases of breast cancer in men compared with 180 300 in women.[2] The median age of diagnosis of 55 years in men is 10 years older than that of woman.

There are some international differences in the incidence rates (**Table 7.1**) and the male to female ratios. In most Western countries the male:female ratio is 1:100,[6] but in Africa the ratios range from 1.4 to 6 per 100 breast cancers diagnosed in women. For example, in Zambia men make up 15% of all breast

High incidence	Low incidence
Recife, Brazil 3.4	Cali, Columbia <0.1
Prince Edward Island, Canada 1.6	Japan <0.1
San Francisco Bay area 1.3[a]	Singapore <0.1
Non-Kuwaits, Kuwait 1.2	Hungary <0.1
Atlanta, USA 1.1[a]	Senegal <0.2
	Africa Bantu Countries 0.4

[a] Affected black males.

Table 7.1 Calculated international incidence figures for breast cancer in men per 100 000 man years

Countries with decreases in death rate	Countries with increases in death rate
Italy	Portugal
Switzerland	Norway
Finland	UK (Scotland and Northern Ireland)
UK (England and Wales)	Denmark
Germany	Austria
Ireland	
France	

Table 7.2 Comparative European data in age-standardised death rates in breast cancer in men between 1955–59 and 1985–89

cancer cases.[6,7] The Bantu African speaking countries also have this greater male:female ratio and this propensity is also seen in Angola, Cameroon, the Ivory Coast, Kenya, Malawi, Tanzania and Zambia.[6] A possible explanation includes the relative high oestrogen concentrations as a consequence of cirrhotic liver disease from viral hepatitis, bilharzia and schistosomiasis.[6,7]

The average incidence of breast cancer in men in Europe is 1.0 case per 100 000 man years (**Table 7.2**).[6] The International Union Against Cancer (UICC) has analysed the incidence and death rates of breast cancer in men across Europe between 1955 and 1989.[8] There are subtle trends, but the overall death rates have not altered much in the 27 countries studied. Table 7.2 compares the data from 1955–59 and 1985–89 in countries showing an increase in age-standardised death rates in men with breast cancer.

Italy, Switzerland, Finland, England, Wales and France have shown improvements in age-standardised death rates per million of men aged 24–64 years from 1955–1989. These figures do not correlate with the higher levels of mortality in women with breast cancer especially in England and Scandinavia.[8] There have been stable incidence rates in Finland, Norway and Sweden but a 1% per year increase in Denmark. Better diagnosis and reporting may be part of the explanation, but this increase is real and is currently unexplained.[9]

The similarities and differences between breast cancer in the two sexes are compared and contrasted in **Table 7.3**.[10]

Aetiology/risk factors

The majority of men with breast cancer have no easily identifiable direct genetic or environmental cause. **Table 7.4** summarises the putative factors identified so far in the aetiology of this rare disease.

	Men	Women
Incidence	Stable (1 case per 100 000 man years)	Increasing in some Western countries
% of all breast cancer cases	0.87	99.13
% of all cancer cases	0.2	23
Age	Linear increase	Bimodal
Median age (years)	65 (rare <40)	55
Screening mammography	No role	Proven efficacy
Side prevalence	L>R	L>R
Nipple discharge	Common and significant	Uncommon; rarely malignant
Bilateral synchronous breast cancer (%)	1.4	2–5
Skin ulceration (%)	10	Rare; often a late sign
Nipple involvement (%)	80	<10
Nodal positivity at diagnosis	60	30
Histology	Ductal	Ductal 70% Lobular 10% Other 20%
Receptor status		
Oestrogen receptor positive (%)	85	60–65
Progesterone receptor positive (%)	75	50
Genetics		
% cases with genetic basis	20	8–10
% cases *BRCA1* positive	Not associated	5 especially in younger patients
% cases *BRCA2* positive	20	5
Lifetime risk of breast cancer	*BRCA2* positive = 5%	*BRCA1* or *BRCA2* positive = 75–85%
% of spontaneoous new mutations	50% of all *BRCA2* cases	5–10% of *BRCA1* and *BRCA2* cases

Table 7.3 Comparison of the features of breast cancer in men and women[1,6,11,12,15,23,38,39]

Genetic
  Family history—especially if *BRCA2* positivity is proven
  Klinefelter's syndrome (XXY,XYY)
Environmental
  Gynaecomastia—particularly postpubertal or geriatric rather than prepubertal in onset
  Endogenous oestrogen administration—transsexuals, prostate carcinoma treatment, phyto-oestrogens (uncertain)
  Testicular disorders—mumps, orchitis, hyperthermia with blast furnace workers
  Ionising irradiation
  Electromagnetic irradiation from occupational exposure
  Hyperprolactinaemia—pituitary tumours, phenothiazine use
  Occupational factors—blast furnaces, newsprinting dyes

Table 7.4 Aetiological factors implicated in breast cancer in men[15]

Genetic factors

Family history

A family pedigree containing breast cancer patients is a definite risk factor for breast cancer developing in men. The *BRCA1* gene was identified on the 17q21 chromosome in 1994 and *BRCA2* was subsequently discovered on chromosome 13q12–13 in 1995.[11,12] There are now more than 200 different mutations described for *BRCA2* and 100 for *BRCA1*.[4] These mutations are mainly gene deletions rather than gene insertions that lead to the synthesis of nonsense, truncated proteins. The inheritance of *BRCA1* and *BRCA2* is of an autosomal dominant pattern.[4] It is now estimated that 20% of men with breast cancer have a *BRCA2* mututation of chromosome 17.[13,14] Interestingly, half those identified are *de novo* mutations without any family history.[13] In comparison spontaneous and directly inherited mutations in *BRCA1* and *BRCA2* are thought to account for only 10% of all women with breast cancer[11] and 33% of those diagnosed between the ages of 20 and 30 years.[4]

Breast cancer in men is only rarely associated with *BRCA1* (<1% of all cases) and is most commonly associated with *BRCA2* in genetically linked families.[4] Determining *BRCA2* status in families with men with breast cancer is a useful genetic marker and may determine the advice given to these patients and their relatives. The absolute lifetune risk of *BRCA2* carriers has not been determined.

No prospective randomised trials have been performed on chemoprevention in male *BRCA2* carriers. The lower overall lifetime breast cancer risk of 5% for *BRCA2*-positive men makes prophylactic mastectomy a more difficult option to support compared with *BRCA1*- or *BRAC2*-positive women with a risk of 70–85%.[4,15]

Currently there are no effective proven pharmaceutical or surgical prophylactic strategies with long-term follow-up for men with a proven *BRCA2* mutation.

If a *BRCA2* carrier develops unilateral disease then bilateral mastectomy could be considered as a reasonable treatment option given that the predisposition is bilateral. In Iceland there is one specific mutation called 999del5 in the *BRCA2* gene that is present in 40% of families with a male member with breast cancer.[13,14] This makes predictive genetic testing easier in this country as the *BRCA2* gene mutation can be localised easily in 40% of cases. The remaining 60% would undergo a full gene analysis for *BRCA2*. In Sweden 20% of patients have a positive-*BRCA2* mutation,[4] but only half of these patients have a positive family history, implying that there is another mutation present. The absence of a family history does not negate the possibility of a *BRCA2*-positive inheritance pattern.[16]

BRCA2-positive patients have a significantly increased risk of developing other malignancies including colorectal, ovarian and prostate cancer and melanoma, but the percentage risk for another visceral malignancy is not currently defined.[17]

Klinefelter's syndrome

Klinefelter's syndrome is thought to increase the lifetime risk of breast cancer by 20–65-fold above the general male population,[15,18–20] and the rare case reports of lobular carcinoma in situ (LCIS) and lobular cancer have been reported in such patients.[19] Gynaecomastia is very common in those with Klinefelter's syndrome but is not thought to be an independent predisposing factor for cancer as those patients without gynaecomastia have also developed the disease. The lifetime risk of developing cancer in those with Klinefelter's syndrome may be as high as 3–6% and therefore probably does not justify prophylactic mastectomy.[18–20]

Environmental factors

Hormonal status

Gynaecomastia is a common disorder and occurs in neonates, adolescents and adults. Hormonal imbalance may be an aetiological factor, although most patients have no detectable deficiency of serum androgen concentration or an increased oestrogen concentration.[21,22] Any relative imbalance of the androgen/oestrogen ratio is difficult to prove as serum assays in these patients have given conflicting results.[1,23] Finasteride treatment for patients with prostate cancer is associated with gynaecomastia but its causative relationship with breast cancer is non-existent.[24]

Oestrogen therapy

Oestrogen administration for those with metastatic prostatic cancer and oestrogen therapy in transsexuals may be aetiological factors,[25] but the number of patients with prior oestrogen therapy was only 3 of 487 in one series.[23] Oestrogen stimulates the acini and lobules in the male breast but the sequence of ductal carcinoma in situ (DCIS) to invasive ductal cancer or LCIS to invasive ductal or lobular cancer is not established in men.

Clinical presentation

The tumour typically presents as a painless lump and is often associated with discharge from an ipsilateral nipple but can also present as a locally advanced disease. The reported features at diagnosis are presented in **Table 7.5**.[1,23,26]

The clinical evaluation of the axilla remains unreliable, with a 1–40% false negative rate and 8–50% false positive rate for metastatic tumour detection.[4]

Skin ulceration is more common in men than it is in women and is not due to Paget's disease but to direct invasion of the epidermis by the cancer.[26]

The time from the initial index symptom has progressively declined from 18–21 months in the 1950s to 1–5 months in the 1990s.[1,23,26] A delay of greater

	Clinical feature	Frequency (%)
History	Painless mass	74–97
	Bloody nipple discharge	4–15
	Family history for breast cancer	5–23
Examination	Nipple retraction	7–38
	Paget's disease	1–7
	Skin/nipple ulceration	10–27
	Fixity to pectoralis muscle	3
	Fixity to skin	14–22
	Palpable axillary nodes	40–55
	Metastatic symptoms	Excluded from the analysis
Diagnosis	Fine needle aspiration alone	8
	Open biopsy	92
	Mammography	58 mass alone
		26 architectural change
		8 microcalcification
	Ultrasonography	55–76

Table 7.5 Frequency of features of breast cancer in men at presentation

than 6 months was an independent variable for worse prognosis, but whether the staging of diseases was matched was not clear, given the discrepancy of time to presentation for these groups.[1,26]

The sites of metastases of breast cancer in men include locoregional (chest wall), lung, liver, bony axial skeleton and the CNS. The most common site of relapse after primary definitive treatment in Borgen's group of 104 patients was bone (83%) and lung (15%).[27,28] Locoregional relapse occurred in 4.8% of patients and most commonly came from the initial node-positive group in 70% of cases.[27,28]

Differential diagnoses

Only 3–7% of men presenting for assessment of a breast mass will subsequently have cancer.[29] The differential diagnosis of a breast mass in men is given in **Table 7.6**.[30]

Pathology

Histologically the breast in men resembles the prepubertal breast in women, with several small ducts in collagen stroma and very few lobules. The terminal duct and lobule unit (TDLU) is thus poorly or not developed in the breast in men, and this is the reason for the relative infrequency of LCIS and invasive lobular cancers in men with breast cancer[15] The ageing male's 'andropause' or

	Gynaecomastia	Breast cancer
History	Predisposing history—alcohol, drugs, steroids	Positive family history for breast cancer in men
		Known *BRCA2* positivity
	No nipple discharge	Bloody nipple discharge
Examination	Bilateral symmetrical retroareolar masses	Unilateral asymmetrical hard mass
	No ulceration	Ulceration
	No fixity to skin or muscle	Fixity to adjacent structures
	No axillary lymphadenopathy	Axillary lymphadenopathy
Diagnosis by mammography	Bilateral retroareolar masses with smooth edges and no suspicious microcalcification	Rarely in midline
		Typical features of breast cancer in women

Table 7.6 Gynaecomastia versus breast cancer in men[7]

absolute hyperoestrogenism allegedly stimulates the TDLU. In a series of men with DCIS there were no patients taking exogenous oestrogen. The larger retroareolar ducts may give rise to DCIS without this hormone-induced cellular differentiation in men.[31]

Histology

A wide spectrum of benign and malignant disease occurs in the breast of men (**Table 7.7**).

Benign disorders

True or pseudo-gynaecomastia is the main differential diagnosis of a breast lump in a man. Cancer is a realistic differential diagnosis in elderly men with apparent gynaecomastia, but cancer rarely occurs before 40 years of age. Benign breast cysts in men are uncommon at any age, and the presence of a cyst should alert the clinician to the diagnosis of malignant cystic papillary cancer.[30] Fibroadenoma is very uncommon but is associated with oestrogen, spironolactone or chlordiapoxide therapy.[29]

Malignant disorders
Pure DCIS

Pure DCIS makes up 5–15% of all cancers in men.[32] It presents as a lump and not as a mammographic abnormality as is the case in women in the screening programme. DCIS with and without invasive cancer occurs in men.[31]

The usual subtypes of DCIS occur in men as they do in women: papillary, cribriform, solid, micropapillary and comedo. In one series of 114 patients there were no cases of high-grade comedo DCIS without an associated invasive

Pathology	Histological types
Benign conditions/tumours	Gynaecomastia—nodular, dendritic, glandular Pseudogynaecomastia—obesity related Lipoma Papillomatosis Fibroadenoma Benign cystosarcoma phylloides Duct ectasia Fat necrosis
Malignant tumours *Carcinoma*	Ductal carcinoma in situ Papillomatosis Invasive ductal Invasive lobular Tubular Mucinous Medullary Oncocytic Inflammatory Intracystic papillary Neuroendocrine Small cell Paget's disease
Sarcoma 1–8% of all men with breast cancer	Spindle cell Fibrosarcoma Malignant cystosarcoma phyllodes Leiomyosarcoma
Other	Primary skin tumours—basal cell carcinoma, small-cell carcinoma, melanoma Lymphomas
Metastatic	Contralateral breast malignancy Melanoma Prostate Lung

Table 7.7 Histological subtypes in the breast of men[30]

cancer.[31] The clinical, genetic and pathological implications of this are uncertain. The percentage of men with DCIS that develop cancer is unknown, but one study found no differences between pure DCIS and DCIS associated with invasive cancer with respect to race, age, laterality or presenting symptoms.[31]

Invasive ductal cancer

The most common cancer in men is invasive ductal cancer. Lobular cancer is very rare and Paget's disease is associated with invasive breast cancer far less commonly in men than it is in women, with only 40 cases reported in the literature.[26] The incidence of an underlying invasive carcinoma in men with Paget's disease is 100%. ER positivity in Paget's disease in men is the same as it is in invasive cancer and the surgical and medical strategies are exactly as for the management of invasive disease.[33]

Sarcomas

Breast sarcomas occur in up to 8% of reported series of male breast cancer and their management and assessment is similar to the counterpart in women.[1,2]

Metastatic lesions

Metastasis to the breast is uncommon but it may be the first indication of an occult extramammary malignancy.[34] Metastatic lesions in the breast mimic benign and malignant conditions and the diagnosis is achieved by FNAC or core biopsy. Tumour-specific immunohistochemistry, such as acid phosphatase, allows the diagnosis of metastatic prostate cancer.

Receptor status

The reported expression of cellular receptors and their frequency are shown in **Table 7.8**.

Receptor types

The ER was first identified in a man with breast cancer in 1974.[35] The ER status of breast cancers in men is 85% compared with that in women of 60%.[1,23] There is no increase in ER positivity with age as there is in women and ER positivity is independent of age.[36] This has significant implications for endocrine manipulation and tamoxifen therapy. Patients with ER levels less than 30 fmol ng^{-1} of protein did not respond to hormonal manipulation,[37] and ER positivity is taken as greater than 5 fmol ng^{-1}.[38,39] The role of endocrine therapy in patients with ER-negative tumours is currently not defined.

Cellular receptors investigated	Positive rate (%)
Oestrogen	85–91
Progesterone	60–96
Androgen	50–95
Bcl-2	94
Cyclin D	58
CerbB2	41
MIB-1	38
HER-2/neu	29
p53	21
Glucosteroid	50
Epidermal growth factor	76

Table 7.8 Receptor status in men with breast cancer[41]

Progesterone receptor (PgR) positivity occurs in 60–94% of tumours and the clinical implications of this are currently limited. PgR positivity is taken as greater than 15 fmol ng^{-1}.[39,40]

Androgen receptor (AR) positivity occurs in 50–95% of tumours, and further work on antiandrogen therapies may have therapeutic implications.[2,41]

Other prognostic gene products

BCL-2 is part of a large protooncogene family responsible for cellular apoptosis, and 94% of breast cancers in men express this marker which correlates with ER positivity and response to tamoxifen. BCL-2 levels increase with tamoxifen therapy.[36]

Cyclin D$_1$, which is involved with cyclin-dependent kinases and regulates the cell cycle into the S phase, is expressed in 41% of tumours. Over-expression is thought to have a positive effect on cell cycling and therefore a negative prognostic outcome, but the converse is true. Cyclin D$_1$ negativity is associated with a shorter disease-free interval, and the reason is not clear.[36]

HER-z/c-erbB2 positivity is associated with a higher node positivity rate (41% v 33%) and hence a worse prognosis. (It is proposed that HER-z/c-erbB2 positivity may become an independent indicator for cytotoxic chemotherapy in those with node-negative tumours.

MIB-1 antibody is directed against Ki-67, which is a proliferation-associated antigen expressed in the Go phase of the cell cycle. It is considered an adverse prognostic marker.

HER-2 is a cell surface growth factor receptor of the tyrosine kinase group, which is positive in 29% of breast cancers in men and associated with an adverse prognosis. HER-2-positive tumours tend to be ER negative, with positive lymph nodes.[36]

A $p53$ mutation on the short arm of chromosome 17 is a common finding in different human malignancies.[36] Twenty-one per cent of cancers are $p53$ positive, found by using a sensitive polymerase technique. Conflicting data exist on the effect of $p53$ positivity on overall survival and disease-free intervals.

Glucocorticoid receptor positivity is 50%, but the therapeutic implications of this are unknown.[2] Epidermal growth factor receptors are positive in 76% of breast cancers in men.[2]

Serum tumour markers

There is uncertain significance and unproven effectiveness in serial measurements of CA15-3 and carcinoembryonic antigen (CEA) in men with breast cancer preoperatively or as part of follow-up surveillance.[2]

DNA ploidy status and mean S phase fraction analysis

Nuclear ploidy is a recognised feature of a tumour's disordered mitosis and contributes to the cellular malfunction leading to malignant cell change and metastasis.[38,41] One study has shown that DNA aneuploidy has no correlation with tumour size and no effect on axillary nodal positivity or 5-year survival rates in 32 men with breast cancer. A study from Iceland showed that 43% of tumours were diploid and 57% were aneuploid.[41] The S phase fraction, which indicates cycle doubling time, was similar between men and women patients at 7.2%, and aneuploidy was not an independent prognostic factor.[38,41]

Prognostic factors and survival rates

Tumour size and nodal status are independent prognostic factors but ulceration and fixity are not. Low-grade tumours and ER positivity are thought to afford a better prognosis in men with breast cancer, but the strongest independent prognostic indicators are tumour size and axillary node positivity (**Table 7.9**).[20,21] Tamoxifen has had a dramatic impact on the survival data when the stage subgroup analysis is reviewed. Data from the 1992 world overview showed that 5-year survival with tamoxifen was 56% compared with 25% without tamoxifen in stage 2 and 3 disease.[29,39,40]

	Better prognosis	Worse prognosis
History		
Time to presentation (months)	<6	>6
Age	No effect	No effect
Examination		
Ulceration	Not present	Present
Tumour size	<2 cm (Jaeyismi)	>5 cm
Axillary nodal involvement	Negative	Positive
Involved nodes	1–4	>4
Pathology		
Stage at diagnosis	1 and 2	3 and 4
Tumour grade	1 or low grade	3 or high grade
Histological type	DCIS/LCIS	Invasive ductal
	Medullary	Inflammatory
	Tubular	Paget's disease
	Papillary	
Lymphovascular invasion	Absent	Present
Oestrogen receptor status	Positive	Negative
cerbB2 status	Negative	Positive

DCIS, ductal carcinoma in situ; LCIS, lobular carcinoma in situ.

Table 7.9 Factors in prognosis in men with breast cancer[7]

Tumour size/stage

Survival stage-for-stage (TNM) is equivalent for men and wome
cancer.[15,23,39,42,45,47] The comparison of survival data is difficult owing
surgeons, differing operations, uncorrected non-cancer death rates and th
ing use of endocrine therapies. The 5-year survival for tumours less than
diameter was 94%, 1–4 cm, 80% and these greater than 4 cm, 40%.[43,44] The i
pretation of survival data is affected by the inclusion of those patients with stage
disease (making up 17% of one series) and improved overall survival data. The
5-year survival of patients with stage 0 disease was 100%.[27]

Axillary nodal status

The number of nodes (0, 1–3, >4) that are positive has been analysed as an
independent prognostic factor with differing average lifespans.[1] The 10-year
survival for node-negative disease was 84%, for one to three positive nodes was
44% and for those with more than four positive nodes was 14%.[43] In women
the effect is obvious, with a significant reduction in overall survival rates from
37% to 13% at 10 years in those undergoing mastectomy with 1–3 nodes and
more than 4 nodes involved.[43] In men, the nodal load with the larger tumour is
more often the critical prognostic factor and not the size of the tumour itself.

Table 7.10 shows that node positivity is a critical factor in survival and
recurrence and should be a marker of adjuvant postoperative therapy as this is a
high risk group for locoregional and distant relapse.

Occult nodal micrometastases can be detected with immunohistochemistry
in as many as 20% of women with apparent node-negative breast cancer, and
these patients have a worse prognosis. This technology has not been applied to
men with breast cancer and it may impact on the prescription of adjuvant
therapy.[44]

Diagnostic techniques

FNAC

There are few articles assessing the role of FNAC in breast masses in men.[28,45]
But the standard features of malignancy are noted: cellularity, lack of cellular

	5-year relapse-free survival (%)	5-year actual survival (%)
Node positive	30	60
Node negative	87	100

Table 7.10 Survival data of 104 cases of men with breast cancer dependent on axillary node positivity

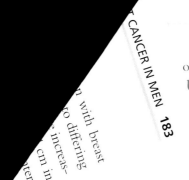
onomorphism, anisonucleosidosis, eosinophilic macronucleoli,
lasmic ratio, mitotic rates and nuclear membrane irregularity. The
ures of gynaecomastia include smooth nuclear membranes, cohesive
population and the absence of macronucleoli. FNAC is an estab-
al part of the initial assessment of the breast mass in men, but the
ettering has only an 8% preoperative diagnosis rate using FNAC
h a 92% open biopsy rate before definite surgery.[26]

Mammography

Adequate bilateral mammography can be technically difficult in men owing to
the relative paucity of breast tissue.[30] The standard craniocaudal and medial/
lateral oblique views are attempted. Given the technical difficulties, a reverse
view is sometimes indicated.[30] Nipple markers may be used when the craniocaudal view cannot visualise the nipple to the most anterior part of the
mammographic image.

The typical mammographic features of breast cancer in men are similar to these
in women and include a mass lesion, architectural distortion, microcalcification,
skin thickening, nipple inversion, spiculation and axillary lymphadenopathy.

Ultrasonography

The typical ultrasonographic features of breast cancer in men include an hypoechoic poorly defined mass with posterior acoustic shadowing, loss of normal
tissue planes and a deeper than wide lesion, and there may be associated pathological axillary lymphadenopathy with nodal cortical/medullary definition
loss.[15]

Magnetic resanance imaging

Therole of magnetic resanance imaging (MRI) is uncertain and is being
investigated.

Ductography

Ductography is outmoded as an imaging modality.

Computed tomography

Computed tomography (CT) is reserved for the detection of metastatic disease
of the CNS, chest and liver.

Bone scan

Bone scanning is used to detect metastatic disease in patients with symptomatic bone pain on presentation.[31]

Treatment of the primary tumour

Surgery

Surgical resection remains the most important and effective treatment modality for breast cancer in men.

Open biopsy

There should be little need for an open diagnostic biopsy of a breast mass in a man. A preoperative core biopsy under local anaesthetic should be standard preoperative assessment in the management of a suspected carcinoma.

Modified radical mastectomy and axillary node clearance

Many operations of varying degrees of radicality have been advocated for treatment of breast cancer in men. Halsted's radical mastectomy, modified radical mastectomy with axillary node clearance and simple mastectomy with wide local excision/lumpectomy have all been advocated.[1,23] There is little role for Halsted's procedure. Direct and/or extensive muscle involvement with a locally advanced cancer may dictate preoperative neoadjuvant therapy before rather than after radical surgery.[23,46] A modified radical mastectomy with a level 1 and 2 axillary dissection is the most commonly performed operation reported in the literature. There seems little role for breast conserving surgery as the cosmetic and psychological advantages are not as strong in men. Men do not seem to attach the same significance to the loss of a nipple/areola as do women. The usual proximity of the tumour to the areola/nipple complex in the male breast would usually mean nipple sacrifice as a preferred oncological procedure to minimise locoregional recurrence. There seems to be little requirement for 'lumpectomy' except in elderly men with a contraindication for general anaesthesia.

The relative increased risk of ulceration and pectoralis chest wall fixation may have clouded the correct clinical management decisions. In men, preoperative radiotherapy has not been prospectively studied as a downsizing technique and neither has the optimal timing of surgery after preoperative radiotherapy. Primary cytotoxic chemotherapy in women has allowed down staging of some tumours and a move from mastectomy to breast conserving surgery in selected cases, although no survival advantage has been demonstrated with primary chemotherapy.[47] The role of preoperative chemotherapy in men has not been prospectively analysed but would require a multicentre trial to determine the results. The role of preoperative primary endocrine chemotherapy has not been evaluated in men.

Management of the axilla

The likelihood of histologically positive nodes in most series of men with breast cancer is 60% compared with a histologically positive axilla rate of 30% in women. The role of sentinel node biopsy in men has not been investigated, but over-treatment of the axilla is a weaker argument in men compared with women owing to the higher rate of node positivity.

The role of primary radiotherapy in the surgically untreated axilla in men is currently uncertain.

Contralateral disease

The role of contralateral prophylactic mastectomy is not a great issue in men owing to the relative low rates of synchronous and metachronous breast tumours. It is uncertain whether *BRCA2* carriers have the same incidence of metachronous breast tumours and whether this advice applies more strongly to this subset of patients, given that their lifetime risk of breast cancer is only 5%.[1]

Chest wall reconstruction

Reconstruction is important when there are large defects after surgery for recurrent or locally advanced cancer. Ipsilateral latissmus dorsi myocutaneous flaps based on the thoracodorsal vascular pedicle and rectus abdominis flaps have both been used in this setting.

Tamoxifen

Tamoxifen has been used in primary, adjuvant and chemopreventive settings. In men with breast cancer the ER status is independent of age. Its mode of action is as an oestrogen agonist and antagonist as in women. The effect of tamoxifen on serum oestradiol, progesterone and testosterone concentrations in men is not clear.[39,40] Fifty-one per cent of all men will show some clinical response with tamoxifen, independent of ER status. The response rate is 71% if the tumours are ER positive.[15] No clinical response occurs with tamoxifen in 28% of patients. There is no information showing whether ER status changes between *in situ* and invasive disease in men or whether the status of metastatic disease changes from that of the primary breast lesion.

PgR status is not a useful clinical indicator of endocrine responsiveness is male breast cancer. The reported side effects of tamoxifen in men are alopecia, neuropsychiatric symptoms, depression, skin rashes, hot flushes, weight gain, insomnia, decreased libido and reversible impotence.[2] Exact rates of thromboembolic events have not been quantified. These side effects may explain why non-compliance rates can be as high as 20% after 12 months of tamoxifen therapy.[48] One advantage of tamoxifen is the relative few drug interactions, but warfarin dosage needs to be decreased owing to inhibition of the hepatic enzyme p450.[49] Tamoxifen is a useful drug if the patient is unfit for cytotoxic chemotherapy. There are three main uncertain areas with tamoxifen use in men:

1. Its role in men with ER-negative tumours
2. The duration of treatment[40]
3. Tamoxifen resistance is unstudied and poorly understood[49]

Some representative data of tamoxifen's effect on disease-free interval and 5-year survival data are shown in Tables 7.11 and 7.12.

Progesterones

Megestrol acetate and medroxyprogesterone may provide partial responses for those with advanced disease, but the side effects of dyspepsia and fluid retention limit their use.[3]

Luteinising hormone-releasing hormone agonists (Buserelin and Goserelin)

Buserelin is an analogue of gonadotrophin-releasing hormone that initially increases and then reduces gonadal steroidogenesis, causing a reversible chemical castration. It is used mainly in men with metastatic prostate cancer. It is con-

Procedure	Clinical response rate (%)
Tamoxifen therapy	71 if oestrogen receptor positive
Orchidectomy	80 (4–46 months)
Adrenalectomy	80 (15 months)
Hypophysectomy	56 (6–20 months)

Table 7.11 Response rates of tamoxifen versus surgical endocrine therapies[2]

	5-year disease-free rate (%)	5-year survival rate (%)
Placebo (n=39)	44	44
Tamoxifen (n=130)	66	61

Table 7.12 Stage 2 and 3 disease in men with breast cancer with tamoxifen[2,40]

sidered a medical 'androgen-ectomy.' One case report describes a dramatic response to nasally inhaled Buserelin 0.4–1.2 mg in a patient with bilateral pulmonary metastases. The side effects are minimal, with good pharmaceutical tolerance.[50]

Flutamide

Buserelin's use with the non-steroidal antiandrogen Flutamide (250 mg t.i.d.) has been encouraging.[51] Partial response and stable disease for 12 months or more has been seen with this combination. Side effects include hot flushes, decreased libido and impotence.

Cyproterone acetate

Cyproterone acetate has been used in patients with metastatic disease because of its antiandrogenic and pronounced progestational properties. The slight decrease in follicle stimulating hormone and luteinising hormone concentration with a decrease in testosterone and oestradiol concentrations have poorly correlated with clinical response. It may have a role after relapse on tamoxifen at a daily dosage of 100 mg.[52]

Aromatase inhibitors

Aromatase inhibitors (Anastrazole, Letrozole and Exemestane) hold much promise as a second-line endocrine therapy in patients with metastatic disease.

Antiprolactin agents

The speciality of pharmaceutical intervention with anti prolactin agents is uninvestigated. The range of endocrine therapies is summarised in **Table 7.13**.

Cytotoxic chemotherapy

There are no double-blind, prospective current trials in men but multiple combinations of agents will be used in preference to single agents as in the treatment of women with similar disease stages. Some studies show some survival and disease-free interval advantages with chemotherapy in men, but these are unrandomised and the results are difficult to interpret.[2]

Current indications for cytotoxic chemotherapy include:

- Postoperatively in those who are axillary node-negative with high-grade tumours and those with lymphovascular invasion, node-positive disease or

Endocrine treatments	Drugs
Adjuvant	Tamoxifen
Metastatic	Tamoxifen
	Progesterones
	LHRH agonists—Buserelin/Goserelin
	Flutamide—non-steroidal antiandrogen agent
	Cryproterone acetate
	Aromatase inhibitors—Arimidex, Anastrozole
	?Prolactin antagonists

LHRH, Luteinising hormone-releasing hormone.

Table 7.13 Endocrine drugs used in men with breast cancer

ER-negative disease independent of nodal status. Two standard adjuvant chemotherapeutic regimens used at the Royal Marsden Hospital are:

i   5-Fluorouracil (5-FU) 600 mg m^{-2} i.v.

with epirubicin 60 mg m^{-2} i.v.

with cyclophosphamide 600 mg m^{-2} i.v.

every 21 days.

ii   Adriamycin 60 mg m^{-2} i.v.

with cyclophosphamide 600 mg m^{-2} i.v.

every 21 days.

- Preoperatively as neoadjuvant therapy for a locally advanced (T4) inflamatory carcinoma.[1,2,23]

- *Metastatic disease*

There are at least 27 different combinations of cytotoxic chemotherapeutic agents reported in the literature, but the outcomes are purely anecdotal and do not form part of any prospective, randomised or double-blind trials. The disease-free and survival comparisons are impossible to compare meaningfully. Some of the agents used are show in **Table 7.14**.[53]

Ketoconazole acts as an oral, imidazole antifungal agent and produces prolonged inhibition of adrenal and testicular androgens. It has been used anecdotally in patients with stage 4 metastatic skeletal disease, producing partial responses.[54]

Radiation therapy

The indications for external beam radiotherapy are:

- Adjuvant postoperative therapy to the chest wall, the internal mammary chain and the supraclavicular fossa for those whose axillary node positive margins are close/incomplete, or in those with locally advanced disease

Single agents
Melphalan
5-Fluorouracil (5-FU)
Cyclophosphamide
Thiotepa
Methotrexate
Chlorambucil
Vinblastine
Mitomycin-C
Ketoconazole

Double agents
Bleomycin and vincristine
Actinomycin and chlorabucil
Cyclophosphamide and 5-FU
Doxrubicin and vincristine
Cyclophosphamide and prednisolone
Lomustine and doxrubicin
Methotrexate and thiotepa
5-FU and prednisolone

Triple agents
CMF = Cyclophosphamide, methotrexate and 5-FU
FAC = 5-FU, doxrubicin and cyclophosphamide
Lomustine, vincristine and doxrubicin

Four agents or more
FAC and BCG (Bacille Calmette–Guerin vaccine)
FAC, BCG and levamisole
CMF and doxrubicin
CMF and vincristine (CMFV)
CMF and medroxyprogesterone
CMFV and medroxyprogesterone
5-FU, cyclophosphamide, methotrexate, testosterone and decadron

Table 7.14 Chemotherapy agents used in men with breast cancer[7]

- In a preoperative neoadjuvant setting in patients with a locally advanced tumour
- Metastatic disease, for example, CNS metastatic space-occupying lesions and metastatic spinal cord compression
- Advanced disease of the chest wall for palliation when patients are unsuitable or unfit for surgery
- Management of the axilla as primary therapy/post-sentinel node biopsy.

These indications are not validated in any prospective randomised trial.

The use of postoperative radiotherapy varies from 3–80% of patients in different centres (**Table 7.15**).

Radiotherapy techniques have now improved, and the skin, pulmonary and cardiac complications are minimised by using preoperative computer-aided field planning and skin burn management techniques.[55] The largest advantage in the

First author (reference)	Years	No of men receiving radiotherapy (%)
Ribeiro[39]	1971–83	53 of 76 (70)
Guinee[43]	1965–86	245 of 308 (80)
Donegan[1]	1953–95	44 of 137 (32)
Carmalt[15]	1958–96	8 of 30 (27)
Borgen[28]	1975–90	3 of 104 (3)

Table 7.15 Incidence of different centres use of radiotherapy in men with breast cancer

use of radiotherapy is the reduction in locoregional recurrence.[55] One option is to use radiotherapy for chest wall and supraclavicular regions in patients with high-grade primary tumours with nodal involvement after modified radical mastectomy and level 2 nodal clearance. The presence of extranodal extension in the axillary specimen may be a more controversial indication for ipsilateral axillary and supraclavicular radiotherapy despite the increased rate of lymph-oedema that can occur.

The downstaging of locally advanced chest wall disease with preoperative adjuvant therapy is yet to be defined. Radiotherapy of the ipsilateral internal mammary chain is recommended in addition to the usual radiotherapy fields.[2]

The role of postoperative axillary radiotherapy after a negative sentinel-node biopsy without axillary dissection is not understood. This is unlikely to be clarified as the 60% node positivity in men with breast cancer negates the reasons and advantages for men having sentinel-node biopsy. Radiotherapy in patients with metastatic disease to the CNS, especially if they have raised and symptomatic intracranial pressure, has a proven benefit. Radiotherapy is also of benefit in the treatment of metastatic extradural and intradural disease, especially if there is imminent spinal cord compression.

Postoperative chest wall radiotherapy does not affect survival,[1] but many of these studies are more than 15 years old.

Psychological effects

There has been no investigation of the psychological impact of the diagnosis of breast cancer on men and their families. Rates of anxiety and depression have been characterised in symptomatic and screened women.[47] Such a study needs to be done in men. The psychological implications of genetic testing and *BRCA2* positivity in these families remains largely unexplored.

References

1. Donegan WL, Redlich PN. Breast cancer in men: special problems in breast cancer therapy. Clin North Am 1996; 76: 343–63.

2. Ravandi-Kashani F, Hayes TG. Male breast cancer: a review of the literature. Eur J Surg 1998; 34: 1341–7.

3. Bezwoda WR, Hesdorffer C, Dansey R *et al.* Breast cancer in men. Clinical features, hormone receptor status and response to therapy. Cancer 1987; 60: 1337–40.

4. Rahman N, Stratton MR. The genetics of breast cancer susceptibility. Ann Rev Genetics 1998; 32: 95–121.

5. Winchester DJ. Male breast carcinoma. A multiinstitutional challenge. Cancer 1998; 83: 399–400.

6. Sasco AJ, Lowenfels AB, Pasker-De Jong P. Epidemiology of male breast cancer (Review). A meta-analysis of published case control studies and discussion of selected aetiological factors. Int J Cancer 1993; 53: 538–49.

7. Bhagwandeen SB. Carcinoma in the male breast in Zambia. East Africa Med J 1972; 49: 89–93.

8. Vecchia CL, Levi F, Lucchini F. Descriptive epidemiology of male breast cancer in Europe. Int J Cancer 1992; 51: 62–6.

9. Ewertz M, Holmberg L, Karjalainen S *et al.* Incidence of male breast cancer in Scandinavia 1943–1982. Int J Cancer 1989; 43: 27–31.

10. Willsher PC, Leach IH, Ellis IO *et al.* A comparision of male breast cancer with female breast cancer. Am J Surg 1997; 173: 185–8.

11. Foulkes WD. BRCA1 and BRCA2: penetrating the clinical arena. Lancet 1998; 352: 1325–6.

12. Wooster R, Neuhasen SL, Mangion J *et al.* Localisation of a breast cancer susceptibility gene to chromosome 13q 12–13. Science 1994; 265: 2088–90.

13. Gogosh H, Sacks NPM. Hereditary breast cancer – a review. Cancer J 1998; 3: 35–48.

14. Thoralacius S, Struewing JP, Hartge P *et al.* Population based risk of breast cancer in carriers of BRCA2 mutation. Lancet 1998; 352: 1337–39.

15. Carmalt HL, Mann LJ, Kennedy CW *et al.* Carcinoma of the male breast: a review and recommendations for management. Aust NZ J Surg 1998; 68: 712–5.

16. Haroldsson K, Loman N, Zhang Q–X *et al.* BRCA2 germ line mutations are frequent in male breast cancer patients without a family history of the disease. Cancer Res 1998; 58: 1367–71.

17. Neugut AI, Murray TI, Lee WC *et al.* The association of breast cancer and colorectal cancer in men. Cancer 1991; 68: 2069–73.

18. Axelsson J, Anderson A. Cancer of the male breast. World J Surg 1983; 7: 281–7.

19. Sanchez AG, Villanueva AG, Redondo C. Lobular carcinoma of the breast in a patient with Klinefelter's syndrome. A case with bilateral, synchronous, histologically different breast tumours. Cancer 1986; 57: 1181–3.

20. Vetto J, Jur S–Y, Padduch D *et al.* Stages at presentation, prognostic factors and outcome of breast cancer in males. Ann J Surg 1999; 177: 379–83.

21. Cassagrande JT, Hanisch R, Pike MC *et al.* A case control study of the male breast cancer. Cancer Res 1988; 48: 1326–30.

22. Kessler LRS II. Selected aspects of breast cancer aetiology and epidemiology. Proc Am Assoc Cancer Res 1980; 21: 72.

23. Crichlow RW, Galt SW. Male breast cancer: strategies for the 1990s II. Clin North Am 1990; 70: 1165–77.

24. Green L, Wysowski DK, Fourcroy JL. Gynaecomastia and breast cancer during finasteride therapy. New Engl J Med 1996; 335; 823.

25. Wilson SE, Hutchinson WB. Breast masses in males with carcinoma of the prostate. J Surg Oncol 1976; 8: 105–112.

26. Joshi MG, Lee AKC, Loda M *et al.* Male breast carcinoma: an evaluation of prognostic factors contributing to a poorer outcome. Cancer 1996; 77: 490–8.

27. Borgen PI, Wong GY, Vlamis V *et al.* Current management of male breast cancer: A review of 104 cases. Ann Surg 1992; 215: 451–9.

28. Borgen PI, Senie RT, McKinnon WM *et al.* Carcinoma of the male breast. Analysis of prognosis compared with matched female patients. Ann Surg Oncol 1997; 4: 385–8.

29. Bhagat P, Kline TS. The male breast and malignant neoplasms. Diagnosis by aspiration biopsy cytology. Cancer 1990; 65: 2338–41.

30. So G, Chantra PK, Wollman JS *et al.* Chapter 28. In: The male breast diagnosis and diseases of the breast. Bassett, Jackson, Jahan, Philadelphia: WB Saunders, 1997.

31. Hittmair AP, Liniger RA, Tavassoli FA. Ductal carcinoma in situ (DCIS) in the male breast. A morphological study of 84 cases of pure DCIS and 30 cases of DCIS associated with invasive carcinoma—a preliminary report. Cancer 1998; 83: 2139–49.

32. Memon MA, Donohue JH. Male breast cancer. Br J Surg 1997; 84: 443–5.

33. Serour F, Birkenfeld S, Amsterdam E *et al.* Paget's disease of the male breast. Cancer 1998; 62: 601–5.

34. Cangiarelli J, Fraser Symanns W, Cohen JM *et al.* Malignant melanoma metastatic to the breast. A report of 7 cases diagnosed by fine needle aspiration cytology. Cancer (Cancer Cytopathology) 1998; 84: 160–3.

35. Wittliff JL. Specific receptors of the steroid hormones in breast cancer. Semin Oncol 1974; 1: 109–18.

36. Rayson D, Erlichman C, Suman VJ *et al.* Molecular markers in male breast cancer. Cancer 1998; 83: 1847–955.

37. Everson RB, Li Fp, Fraumeni JF *et al.* Familial breast cancer. Lancet 1976; 1: 9.

38. Gattuso P, Reddy VB, Green L *et al.* Prognostic significance of DNA ploidy in male breast carcinoma. A retrospective analysis of 32 cases. Cancer 1992; 70: 777–80.

39. Ribeiro GG. Male breast carcinoma—a review of 301 cases from the Christie Hospital and Holt Radium Institute, Manchester. Br J Cancer 1985; 51: 115–9.

40. Ribeiro G, Swindel R. Adjuvant tamoxifen for male breast cancer (MBC). Br J Cancer 1992; 65: 252–4.

41. Jonasson JG, Agnarsson BA, Thoralacius S *et al.* Male breast cancer in Iceland. Int J Cancer 1996; 65: 446–9.

42. Papadoupoulos T, Hayes PR, Danil J *et al.* Male breast cancer. Aust NZ J Surg 1997; suppl 1: A6.

43. Guinee VF, Olsson H, Moller T *et al.* The prognosis of breast cancer in males. A report of 335 cases. Cancer 1992; 71: 154–61.

44. Cote RJ, Peterson HF, Chaliwun B *et al.* Role of immunohistochemical detection of lymph node metastases in management of breast cancer. Lancet 1999; 354: 896–900.

45. Gupta RK, Naren S, Simpson J. The role of FNAC in the diagnosis of breast masses in males. Eur J Surg Oncol 1988; 14: 317–20.

46. Jaiyesimi IA, Buzdar AU, Sahin AA *et al.* Carcinoma of the male breast. Ann Intern Med 1992; 117: 771–7.

47. Dixon M, Sainsbury R. Male breast cancer. In: Handbook of diseases of the breast, 2nd edn. Edinburgh: Churchill Livingstone, 162–3.

48. Moredo Anelli TF, Anelli A, Tran K *et al.* Tamoxifen administration is associated with a high rate of treatment limiting symptoms in male breast cancer patients. Cancer 1994; 74: 74–7.

49. Kent Osborne C. Tamoxifen in the treatment of breast cancer. New Engl J Med 1998; 339: 1609–18.

50. Vorobiof DA, Falkson G. Nasally administered Buserelin inducing complete remission of lung metastases in male breast cancer. Cancer 1987; 59: 688–9.

51. Doberauer C, Niederle N, Schmidt CG. Advanced male breast cancer treatment with the LH-RH analogue Buserelin alone or in combination with antiandrogen Flutamide. Cancer 1988; 62: 474–8.

52. Lopez M. Cyproterone acetate in the treatment of metastatic cancer of the male breast. Cancer 1985; 55: 2334–6.

53. Patel H, Buzdar AU, Hortobagyi GN. Role of adjuvant chemotherapy in male breast cancer. Cancer 1989; 64: 1583–5.

54. Feldman LD. Ketoconazole for male metastatic breast cancer. Ann Int Med 1986; 104: 123.

55. Huddart RA, Yarnold JR. The principles of radiotherapy. In: Kirk M, Mansfield A, Cochrane J (eds). Clinical surgery in general RCS course manual, 2nd edn. Edinburgh: Churchill Livingstone, 1996: 239–49.

56. Adami HO, Holmberg L, Malker B *et al.* Long term survival in 406 males with breast cancer. Br J Cancer 1995; 52: 99–103.

57. Gough DB, Donohue JH, Evans MM *et al.* A 50 year experience of male breast cancer: is outcome changing? Surg Oncol 1993; 2: 325–33.

58. Wick MR, Sayadi H, Ritter JH *et al.* Low stage carcinoma of the male breast. A histological, immunohistochemical and flow cytometric comparision with localised female breast carcinoma. Am J Clin Pathol 1999; 111: 59–69.

8 Breast abscess and breast inflammation

Peter Malycha

Inflammatory breast disease

Breast abscess and breast inflammation come under the heading of benign breast disease and are rarely addressed at scientific meetings, where malignancy and new technologies dominate the agendas. They are nonetheless common and a source of significant morbidity. The type, degree and extent of inflammatory breast diseases differ in various communities but have the greatest impact in the developing countries.

- *Lactational mastitis* is common but rarely progresses to require referral to a surgeon.
- *Lactational breast abscess* is a serious health problem, particularly in the developing world. Standards of living and availability of health services may explain the variation with regard to its incidence. Early intervention and drainage under ultrasound guidance may avoid parenchymal breast damage. Most women can continue to breast feed after treatment.
- *Tuberculosis* remains a cause of breast infection in endemic areas but is rarely seen in developed countries. Its differentiation from malignancy remains a diagnostic problem.
- *Non-lactational pyogenic abscesses* of the breast are similar to those found in other soft tissues. They should be treated according to the causative agent. The abscesses associated with periductal mastitis are different and are addressed separately.
- *Duct ectasia* is common and mostly asymptomatic but can cause persisting nipple discharge. Its aetiology is unknown and is a separate entity from peridutcal mastitis.
- *Periductal mastitis* is less common than duct ectasia and has been charac- terised in descriptions mainly from Europe and North America. It is more

common in heavy cigarette smokers. Resulting abscesses and fistulae are difficult to treat and tend to recur.

● *Hidradenitis suppurativa of the axilla* is included here, as the axillary apocrine glands have a common embryological origin with the breast and patients may be referred to a breast surgeon. This is also more common in cigarette smokers.

Anatomy and physiology

Each of the 15 to 20 lobes of the breast has a final draining duct, which enters the base of the nipple to form a lactiferous duct and sinus. Near the nipple surface the sinus terminates at the ampulla, which is lined with stratified squamous epithelium. In the resting adult breast, desquamation of the stratified squamous epithelium plugs the opening, but with lactation this plug is cleared by the milk flow.[1] The ampulla is the common portal for bacteria, which produce mastitis and breast abscesses.

The areola contains apocrine glands as well as Montgomery's tubercles (named after the 19th century Irish obstetrician who described them). Montgomery's tubercles are modified sebaceous and lactiferous glands that lubricate and protect the areola and nipple.

The infective events involving the breast that are described in this chapter arise mostly from these components of the areola and nipple.[2]

Lactational mastitis

The majority of patients with mastitis treated by nurses and general practitioners are breast feeding women. Although the definition of lactational mastitis is vague it means minor infection of the lactating breast that usually settles spontaneously or after local decompression and antibiotic therapy. One reviewer described mastitis as redness and soreness of the lactating breast associated with influenza-like symptoms and a temperature up to 38°C.[3] The incidence of mastitis in Britain in the mid-20th century was 9%.[4] In the USA for the 20 years to 1991 an epidemiological but retrospective study found a 3% incidence of mastitis in the first seven weeks postpartum. This figure remained constant during a period when breast feeding became much more popular.[5] A recent prospective but patient-centred questionnaire estimated the incidence to be 20% using the criteria of redness, soreness, influenza-like symptoms and a temperature above 38°C.[3] Whatever the definition, it is generally accepted that mastitis occurs more commonly when mothers start or stop breast feeding. Even though there is a perception that lactational mastitis is more common in the less experienced prima gravida, parity does not influence the incidence.[5] In one study, 9% of mastitis was bilateral, 14% recurrent and 92% of patients continued to breast feed. When mastitis does not settle, patients are usually referred to surgeons for management. Inflammatory carcinoma is always a part of the differential diagnosis and can produce concern for the general practitioner when the inflamed breast has not responded to conservative treatment.[7]

Breast feeding

It is important, when considering this topic, to consider aspects of breast feeding, as they impact heavily on the management of complications arising from it.

Breast feeding has become an important social and political issue, provided by strong advocacy groups that have grown from local and national bodies to international organisations. The internet has become an important resource for advocacy groups to disseminate information. Surgeons who wish to know what their patients are reading on the internet can access it with key words like 'nursing mothers' association' or 'breast feeding.' Recommendations from these groups are presented in lay terms and not referenced. Overall they offer sensible advice. They advise a high standard of personal as well as breast and nipple hygiene for the pregnant and lactating woman. They recommend that women with cracked nipples gently wash and dry the nipples without scrubbing and that they always avoid locally damaging cleansing agents. It is acknowledged that cracked nipples are a potential source of sepsis, but breast feeding should continue if it does not cause excessive pain. If the mother is unable to continue then resting of the breast and nipple by using hand expression of the engorged breast is recommended. The sources state that engorgement or duct blockage usually responds to massage, gentle expression and cold or warm compresses. It is acknowledged that breast abscesses may develop quickly, and referral to a doctor is advised if conservative measures fail after 12 hours.[8]

The internet may be a bonus for surgeons rather than a hindrance as breast feeding women can access relatively standard information, which is designed to be helpful and not controversial.

Aetiology

Lactational mastitis is usually caused by *Staphylococcus aureus*, which enters via the nipple to colonise the duct, initially in a single segment of the breast. *Staphylococcus epidermidis* and streptococci are found occasionally. Nonetheless, haematogenous spread to the breast by *S. aureus* from a different infective focus should always be considered.

The clinical picture of mastitis varies according to the extent and duration of the inflammation. Signs of local tenderness, knottiness and redness are early signs. When symptoms of early sepsis develop, antibiotics are normally pre-scribed. Antibiotics were prescribed by family doctors in 77% of women, and 68% continued to breast feed. Only one patient was admitted to hospital.[3]

Women with sore and cracked nipples who were feeding an infant of less than 1 month were shown to have a 15% chance of growing *S. aureus* on culture. If the women were not treated with oral antibiotics they had a 12 to 35% chance of developing an abscess. This situation is a potential source for widespread impetigo vulgaris.[9,10]

Some have advocated 'stripping' the breast to evacuate the infected lobe. Mothers were asked to feed their infants from the affected breast and then to lubricate the skin of the breast with a gel to facilitate the stripping action between finger and thumb. Stripping proceeded from the breast and along the full length of the nipple. Pus differs from milk in that it is mucoid, gelatinous, curd-like and does not flow. When pus was obtained it indicated adenitis and when there was no pus, cellulitis. Staphylococci were isolated approximately twice as often in the adenitis group. Each episode of stripping took about 15 minutes. This activity was to be continued until the milk was clear.[6]

Lactational breast abscess

The change from mastitis to an abscess can be subtle and depends on the defini-tion of the former. The early phases of an abscess will be associated with minimal tissue destruction but, with time, this damage becomes greater as the infection extends into the breast parenchyma. Hughes *et al.* advise surgeons to intervene before extensive parenchymal tissue damage occurs.[2]

Stasis of the colostrum or lactose-rich milk within the warm breast offers a medium for bacterial growth. An abscess may form over hours or days, with the classic features of swelling, redness, local pain and a reduced ability or an in-ability to feed from the affected breast. Fever with rigors often occurs within hours of local symptoms becoming apparent. *S. aureus* can come from maternal autoinfection or from the skin and mouth of the baby. Historically, 'pemphigus neonatorum' was a common source of epidemic puerperal mastitis and breast abscesses in nurseries.[11]

Abscesses may arise in any lobe of the breast, with the presenting features varying according to site. When the abscess is subcutaneous, oedema of the skin and cellulitis will be visible signs. When deeper within the breast, cutaneous manifestation may occur later, although the relatively rapid progress of a staphy-lococcal abscess can be expected to produce skin redness and oedema within 12 to 24 hours. A neglected abscess, superficial or deep, will cause extensive parenchymal loss and normally 'point' to the skin as a fluctuant mass, with eventual skin ulceration and perforation. Occasionally, deep abscesses can penetrate into the pectoral muscles and to the chest cavity.[2]

Early or deep abscesses may be difficult to detect clinically. An awareness of the possibility of a lactational breast abscess from the presenting clinical signs and symptoms should encourage the clinician to perform ultrasonography to demonstrate the lesion.[12]

Once a lactational abscess is established, symptoms of septicaemia with high fever and rigors may occur. The neutrophil white count will be raised and blood cultures may be positive, usually showing *S. aureus*.

Treatment

Expression of pus from the nipple or aspiration of pus from the abscess should be performed for immediate culture of organisms. Antibiotic sensitivity must be requested (**Fig. 8.1**).

O'Hara *et al*. reported 19 successful aspirations of abscesses in 22 patients. Eighteen of 53 patients with clinically suspected abscesses had no abscess on ultrasonography, and these all settled with antibiotics. It may be better to describe this condition as mastitis.[13]

Repeated needle aspiration together with appropriate antibiotic use should be continued until the abscess resolves. Ultrasonography should be used not only to diagnose an abscess but to assess resolution. Drainage by insertion of a percutaneous catheter is similar to the method for draining deep visceral abscesses, and it has the advantage of allowing continuous drainage and irrigation, if that proves necessary.[14]

When formal drainage is required, incision is usually made over the abscess to evacuate the pus and debris of involved parenchyma. Inframammary fold drainage may have a more pleasing aesthetic result—as judged by the patient.[15]

Postoperative care

If suckling can continue it is the best way to achieve decompression of the breast, and it is reasonable for this to resume as soon as comfort allows. The affected breast should be decompressed by manual or mechanical means if suckling cannot continue. In 1976 an editorial in the *British Medical Journal* encouraged the continuation of breast feeding as infants experience no ill effects from feeding from the affected breast.[16] Others found a positive correlation between the incidence of diarrhoea, colic, rash and thrush in the infant when its mother was taking antibiotics.[6]

The concern of both doctor and patient may be hard to allay as unsupported evidence relating to the risk of neonatal staphylococcal pneumonia or lung

Figure 8.1
Ultrasound.
(a) Needle in
abscess cavity.
(b) Post-aspiration
film.

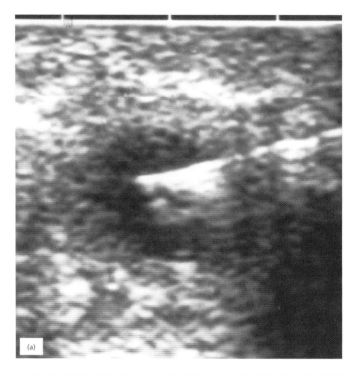

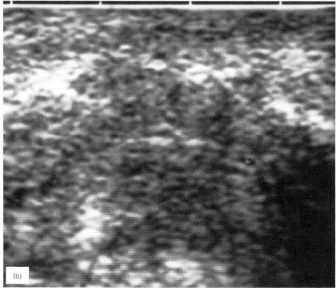

abscesses with breast feeding is still abroad. The concern regarding litigation will make surgeons cautious about advising patients to resume feeding while the breast remains acutely inflamed. A large lactational breast abscess that requires open drainage and packing will have to be left to granulate and heal. As a breast abscess involves a similar pathological process to any other soft tissue abscess it should not require postoperative antibiotics. The rationale for continued usage is that the breast remains engorged with milk and remains an ideal site for colonisation. If breast feeding cannot continue or the patient wishes to stop, suppression of lactation may be necessary. Cabergoline is considered to be the most effective suppressant available. It is effective as a single dose. Bromocriptine requires a 2-week course and is secreted in the breast milk. It is contraindicated if the mother wishes to resume feeding. The breast should be decompressed as required for comfort. Binding of the breasts to the chest wall and fluid restriction are unnecessary.[17]

Antibiotics

Nearly all lactational abscesses are caused by *S. aureus*. From 165 cultures Efem was able to grow *S. aureus* in 85%, coliforms in 5%, and no organisms in 10%.[18]

After pus has been obtained for culture and antibiotic sensitivities, flucloxacillin or dicloxacillin should be started. The manufacturer's literature should be checked before prescribing antibiotics for a breast feeding mother. Experience suggests that the infant experiences few ill effects, even though manufacturers recommend an alternate method of feeding to avoid possible sensitisation of newborn infants. Flucloxacillin and dicloxacillin have a narrow range of antibacterial activity against coagulase-negative and coagulase-positive *S. aureus*, as well as β-haemolytic streptococci. These are the expected organisms in a lactating abscess.

Clinicians must be aware that methacillin resistant *S. aureus* has been reported.

Patients who are sensitive or allergic to penicillin can be prescribed a cephalosporin. The cephalosporins are active against the bacteria commonly found in lactational breast abscesses but are less specific than flucloxacillin. They are secreted in the milk but are unlikely to have an adverse effect on the infant.

Erythromycin is effective also but the gastrointestinal side effects make it less popular than other antibacterials.

Tetracyclines, aminoglycosides and other antibiotics that are secreted into breast milk are harmful to the child and should be avoided.

Transmission of infection to infant

Clinicians should be aware that transmission of certain infections has been reported from breast milk to infants.

Mother to child transmission of HIV-1 is a leading challenge for public health policy in developing countries. Various risk factors for vertical transmission, including breast feeding, have been identified.[19] In a study from Malawi, Miotti *et al.* found that the risk of HIV infection is highest in the early months of breast feeding, and that this should be taken into account when formulating a breast feeding policy in developing countries.[20] Typhoid abscesses can be seen in developing countries and *Salmonella* is secreted in milk and may be transmitted to infants.[2]

Transmission of herpes simplex virus type 1 (HSV-1) has been reported. Although rare, such infections are associated with significant infant mortality.[21]

Non-lactational abscesses

Non-lactational breast abscesses, other than those associated with periductal mastitis, are treated in the same way as any other abscess arising in soft tissue. Periductal mastitis and abscesses that occur near to the areola are considered to have a different aetiology and are described below.

Abscesses that arise separately from the nipple tend to occur in older women. They are caused by various organisms. Of 29 abscesses, Tan and Low cultured staphylococci from 4, corynebacterium from five and no bacteria from four. These peripheral abscesses, which have no underlying cause, should be treated according to symptoms. On most occasions ultrasound-guided needle aspiration with appropriate antibiotics should be sufficient.[22] Patients who are immunocompromised will be more prone to sepsis in the breast, as elsewhere. Diabetes, HIV infections, general debility, chemotherapy and steroid therapy predispose patients to such sepsis.

Other infections of breast

Tuberculosis

Tuberculosis (TB) of the breast parenchyma is reported regularly from developing countries, where pulmonary and systemic tuberculosis remain a serious problem. In developed countries it is much less common. Over the past 15 years only 28 patients have been reported with TB of the breast in Japan.[31]

Case reports published by breast units in developed countries highlight the dilemma with diagnosis of TB of the breast and its differentiation from cancer. In India, where TB is endemic, the differential diagnosis is also a problem. Studies of 100 patients with TB of the breast found that mammography, fine needle aspiration cytology (FNAC) and excision biopsy achieved a diagnosis in 14%, 12% and 60% of cases, respectively. A lump in the breast, with or without ulceration, was the most common presentation, whereas sinus formation and diffuse nodularity presented less often. Axillary lymphadenopathy was present in one third of patients.[33]

The incidence of TB in different countries varies from 0.025% of breast lesions in Germany to 0.52% of 1152 consecutive mammograms in Saudi Arabia and as high as 3% in India.[32,34,35]

The possibility of TB should always be considered in endemic regions when women present with thickening of the skin and the underlying breast parenchyma, with or without a lump.

Nodular TB, which presents as a painless mass with skin involvement, is much more difficult to differentiate from cancer. On occasion it is associated with sinus formation and sclerosis, producing skin and tissue tethering. Disseminated breast TB is multifocal, with a coalescing abscess involving the whole breast and overlying skin.[33]

Mammography often identifies a change in breast shape and an underlying breast mass. There is usually a sinus track leading to the skin. The mammographic mass has asymmetrical margins and axillary lymph nodes are often involved.[34] Ultrasonography may identify the mass and show a thin, smooth border with heterogeneous indeterminate echoes.[36] FNAC may provide sufficient material for diagnosis of cutaneous lesions, but its inability to identify a specific cytological feature for TB has been a problem. Identification of mycobacterium from a smear is possible.[37]

If mammography and cytology do not provide a diagnosis an open biopsy for conventional histopathology or for identification of acid-fast bacilli will be necessary.

More sophisticated investigations with computed tomography (CT),[38] magnetic resonance imaging (MRI), nuclear scanning and polymerase chain reaction (PCR)[32] have been reported. Most cases of TB occur in developing countries where these technologies may not be readily available and the final diagnosis may depend on the identification of acid-fast bacilli from breast aspirates or biopsy specimens.

Treatment is by appropriate medications and, where breast deformity is produced by sclerosis, mastectomy and, where feasible, reconstruction.[2]

Breast feeding may continue as most antitubercular drugs seem to have no ill effect on infants. The current first-line drugs such as isoniazid, rifampicin, ethambutol and streptomycin seem to be safe, with milk secretion rates between 0.05% and 28%.[39]

Traumatic abscesses

Local infection is associated with trauma and foreign bodies. Penetrating injuries should be treated on merit with careful debridement and removal of foreign bodies. Cosmesis is important, and attention should be paid to surgical technique.

Seat belt trauma is common, mostly causing bruising but on occasion fat necrosis and inflammation of the underlying breast. This is not due to infection or sepsis.

Infection around prostheses

A prosthesis is a foreign body and has an infection rate of around 1%, which is about the same as surgery in general.[2] Prevention of infection is important. Attention to surgical technique and sterility is mandatory. Peroperative broad-spectrum antibiotics are advocated. Tetracycline lavage of the wound and prosthesis has been advocated by some, but this is probably unnecessary and may lead to drug sensitivity.

When postoperative infection occurs after insertion of a prosthesis it may be possible to leave the prosthesis *in situ* and to treat the patient with antibiotics. Advice from an infectious diseases specialist is recommended. When infection is established and non-responsive to treatment the prosthesis should be removed and the wound allowed to settle.

Staphylococcal infections tend to recur when prostheses are replaced. The patient should be counseled accordingly.

Infection after breast reduction

The reduction of large breasts involves removal of a large amount of fat with resultant fat necrosis and seroma formation. Opportunistic infections can occur in the seroma or at the healing edge of the wound. Peroperative and postoperative prophylactic antibiotics are recommended. Patients must stop smoking before breast reduction.[23]

Postirradiation breast abscesses

Breast conservation for early breast cancer is usually followed by breast irradiation. A 6% infection rate has been reported, and some as delayed infection, with a mean time from surgery of 5 months.[24] This differs from the experience of most surgeons but is a problem that should be kept in mind when advising patients.[24]

Chemotherapy/radiotherapy breast inflammation

The intense non-infective inflammatory response seen particularly when radiotherapy and chemotherapy are used together can be avoided in most patients by separating these treatment modalities. The inflammatory response is particularly marked when radiotherapy is used in conjunction with anthracyclines. Other chemotherapeutic agents may also be contributory.[25]

Granulomatous mastitis

Kessler and Wolloch described granulomatous mastitis in 1972 and appreciated that it was not associated with any infective process or tuberculosis.[26] Recently the emphasis has been on diagnosis. Cytology has proved difficult because it is nearly impossible to separate a non-specific granulomatous lesion from tuberculosis (**Fig. 8.2**). Some say that the term granulomatous mastitis should be avoided in cytology reports and substituted by non-committed terms such as a granulomatous lesion of the breast.[27]

Mammographic and ultrasonographic appearances of granulomatous mastitis were assessed in nine women. Granulomatous mastitis can mimic breast carcinoma clinically and mammographically. The sonographic appearances of multiple, often contiguous tubular hypoechoic lesions that are sometimes associated with a large hypoechoic mass should suggest the possibility of granulomatous mastitis.[28]

The consensus with regard to aetiology is that granulomatous mastitis is an autoimmune disease. However in a condition as rare as this it is not possible to be dogmatic regarding management. Specific granulomatous mastitis cannot always be distinguished from peripheral periductal mastitis. Local excision of the mass in continuity with a central duct excision under appropriate antibiotic control has been the basic treatment. Subsequent prolonged high-dose steroid medication may be required and if recurrence occurs further surgery. In the past periductal mastitis was misdiagnosed as tuberculosis and now it is being misdiagnosed as idiopathic granulomatous mastitis.[29]

Dermatitis artifacta

Surgeons should be aware of this condition when wounds do not heal and no reason can be found.

Psychiatric consultation should be sought if the diagnosis is considered likely or confirmed. Further surgery should be deferred until professional help has been obtained. Most factitial disorders are self-limiting and have a good prognosis.

Neonatal breast abscesses

Breast abscesses can occur in neonates. Care should be taken to avoid damaging the breast bud as it affects breast development. The abscess can usually be treated

Figure 8.2
Granulomatous mastitis (low power and high power). Breast lobule replaced and partly destroyed by non-caseating granulomatous inflammation with giant cells. Courtesy of Dr John King, King & Mower Pathology, Adelaide, Australia.

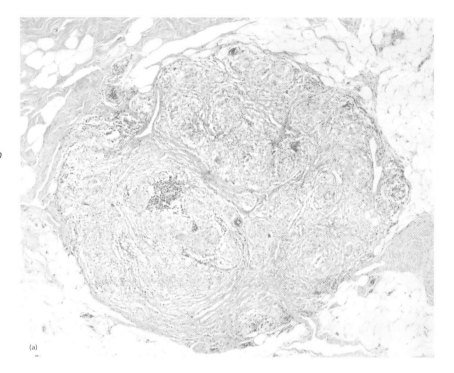

(a)

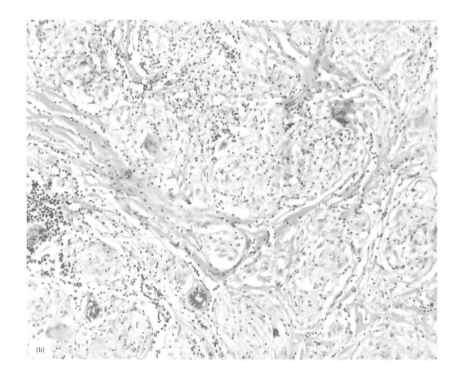

(b)

Breast abscesses can occur in neonates. Care should be taken to avoid damaging the breast bud as it affects breast development. The abscess can usually be treated by aspiration and antibiotics. Staphylococcus can be identified in 85% of cases.

In the rare case when incisional drainage is required the incision should be made at the areola edge to avoid the breast bud.[30]

Other infections of breast

Occasional reports of rare breast infections by unusual organisms continue to appear. Breast involvement by leprosy has been reported as part of the general manifestation of the disease, and mycobacterial infections have been reported in association with breast augmentation.[2]

Hydatid disease

Hydatid disease is of historical and contemporary interest. Ouedraogo reported 20 patients with breast hydatid in Tunisia between 1969 and 1982,[40] and case reports continue to be published, some indicating the difficulty in differentiating the disease from carcinoma.[41]

Hydatid may involve the breast alone or be part of systemic infection. Calcification in the cyst wall is usually seen. Ultrasonography and aspiration have identified hydatid on occasion, but this would seem to be unnecessary for diagnosis. Local excision is curative if the disease is localised to the breast.

Schistosomiasis, cysticercosis and guinea worm

Schistosomiasis, cysticercosis and guinea worm can all affect the breast. Schistosomiasis can be difficult to differentiate from cancer.

Brucellosis

Brucellosis is common in dairy herds, from whence extensive scientific literature arises, but it is rare in humans. It responds to a combination of trimethoprim/sulphamethoxazole and doxycycline.[42] It can be an important zoonosis in some countries—e.g. it is an endemic infection in Turkey. The clinical features can lead to difficulties in diagnosis. The disease may occur in pregnancy and may produce bilateral breast abscesses.[43]

Actinomycosis

Actinomycosis of the breast can occur as part of a general or systemic actinomycotic infection. Infection generally presents as a lump and the differential diagnosis is from carcinoma. Treatment involves drainage of the lesion and appropriate antibiotic therapy.[44]

Filarial infections

Filarial infections are reported from endemic areas, mostly in Asia. The adult worm may appear at the nipple or produce a granulomatous mass.

Mycotic infections

Clinical experience suggests that the incidence of mycotic infections affecting breast is very low. A number of fungi have been associated with breast disease and they *usually* present as a mass. Blastomycosis has been the most commonly reported mycotic infection. Other rare mycotic infections of the breast include pityrosporum, cryptococcus, aspergillosis and histoplasmosis.[2]

Candida infections

Anecdotal evidence suggests that breast feeding mothers may develop candida infections of the nipple from an oral infection of the suckling child, and this may be the cause of nipple pain. However, this has not been supported by careful examination of the milk of breast feeding mothers.[37] As anticipated, the aetiology of candida infections is related to factors such as long-term antibiotic use by the mother or child, nipple trauma and maternal vaginal thrush. Candida is found more commonly in children whose mothers have symptomatic candida infections.[37]

The treatment of candida of the nipple involves ridding the baby of oral thrush and using topical antifungal applications to the nipple.

Duct ectasia and periductal mastitis

It has taken more than 70 years to reach a point where duct ectasia and periductal mastitis are considered separate entities (**Table 8.1**).

The sequence of research into these benign conditions has been reported by Hughes, Mansell and Webster in their book '*Benign Disorders and Diseases of the Breast*', and they have played a very significant part in increasing the understanding of these conditions.[2]

In the past 25 years the duct ectasia story has been reappraised. Hughes *et al.* introduced the concept of ANDI (aberrations of normal development and involution) and claimed that most benign breast disease arose from minor

Duct ectasia	Periductal mastitis
Author	Term used
Bloodgood	Varicocoele tumour
Cheatle	Plasma cell mastitis
Luska	Lactiferous duct fistula
Haagensen	Duct ectasia
Hughes & Mansel	The ANDI concept
Dixon & Bundred	Separation of duct ectasia from periductal mastitis
Dixon & Bundred	Smoking and periductal mastitis

Table 8.1 Salient events in the development of current concepts of duct ectasia

aberrations of normal processes of development, cyclical activity and involution. ANDI replaced the concept of normal disease, with a spectrum of conditions ranging from normal to disease. In this concept duct involution with dilation and sclerosis is normal. Duct ectasia with nipple retraction is an aberration whereas periductal mastitis with abscess and fistula is a disease.[2]

Subsequently Dixon and Bundred developed the concept that duct ectasia and periductal mastitis are separate entities. Duct ectasia is now considered to be an involutionary and age-related condition in the breast not often associated with significant clinical problems. On the other hand, periductal mastitis is considered to be a pathological, inflammatory disease found more commonly in younger women who smoke leading to abscess formation and fistula.

In 1996 Dixon *et al.* carried out a prospective survey of 14 225 patients in a study designed to determine the relationship between duct ectasia and periductal mastitis. Of the 139 patients with the clinical diagnosis of perductal mastitis, 70% had a history of previous periductal mastitis. By comparison only 1% of patients with the clinical diagnosis of duct ectasia had had periductal mastitis. These findings were highly significant.[45]

Cigarette smoking and periductal mastitis

In 1992 Bundred *et al.* reported a retrospective 11-year review of 85 patients with non-lactational abscesses and found that women who smoked cigarettes were more likely to experience recurrent abscesses and fistulae than women who did not smoke.[46]

Smoking was therefore important in the natural history of non-lactational breast abscesses and may predispose a woman to anaerobic infections and the development of mammary fistulae. Smoking was associated with increased squamous metaplasia within the lactiferous duct and seemed to have a direct and toxic effect on the mammary ducts.[47]

The most recent and supportive evidence to implicate smoking was the prospective study by Dixon *et al.* of over 14 000 Edinburgh women. They found a highly significant relationship between smoking and inflammatory conditions of the nipple and areolar complex but not duct ectasia.[45]

In the year 2000 there now seems to be enough evidence to finally separate the entities. Duct ectasia is a relatively innocuous, age-related and involutionary dilation of the ducts of the breast. The more problematic periductal mastitis is associated with abscess formation and fistulae and is strongly associated with cigarette smoking in younger women.

In 1986 Browning *et al.* reviewed 1256 patients undergoing routine breast surgery. They found mammary duct ectasia in 4.2% of women with symptoms and 8.1% of women without symptoms.[48] This and other work led to the conclusion that duct ectasia occurs increasingly with age, and may be found in one half of women at 60 years. Even though common it causes few problems and has been reported to be present in 4 to 5% of women with symptoms.

Incidence

Dixon *et al.* reported the incidence of duct ectasia and periductal mastitis to be 1–2% of symptomatic breast patients. At that stage they considered the two conditions to be part of a common syndrome.[49]

When reporting on the activities of an Australian multidisciplinary breast clinic for symptomatic women Bochner *et al.* found that only 5.9% of 686 patients presenting over a 9-month period had nipple problems. None of these women had major periductal sepsis, abscesses or fistulae.[50]

In New Zealand a higher incidence of mammary fistula was noted in Melanesian women from the Pacific Islands. These reports suggest that the incidence of this relatively morbid problem varies from centre to centre. In the Northern latitude of the UK it seems to be prevalent and constitutes 1 to 2% of symptomatic breast disease. Earlier reports from Haagensen suggest it is much less common in the USA. Bochner *et al.* found none in a busy Australian clinic for symptomatic women.[50]

The aetiology of duct ectasia and periductal mastitis seems to be firmly linked with cigarette smoking, and if Collins is correct it occurs more often in more socially deprived populations.[53] Other environmental or socioeconomic factors have not yet been identified.

Those surgeons who treat many women with breast problems but see very little symptomatic inflammatory disease will observe expectantly.

Bacteriology

Duct ectasia

Asymptomatic duct ectasia seen at operation is considered by many surgeons to be sterile, but this may not be the case. Bundred *et al.* isolated bacteria from

62% of such patients, which they separated from those who presented with abscesses and those with fistulae. Both anaerobic and aerobic bacteria were isolated and the organisms included *S. aureus*, bacteroides, enterococci and anaerobic streptococci.[51] Similarly, Dixon *et al.* reported isolation of pathogens from 62% of patients with ectasia.[52]

It is believed to be these bacteria in the dilated duct that cause the inflammation which is, in duct ectasia, limited to the duct wall.

Periductal mastitis and associated abscesses and fistulae

Non-lactational breast abscesses have been found to contain many differing bacteria.

Walker *et al.* performed a prospective study of 29 patients with non-lactational breast abscesses. They aspirated material and cultured it anaerobically and aerobically for up to 14 days.[53] Of the 108 bacterial strains recovered, 32 were anaerobes and five aerobes. The overall anaerobic recovery was twice that for aerobes. Coagulase-negative staphylococcus constituted 60% of the aerobes, with peptostreptococci making 47% of anaerobes. The commonest organism grown from these abscesses was *S. epidermidis* (60%) with *S. aureus* only 8%. Many of the organisms cultured were commensals of mouth and vagina rather than gut.[52]

Other reports of opportunistic infections isolated *Peptostreptococcus magnus*, which produces enzymes that encourage the burrowing activities seen in periareolar abscesses. The possibility of anaerobic migration to the breast by these organisms commonly found in the female genital tract are a potential source of sepsis. This would explain the association between the bacteria associated with subareolar abscesses and those found in the mouth and vagina.[2]

Clinical presentation

Duct ectasia

In duct ectasia, the ducts tend to be most dilated and affected near the nipple. The duct diameter, which should be between 0.5 and 1 mm, can be five times wider than normal.

In clinical practice middle-aged or older patients may present with a spontaneous nipple discharge from one or more ducts, with occult or macroscopic blood staining in 50% of patients.

At operation the viscous thick white to green coloured fluid is often seen when the ducts near the nipple are transected. The ducts can be confused with breast cysts. The fluid within ectatic ducts is thicker and often like toothpaste, whereas cysts usually contain thin watery fluid varying from clear amber to brown, green or even black. When first seen by a surgical trainee their immediate response is to conclude that they have entered an abscess cavity.

Patients often express fluid from the nipple to see if the discharge is still present and attend a surgeon after a period of waiting. They are best advised to stop this activity as spontaneous discharge of embarrassing quantity is uncommon.

On histological section the inflammatory process is seen in association with duct wall scarring and thickening (Fig. 8.4). The material in ectatic ducts is amorphous and represents cellular debris and fatty acid crystals. It may be packed with inflammatory and colostrum cells, which are probably macrophages or myoepithelial cells.[2]

Cytology from a nipple smear will not be particularly helpful but may differentiate between ectatic fluid and an intraduct papilloma.[52] With more long-standing symptoms the nipple can be pulled inwards and often shows a transverse crease (Fig. 8.4). The skin of the breast adjacent to the areola can be dimpled or tethered. Very few women require treatment for duct ectasia.

Periductal mastitis

Patients with early periductal mastitis present with redness or swelling near the areolar complex that has developed over a week or two. It often settles spontaneously or with prescribed antibiotics, but whether antibiotics are required in the early stages is unclear. The patient often attributes the redness to a local injury such as an insect bite. If the inflammation does not settle a chronic mass with induration may develop, and from this presumed septic focus the complications of abscess and/or fistula may occur.

Figure 8.3
Excision of fistulous tract in mammary fistula.

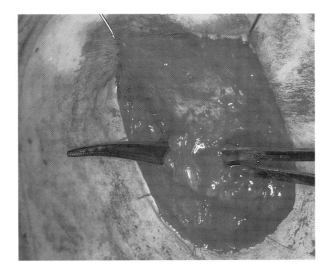

Figure 8.4
Duct ectasia (high power and low power). Dilated duct surrouded by fibrosis and inflammatory cell infiltrate, filled with foam cells and debris. Courtesy of Dr John King, King & Mower Pathology, Adelaide, Australia.

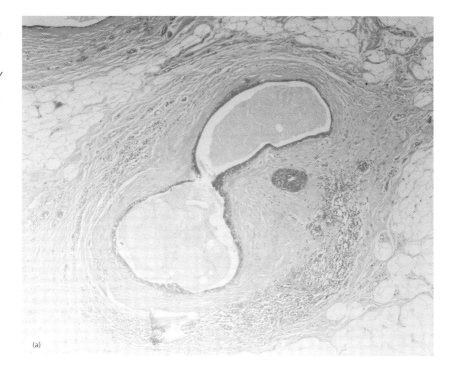

(a)

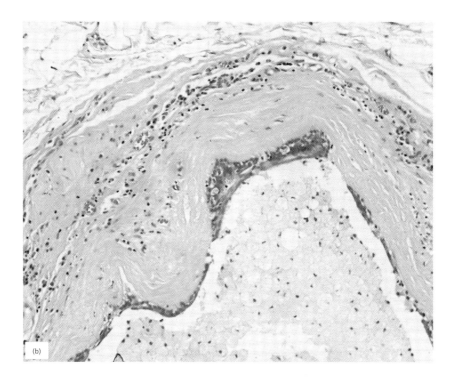

(b)

Abscess formation

A non-lactational periductal abscess presents as a raised reddened lesion adjacent to the areola but not usually extending into it. The underlying abscess may be small and undetectable clinically but visible ultrasonographically.

Mammary duct fistula

Fistula formation is an extension of the periductal mastitis complex and presumed to be a later stage and associated with retractional scarring of the nipple.[54] The fistula opening is usually found at the areola edge. When healed it will be locally indurated, but when open it will be granulating and discharging pus.

Investigations

Duct ectasia

Mammography to assess the subareolar and periductal component of the breast is difficult to visualise. When there is nipple retraction, tethering or skin thickening it is even more difficult. Occasionally dilated ducts may be seen on plain mammography. Extensive microcalcification within ducts that is mammographically diagnostic of duct ectasia is found quite commonly. The microcalcification will often be reported by the radiologist as benign plasma cell mastitis. Duct ectasia and plasma cell mastitis are often included under the same heading in radiological teaching. The condition results from extravasation of intraductal secretions, causing a periductal sterile chemical inflammation. Periductal fibrosis and intraductal and/or periductal calcifications are the final results. The calcifications may be located in or around the dilated duct or in the duct wall.

Periductal calcification is revealed as a calcified ring outside a dilated duct where the lumen is well seen. When it extends along the duct it can appear oval or elongated.

Intraductal calcifications are seen as filling segments with uniform, linear, often needle-like or branching calcifications.

Differentiation of the benign intraductal calcifications associated with 'plasma cell mastitis' (duct ectasia) can be easily separated from the malignant type, casting calcifications of intraductal carcinoma. The calcifications of plasma cell mastitis (duct ectasia) have a high and uniform density and a generally wider calibre and tend to follow the course of the normal ducts to the nipple.[55]

When the calcifications are multiple, bilateral and oriented toward the nipple it is likely to be due to duct ectasia or possibly periductal mastitis.

Galactography or ductography may be useful for patients with a single-duct discharge to exclude a papilloma but is inappropriate for multiple bilateral duct discharge (**Fig. 8.5**).

Figure 8.5
Ductogram: duct ectasia with dilated periareolar ducts. Courtesy of Dr S Langlois, Royal Adelaide Hospital, Adelaide, Australia.

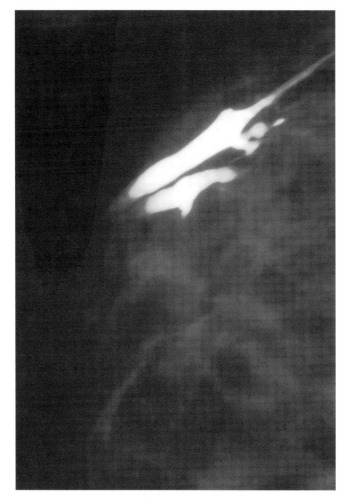

Ultrasonography will identify dilated ducts leading to the nipple. It can also identify microcalcification within dilated ducts that are presumed to be part of a longstanding duct ectasia (**Fig. 8.6**).

Periductal mastitis

When the patient presents with a mass, carcinoma must be excluded. FNAC should be performed. Mammography may be of little value in a younger woman but ultrasonography can readily identify an abscess requiring drainage. Aerobic and anaerobic bacteria should be cultured from the fluid or pus aspirated. An open biopsy may be needed to exclude cancer.

Figure 8.6
Ultrasound of dilated periareolar duct (duct ectasia). Courtesy of Dr S Langlois, Royal Adelaide Hospital, Adelaide, Australia

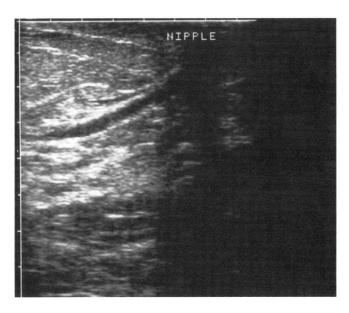

Management

Duct ectasia

Surgery for treatment is rarely needed and observation with clinical review is required. In younger patients, serum prolactin concentration should be measured to exclude a pituitary adenoma. Unilateral disease cannot be attributed easily to a pituitary cause.

Surgery may be needed if the nipple discharge persists and particularly if it is bloodstained and concerns the patient. The ectatic disease can be excised as the ducts reach the nipple or more formally by excision of the rertro/areola duct complex. Antibiotic cover against possible contaminants is probably worthwhile.

Periductal mastitis

When patients present with a mass, carcinoma must be excluded. A palpable or ultrasonographically detected abscess can be drained by needle aspiration and treated with appropriate antibiotics. When pus or tissue fluid is aspirated it should be cultured and antibiotic sensitivities obtained. A smear of this fluid should be sent for cytological assessment, particularly if no pus is obtained.

Management will be determined by the extent of the septic process and will require antibiotic therapy. Appropriate antibiotics alone may be sufficient for localised inflammation without abscess formation. Broad-spectrum antibiotics to cover both anaerobes and aerobes will be necessary. Augmentin, with its relatively broad spectrum against Gram-negative and Gram-positive organisms as well as anerobes can be used or, alternatively, a cephalosporin with metronidazole for penicillin-sensitive patients. Clindamycin is an alternative antibiotic, but should be used as a second-line medication and only after organisms have been identified.

Large or recurrent abscesses may be better treated by formal incision and drainage, but the majority can be handled more conservatively with repeated aspiration and antibiotics.

Fistulae

Good results can be obtained from less radical dissection with fistulotomy and primary closure or fistulectomy and allowing the wound to granulate. More advanced or chronic disease probably benefits from fistulotomy.[60]

The fistulous track may be identified by ultrasonography, and the extent of surgery may be less when the tract can be followed more easily from its opening at the skin to the duct of origin. This may not be a direct line as the fistula can arise in the lactiferous sinus and track indirectly to the area of discharge. As in any fistula, adequate excision of the track is necessary. The incision can be kept to the areola edge without compromising the nipple itself.

When fistulae become chronic or complicated by recurrent abscess, excisional surgery will be necessary, particularly if the fistulae are recurrent. The best method comes from the eponymous Hadfield's operation even though it was originally reported by Urban in 1963.[57,58]

The conventional Hadfield operation involves the disconnection and full removal of the subareolar ducts from the nipple with removal of a core of breast tissue from the nipple down to the fascia over pectoralis major. Although this procedure has a good reputation for curing the nipple discharge, 28% will require further surgery, mostly as a result of sepsis. Careful cosmetic closure, preferably with monofilament non–absorbable subcuticular suture, can produce a good result.

The centres with most experience indicate that they have more success than the occasional operator, which, in itself, is not surprising. The recurrence rate varied from 2 to 16%.[59,60]

When a circumareolar incision is made to gain access to the subareolar plate and to disconnect the lactiferous sinuses from the nipple some desensitisation of the nipple may occur. A depression beneath the nipple can be difficult to prevent particularly when the tissues inferior to the nipple are already tethered or hollowed.

In patients who have a scar and retraction of the nipple, release of the scar tissue can improve cosmesis but it will not allow spontaneous eversion of the nipple. A formal cosmetic repair will be necessary but should not be done in the presence of infection.

Patients should stop smoking before an operation is offered and when performed the operation should be under appropriate antibiotic cover.

Bilateral Disease

The real incidence of bilateral disease is not clear. It is associated with cigarette smoking and may occur in up to 20% of patients.

Rare periductal inflammation

Neonatal periductal inflammation, with or without ectasia, is seen on occasions.[61]

Duct ectasia and periductal mastitis does occur in males and is also associated with smoking.[62]

Axillary hidradenitis suppurativa

Hidradenitis suppurativa is a recurrent suppurative disease manifested by abscess, fistulae and scarring. It predominantly affects young women, with a prevalence of between 0.3% and 4% of the population in developed countries.[66]

It was considered to be a disease of the apocrine glands but is now known to be a complex inflammatory event involving the terminal epithelium of which the apocrine glands are a minority. Nonetheless it occurs in the apocrine gland-bearing areas, the axilla, areola, groins and anogenital regions (**Fig. 8.7**).

Breast surgeons may see patients with axillary hidradenitis suppurativa because of the close anatomical and embryological association between the axilla and breast. Some have found that infected apocrine glands made up a minority of primary and secondary disease in the infected skin element.[63] It has been suggested that follicular occlusion by keratinous material with subsequent active folliculitis leads to destruction of the skin and subcutis.[64] Secondary axillary lymphadenopathy may be evident clinically or seen on mammography or ultrasonography.

Cigarette smoking may be an aetiological factor in hidradenitis and is not a vascular or neoplastic consequence. Ceasing smoking should be part of management.[65]

Incidence

Jemec *et al.* found an incidence of hidradenitis suppurativa of 4% in healthy, unselected Danish members of the public.[66]

Axillary hidradenitis was less common than genitofemoral hidradenitis and gender difference was noted in those with axillary disease. Hidradenitis occurred

Figure 8.7
Hidradenitis suppurativa (low power and high power). Axillary skin with apocrine sweat glands showing suppurative inflammation and foreign body reactions in glands and deeper tissues. Courtesy of Dr John King, King & Mower Pathology, Adelaide, Australia.

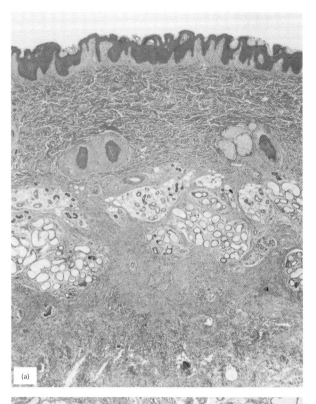

(a)

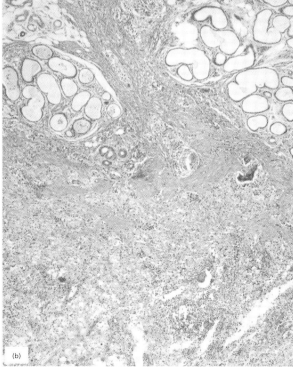

(b)

more commonly than expected and this low-grade disease had a significant impact on general health. The previously implied associations between hidradenitis and the menstrual cycle or oral contraceptive usage could not be confirmed.[67]

Bacteriology

Jemec *et al.* found *S. aureus* and *S. epidermidis* in only 8% and 11% of abscesses.[66] Others were more successful in identifying bacteria, with aerobic and facultative organisms isolated in 35% of abscesses, anaerobic bacteria in 41% and mixed in 24%. The organisms were as varied, as those in periareolar abscesses seen in periductal mastitis.[68]

The association of these two conditions is fostered by the knowledge that the apocrine glands are common to the axilla and the areola and that smoking seems to be contributory to both. Current research, however, does not support this theory.

Treatment

Hidradenitis suppurativa can be a minor problem, that will settle with time or with antibiotics. Broad-spectrum antibiotics, e.g. clindamycin, should be used to cover the variable pathogens.[62]

When the disease is more extensive, with chronic dermal thickening and abscess or sinus formation, it can be disabling. More extensive surgical removal will be necessary to widely but locally excise the apocrine or hair-bearing area of the axilla. The wound can be left to granulate or can be skin grafted. As the lesion is not associated with sebum excretion, retinoids are of no value.[69]

Rarely, sweat gland tumours or breast cancers can occur in or near the axillary skin, simulating hidradenitis suppurativa.

Hidradenitis suppurativa and hyperhidrosis are different conditions, and the former does not not respond to sympathectomy.

Hidradenitis suppurativa can occur in the inframammary groove.[2]

Skin lesions

Epidermoid cysts

Epidermoid cysts are quite commonly in the breast skin. They should be treated on merit. If they should become tender, increase in size, become infected or rupture, local excision of the cyst and surrounding capsule is recommended.

Inflammation of montgomery's glands

Montgomery's glands at the edge of the areola can become enlarged and discharge spontaneously. They rarely become infected, but when problematic simple excision is necessary.

Infection of the inframammary fold

Infection of the inframammary fold is associated with intertrigo. It is a problem, particularly in hot climates and for women with large breasts. Treatment is by local management of the inflamed or infected skin. Drying agents, water-resistant creams and antifungal preparations are useful. Breast reduction may be beneficial.

Basal and squamous cell carcinomas

Inflamed basal and squamous cell carcinomas of the exposed skin of the breast are sometimes seen. They should be excised and treated according to pathology.

Basal cell carcinoma of the nipple

Basal cell carcinoma of the nipple is a rare condition, which occurs in both men and women, usually in old age. It presents as an eczematous and reddened area around the nipple and areola that does not settle. It requires biopsy to exclude Paget's disease of the nipple.[70]

Eczema of the nipple

Eczema of the nipple occurs mainly in young women between 15 and 30 years and is usually bilateral. The cause is unknown, but sensitivities or allergies to clothing should be considered. *Candida albicans* can mimic eczema.[71]

The intermittent course of eczema with severe itching and lack of nipple destruction help distinguish this from Paget's disease. If non-responsive to treatment, biopsy should be performed. Eczema of the nipple in a woman of 40 years or more should be considered to be Paget's disease until proved otherwise.

Hyperkeratosis of the nipple

The skin of the nipple can become thickened, pigmented and covered with coalescing warty growths. It is a rare condition that may be seen in patients who are immunocompromised. It is particularly associated with T-cell lymphoma and in men with carcinoma of the prostate that are being treated with oestrogen.[72]

Nipple rings

These ornaments have become more common in males and females and, as with any foreign body, infection and inflammation can result. There are reports of duct ectasia secondary to trauma from nipple rings with tassels in exotic dancers.[72]

Hidradenitis of the breast

Hidradenitis suppurativa is mostly restricted to the axilla, but has been reported in the inframammary fold. Patients with this condition often have several lesions along the lower border of the breast. As this disease is thought to arise in apocrine glands, it is difficult to be sure that this is the same disease as seen in the axilla. Conservative treatment is best, but excision may be required.[2]

Pilonidal infections

Pilonidal infections have been reported in the periareolar area of the breast in women engaged in sheep shearing (roust-abouts' breast). It has also been reported in dog beauticians and hairdressers. For such women there is now a protective brassiere 'the baa bra!'[73–75]

They occur around the areola where hidradenitis suppurativa is occasionally seen. The presence of hair in the abscess is diagnostic of pilonidal infection.

Mondor's disease

Mondor's disease is an obliterative phlebitis. It can occur in the skin of the breast and axilla. It occurs mainly between 30 and 60 years and affects women three times more commonly than men. The patient may notice a red linear cord running from the breast to the abdominal or axillary skin. Banding of this type is seen commonly in the axilla after surgery. The band can be red and tender but can be expected to settle slowly over weeks. It can restrict shoulder movement.

Seborrhoeic warts

These are commonly seen on or beneath the breast in middle aged and elderly women and often associated with intertrigo.

Rare conditions of the skin

The breast skin is not selected specifically by rare systemic conditions such as calciphylaxis from untreated hyperparathyroidism, pyoderma gangrenosum with inflammatory bowel disease or a variety of auto-immune diseases. Treatment will be directed at the underlying problem.

References

1. Haagensen CD (ed). Diseases of the breast, 3. Philadelphia: WB Saunders, 1986.

2. Hughes LE, Mansell RE, Webster DJT (eds). Benign disorders and diseases of the breast, 2. London: Harcourt, 2000.

3. Kinlay JR, O'Connell D, Kinlay S. Incidence of mastitis in breastfeeding woman during the six months after delivery: a prospective cohort study. Med J Aust 1998; 169: 310–2.

4. Fulton AA. Incidence of puerperal and lactational mastitis in an industrial town of some 43,000 inhabitants. BMJ 1945; 1: 693–6.

5. Kaufmann R, Foxman B. Mastitis among lactating women: occurrence and risk factors. Soc Sci Med 1991; 33: 701–5.

6. Bertrand H, Rosenblood LK. Stripping out pus in lactational mastitis: a means of preventing breast abscess. CMAJ 1991; 145: 299–306.

7. Jaiyesimi IA, Buzdar AU, Hortobagyi G. Inflammatory breast cancer: a review. J Clin Oncol 1992; 10: 1014–24.

8. Olsen CG, Gordon RE Jr. Breast disorders in nursing mothers. Am Fam Physician 1990; 41: 1509–16.

9. Livingstone VH, Willis CE, Berkowitz J. Staphylococcus and sore nipples. Can Fam Physician 1996; 42: 654–9.

10. Livingstone V, Stringer LJ. The treatment of Staphylococcus aureus infected sore nipples: a randomised comparative study. J Hum Lact 1999; 15: 241–6.

11. Walter & Israel. General Pathology, 3edit., 1970.

12. Crowe DJ, Helvie MA, Wilson TE. Breast infection. Mammographic and sonographic findings in clinical correlation. Invest Radiol 1995; 30: 582–7.

13. O'Hara RJ, Dexter SPL, Fox JN. Conservative management of infective mastitis and breast abscesses after ultrasonographic assessment. Br J Surg 1996; 83: 1413–4.

14. Berna JD, Garcia Medina V, Madrigal M et al. Percutaneous drainage of breast abscesses. Eur J Radiol 1996; 21: 217–9.

15. Peters F, Flick-Fillies D. Drainage of puerperal breast abscesses while preserving aesthetic and functional aspects. Geburtsh U Frauenheilk 1991; 51: 901–4.

16. Puerperal mastitis (editorial). BMJ 1976; 1: 920–1.

17. European Multicentre Group for Caberegoline in Lactation Inhibition. Single dose cabergoline v bromocriptine in inhibition of puerperal lactation: randomised double blind multi centre study. BMJ 1991; 302: 1367–71.

18. Efem SEE. Breast abscesses in Nigeria. Lactational versus non lactational. J R Coll Surg Edinb 1995; 40: 25–7.

19. Van de Perre P. HIV and AIDS in Africa: impact on mother and child health. Eur J Med Res 1999; 4: 341–4.

20. Miotti PG, Taha TE, Kumwenda NI et al. HIV transmission through breast feeding: a study in Malawi. JAMA 1999; 282: 744–9.

21. Sullivan-Bolyai JZ, Fife KH, Jacobs JF et al. Disseminated neo natal herpes simplex virus type 1 from a maternal breast lesion. Paediatrics 1983; 71: 455–7.

22. Tan SM, Low SC. Non operative treatment of breast abscesses. Aust NZ J Surg 1998; 68: 423–4.

23. Jorgensen LN, Kallehave F, Christensen E et al. Less collagen production in smokers. Surgery 1998; 123: 450–5.

24. Keiden RG, Hoffman JP, Weese JL et al. Delayed breast abscess after lumpectomy and radiotherapy. Am Surg 1990; 56: 440–4.

25. Taylor ME, Perez CA, Halverson KG et al. Factors influencing cosmetic results after conservation therapy for breast cancer. Int J Radiat Oncol Biol Phys 1995; 31: 753–64.

26. Kessler E, Wolloch Y. Granulomatous mastitis: a lesion clinically simulating carcinoma. Am J Clin Pathol 1972; 58: 642–6.

27. Martinez-Parra D, Nevado-Santos M, Melendez-Guerrero B et al. Utility of fine-needle aspiration in the diagnosis of granulomatous lesions of the breast. Diagn Cytopathol 1997; 17: 108–14.

28. Han BK, Choe YH, Park JM et al. Granulomatous mastitis: mammographic and sonographic appearances. Am J Radiol 1999; 173: 317–20.

29. Hughes LE, Mansel RE, Webster DJT. Benign disorders and diseases of the breasts: concepts and clinical management, 2. WH Saunders 2000.

30. Efrat M, Mogilner JG, Iutjman M et al. Neo natal mastitis diagnosis and treatment. Isr J Med Sci 1995; 31: 558–60.

31. Ohgika K, Horry T. Tuberculosis of the breast. Nippon Rinsho 1998; 12: 3126–8.

32. Diallo R, Frevel T, Poremba C. Lupus vulgaris as the etiology of tuberculous mastitis. Pathologe 1997; 18: 67–70.

33. Shinde SR, Chandawarkar RY, Deshmukh SP. Tuberculosis of the breast masquerading as carcinoma: a study of 100 patients. World J Surg 1995; 19: 379–81.

34. Makanjuola D, Murshid K, al Sulaimani S, Al Saleh M. Mammographic features of breast tuberculosis: the skin bulge and sinus tract sign. Clin Radiol 1996; 51: 354–8.

35. Rangabashyam N, Gnanaprakasam N, Krishnanaraj B et al. Spectrum of benign breast lesions in Madras. J R Coll Edinb 1983; 28: 369–73.

36. Oh KK, Kim JH, Kook SH. Imaging of tuberculosis disease involving breast. Eur Radiol 1998; 8: 1475–80.

37. Thompson KS, Donzelli J, Jensen J et al. Breast and cutaneous mycobacteriosis: diagnosis by fine needle aspiration biopsy. Diagn Cytopathol 1997; 17: 45–9.

38. Chung SY, Yang I, Bae SH et al. Tuberculous abscess in retromammary region: CT findings. J Comput Assist Tomogr 1996; 20: 766–9.

39. Tran JH, Montakantikul P. The safety of antituberculosis medications during breastfeeding. J Hum Lact 1998; 14: 337–40.

40. Ouedraogo EG. Hydatic cyst of the breast. 20 cases. J Gynecol Obstet Biol Report (Paris) 1986; 15: 187–94.

41. Schechner C, Schechner Z, Boss J et al. Echinococcus cyst of the breast imitating carcinoma. Harefuah 1992; 122: 502–3, 551.

42. Al Abedely HM, Halim MA, Amin TM. Breast abscess caused by Brucella melitensis. J Infect 1996; 33: 219–20.

43. Cokca F, Azap A, Meco O. Bilateral mammary abscess due to Brucella melitensis. Scand J Infect Dis 1999; 31: 318–9.

44. Jain BK, Sehgal VN, Jagdish S et al. Primary actinomycosis of the breast: a clinical review and a case report. J Dermatol 1994; 21: 497–500.

45. Dixon JM, Ravisekar O, Chetty U et al. Periductal mastitis and ductal ectasia: different condition with different aetiologies. Br J Surg 1996; 83: 820–2.

46. Bundred NJ, Dover MS, Coley S et al. Breast abscesses and cigarette smoking. Br J Surg 1992; 79: 58–9.

47. Furlong AJ, Al-Nakib L, Knox WF et al. Periductal inflammation and cigarette smoke. J Am Coll Surg 1994; 179: 417–20.

48. Browning J, Bigrigg A, Taylor I. Symptomatic and incidental mammary duct ectasia. J R Soc Med 1986; 79: 715–6.

49. Dixon JM. Periductal mastitis/duct ectasia. World J Surg 1989; 13: 715–20.

50. Bochner M, Kollias J, Gill PG et al. Audit of new presentations to a multidisciplinary symptomatic breast assessment clinic. Submitted for publication.

51. Bundred NJ, Dixon JM, Lumsden AB et al. Are the lesions of mammary duct ectasia sterile? Br J Surg 1985; 72: 844–5.

52. Dixon JM, Anderson TJ, Lumsden AB et al. Mammary duct ectasia. Br J Surg 1983; 70: 601–3.

53. Walker AP, Edmiston CE Jr, Krepel CJ et al. A prospective study of the microflora of nonpeurperal breast abscess. Arch Surg 1988; 123: 908–11.

54. Bundred NJ, Dixon JM, Cherry U et al. Mamillary fistula. Br J Surg 1987; 74: 466–8.

55. Tabar L, Dean PB. Teaching atlas of mammography, 2. New York: Thieme, 1985.

56. Dixon JM, Thompson AM. Effective surgical excision for mammary duct fistula. Br J Surg 1991; 39: 1185–6.

57. Hadfield GJ. Further experience of the operation for excision in the major duct system of the breast. Br J Surg 1968; 55: 530–5.

58. Urban JA. Excision of the major duct system of the breast. Cancer 1963; 16: 516–20.

59. Lambert ME, Betts CD, Sellwood RA. Mamillary fistula. Br J Surg 1986; 73: 367–8.

60. Bundred NJ, Webster DJT, Mansell RE. Management of mamillary fistula. J R Coll Edinb 1991; 36: 381–3.

61. Stringell G. Infantile mammary duct ectasia—a cause of bloody nipple discharge. J Paediatr Surg 1986; 21: 671–6.

62. Brown TJ, Rosen T, Orengo IF. Hidradenitis suppurative. South Med J 1998; 12: 1107–14.

63. Jemec GB, Hansen U. Histology of hidradenitis suppurative. J Am Acad Dermatol 1996; 34: 994–9.

64. Attanoos RL, Appleton MA, Douglas-Jones AG et al. The pathogenesis of hidradenitis suppurativa: a closer look at apocrine and apoeccrine glands. Br J Dermatol 1995; 133: 254–8.

65. Konig A, Lehmann C, Rompel R et al. Cigarette smoking as a triggering factor of hidradenitis suppurative. Dermatology 1999; 198: 261–4.

66. Jemec GB, Heidenheim M, Nielsen NH. Prevalence of hidradenitis suppurative in Denmark. Ugeskr Lager 1998; 6: 847–9.

67. Barth JH, Layton AM, Cunliffe WJ. Endocrine factors in pre- and postmenopausal women with hidradenitis suppurativa. Br J Dermatol 1996; 134: 1057–9.

68. Brook I, Frazier EH. Aerobic and anaerobic microbiology of axillary hidradenitis suppurative. J Med Microbiol 1999; 48: 103–5.

69. Jemec GB, Gniadecka M. Sebum excretion in hidradenitis suppurative. Dermatology 1997; 194: 325–8.

70. Sauven P, Roberts A. Basal cell carcinoma of the nipple. J R Soc Med 1983; 76: 69.

71. Amir LH. Eczema of the nipple and breast—a case report. J Hum Lact 1993; 9: 173–9.

72. Rook, Wilkinson, Ebling. Text Book of Dermatology 6e. London: Blackwell Science, 1998.

73. Gardiner G. Roust-abouts breast. NZ Med J 1994; 107: 494.

74. Banerjee A. Pilonidal sinus of the nipple in a canine beautician. BMJ 1985; 291: 1787.

75. Bowers PW. Roustabouts' and barbers' breasts. Clin Exp Dermatol 1982; 7: 445–7.

9 Provision of care/guidelines and quality assurance

Christopher Wilson
Julie C. Doughty

The establishment of guidelines for patients with breast cancer have their origins in the development of the NHS Breast Cancer Screening Programme (NHSBSP). Prior to the publication in 1992 of *Quality Assurance Guidelines for Surgeons in Breast Cancer Screening*,[1] there were no published guidelines for the management of any surgical condition. These original screening guidelines led to the development of *Guidelines for Surgeons in Symptomatic Breast Disease*[2] which were consensus based. The updated versions of these guidelines are evolving to become more evidence based.

Evolution of guidelines for the management of breast disease

1. **1992** *Quality Assurance Guidelines for Surgeons in Breast Cancer Screening* (revised 1996)[1,6]
2. **1995** Guidelines for referral of patients with breast problems[19]
3. **1995** The training of a general surgeon with an interest in breast disease[10]
4. **1996** Guidelines for surgeons in the management of symptomatic breast disease in the UK (revised 1998)[2,7]
5. **1998** Scottish Intercollegiate Guidelines Network—Breast Cancer in Women[18]
6. **1999** BASO guidelines for the management of metastatic bone disease in breast cancer in the UK.[9]

Breast screening model

The national cervical screening programme, which was established several years prior to the introduction of the breast screening programme, had been plagued with criticism, particularly relating to quality. Those individuals involved in the evolution of the NHSBSP were determined to avoid some of the mistakes made during the implementation of cervical screening. Quality Assurance (QA) had to be a priority as the very notion of the NHSBSP had many critics who believed that the concept of breast screening was flawed and that the programme would fail due to lack of resources. The ability of the NHSBSP to produce modest improvements was based on only the highest quality of the process. Inefficient screening would clearly cause harm by increasing the benign:malignant ratio, resulting in unnecessary anxiety for women and a huge increase in surgical workload. The eventual decision to introduce the NHSBSP was political as each party had supported its introduction in the run up to the 1987 general election. Once the decision had been made, each discipline involved in the development of the NHSBSP was invited to compose specific QA guidelines.

In 1988, faced with understandable scepticism from the surgical community, the British Association of Surgical Oncology (BASO) under the presidency of Professor Harold Ellis sanctioned the setting up of a subgroup of interested breast surgeons to represent their views to the organisers of the NHSBSP. Under the leadership of Professor Roger Blamey the National Surgical Coordination Group for Breast Screening was formed within BASO, which has now developed into the BASO Breast Specialty Group.

This subgroup published the original surgical QA guidelines in 1992, *Quality Assurance Guidelines for Surgeons in Breast Cancer Screening*.[1] The two underlying concepts of the original guidelines were 'quality objectives' and 'outcome measures.' A quality objective is a standard set by surgeons for themselves and their peers, whereas an outcome measure is a defined target to be reached to ensure a surgeon's objective is met. For example, one quality objective is to maximise the number of women accepting the invitation to be screened. To assess whether this objective is being achieved, it is necessary to define an outcome measure. In this case, the outcome measure is defined as '>70% of those women invited to screening should attend' (**Table 9.1**).

Good quality and complete data must be produced by the nominated surgeon in each screening unit, and the agreed standard dataset must be completed each year.

The publication of nationally developed surgical screening QA guidelines represented a real breakthrough in surgical practice. For the first time surgeons had ammunition to extract necessary funding if the realistic and achievable standards could not be met owing to a lack of resources but also allowed units to determine the quality of the care provided. The establishment of national standards had the beneficial effect of pressurising Trusts to provide more surgeons, beds, operating lists and support services.

Category	Quality objective	Outcome measures and targets
General performance of a unit (the surgeon is a member of the whole screening team)	To maximise the number of women accepting the invitation to be screened	>70%
Biopsy	To improve the operative identification of changes producing mammographic abnormalities	>95% of impalpable lesions should be correctly identified at the first localisation biopsy operation
	To maximise the accurate positioning of marker wires in localisation biopsies	>80% of wires should be within 10 mm of the lesion in any plane
	To minimise the cosmetic disadvantage of operative biopsies carried out for diagnostic (not therapeutic) purposes	80% of biopsies that prove benign should weight <20 g (fresh or fixed weight); the surgeon should ensure that the weight is recorded
Treatment	To ensure completeness of excision, when operation for removal of the cancer by breast conservation has been undertaken (by wide local excision, quadrantectomy or segmentectomy)	Specimens must be oriented by the surgeon, and histological examination of the margins should be made. Surgeons should be aware of the report regarding the margin and if necessary re-excise to clear margins
	To minimise the number of repeat operations for therapeutic purposes	90% of operations carried out with a proven preoperative diagnosis of cancer (*in situ* and invasive) should not require a further operation for incomplete excision
	To ensure that all necessary data are obtained for making decisions on adjuvant radiotherapy or adjuvant systemic therapy	Histological node status should normally be obtained on all invasive tumours, either by sampling or clearance
	To ensure appropriate treatment of well differentiated histological node-negative cases	Prophylactic axillary radiotherapy is inappropriate

Table 9.1 Examples of quality assurance guidelines for surgeons involved in breast cancer screening

The guidelines, in conjunction with visits from the Regional Cancer Screening QA Committee, have promoted and strengthened multidisciplinary teamwork between surgeons, pathologists and radiologists, which has in turn led to an improvement in the diagnosis and treatment of both impalpable and palpable breast disease. The implementation of these guidelines also led to an area of surgical practice being open to independent and outside scrutiny, which was previously unheard of.

Development of guidelines for the management of symptomatic breast disease

When the NHSBSP was introduced, it soon became apparent that a double standard of care was being applied to patients with breast disease. Patients with screen-detected cancers were receiving a high standard of care from breast specialists, reinforced by QA guidelines and overseen and audited by a National Screening Coordinator, whereas women presenting with symptomatic breast disease were being offered an unregulated quality of care differing widely between centres.

There was no evidence base available to identify best practice in breast disease, but the lessons of breast screening together with several reports published at this time[3,4,5] demanded changes in the organisation of breast services. These reports identified deficiencies in the quality of care of women with symptomatic breast disease and highlighted the potential advantage of establishing Breast Cancer Units, staffed by multidisciplinary specialists along similar lines to that of breast screening.

In 1993, the BASO Breast Speciality Group embarked on a process of consultation with surgeons, who had an identifiable interest in breast disease, to compose guidelines for the management of women with symptomatic disease. In addition to adopting the organisation of services and QA that is an integral part of the NHSBSP, symptomatic guidelines had to address the problem of the huge number of women who are referred for a specialist opinion who constitute the 'worried well.' Because so many women with breast symptoms understandably imagine they have breast cancer, it was thought crucial that the diagnostic process paid as much attention to those women with benign disease as to those with cancer. Hence, the symptomatic guidelines were designed to emphasise how quality objectives can be measured in the diagnostic process with the establishment of the 'one-stop breast clinic.'

The first symptomatic guidelines, the *Guidelines for Surgeons in the Management of Symptomatic Breast Disease in the UK*[2] were published in 1995 by the National Coordination Group, after detailed consultation with a national workshop consisting of 170 'breast' surgeons, the Cancer Committee of the Royal College of Surgeons of England and the Specialities Board of the Association of Surgeons. Although the guidelines were written by a core of surgeons involved in the management of breast disease, a huge effort was made to consult and allow contributions from all breast surgeons as the success of any set of guidelines would inevitably depend on those using the guidelines having participated in their construction.

Some key outcome measures of the symptomatic guidelines related to the surgeon are listed below.

Preoperative standards

- More than 80% of patients who subsequently prove to have breast cancer should be seen within 2 weeks of receipt of the referral by the unit
- Less than 10% of all new breast patients should have to attend the clinic on more than two occasions for diagnostic purposes
- A breast cancer unit must have a specialist surgeon, radiologist and pathologist with easy access to oncology and radiotherapy services and a breast care nurse
- More than 90% of patients requiring breast cancer surgery should be operated on within 2 weeks of diagnosis
- The benign:malignant operation rate should be 1:10 (operations for nipple discharge, abscess or previously diagnosed fibroadenoma should be excluded)
- Ninety per cent of palpable breast cancers should be diagnosed preoperatively by cytology or core biopsy

Operative

- Ninety per cent of women undergoing conservation surgery should have no more than three operations
- Gross margins should be identified without cutting into the tumour, and all specimens should be oriented
- Patients with involved circumferential margins should not proceed to further adjuvant therapy without having a further surgical excision
- An adequate surgical margin may be defined as that which results in a local recurrence of less than 5% at 5 years
- Node status should be obtained in more than 90% of patients with invasive breast cancers, with a minimum of four nodes being obtained if a sample has been undertaken
- A local excision is not appropriate for extensive or multifocal ductal carcinoma in situ (DCIS)
- Patients with previously diagnosed DCIS should not undergo an axillary clearance

Follow-up

- All patients should be discussed at a formal multidisciplinary meeting to discuss adjuvant therapy
- All patients undergoing breast conservation should receive postoperative radiotherapy

- After breast conservation, mammography should be undertaken every 1–2 years
- Patients should be followed-up for at least 5 years.

Evolution of breast guidelines

Contribution of BASO

The BASO Breast Specialty Group pioneered the development of guidelines in the management of breast disease and have reviewed and updated the screening and symptomatic guidelines and will do so every 2 years.

- *Quality Assurance Guidelines for Surgeons in Breast Cancer Screening.* NHSBSP Publication No. 20. Revised April 1996[6]
- The British Association of Surgical Oncology Guidelines for Surgeons in the Management of Symptomatic Breast Disease in the UK (1998 revision). *European Journal of Surgical Oncology* 1998; 24: 464–76[7]

Whereas the original guidelines were mostly consensus based the revised guidelines are more evidence based, in line with the format used by the Clinical Outcomes Group in *Guidelines for Purchasers—Improving Outcome in Breast Cancer* Leeds: NHS Executive 1996.[8] The authors of the revised guidelines sought to justify scientifically what was written by providing levels of evidence and by assessing the quality of the evidence. This would range from mere professional consensus (low quality) to well structured double-blind controlled trials (high quality).

The process of identifying quality objectives within a set of guidelines has enabled the development of an audit programme. The BASO Breast Cancer Database has been formed, allowing the uniform collection of data that will eventually allow the production of national data for patients with symptomatic breast disease.

- The Guidelines for the Management of Metastatic Bone Disease from Breast Cancer in the United Kingdom[9]

These guidelines herald the development of a new generation of clinical guidelines designed to improve the quality of care for patients in particular clinical situations. The nature of these guidelines will lead to an extension of the multidisciplinary team involved in the care of patients with breast cancer, with medical professionals from a wide variety of disciplines being involved in their care. The BASO Breast Speciality Group has recently developed guidelines for the specific management of metastatic bone disease due to breast cancer.

The past decade has seen advances in the diagnostic and therapeutic evaluation of women with breast disease. However, failure to coordinate the diagnosis and management can result in delays in diagnosis, poor treatment and prolonged suffering for patients. The management of metastatic bone disease was targeted because bone is the commonest site of metastasis and outcomes after bony relapse can vary considerably, with 20% of patients alive at 5 years. During that time each patient will have undergone several interventions by a variety of medical professionals who may or may not have had specialist expertise in that area. Those involved in the management of metastatic bone disease realised the need to extend the multidisciplinary team to include orthopaedic surgeons, physiotherapists and palliative care physicians with a particular interest and training in the management of metastatic bone disease.

The guidelines emphasise that the accuracy and speed of diagnosis of metastatic bone disease is considerably improved if radiologists are empowered to initiate appropriate imaging so that the complete clinical picture can be presented to the multidisciplinary team. The eventual success of the guidelines were thought to depend on the presence of a dedicated orthopaedic surgeon with a specialist interest in metastatic bone disease to bring expertise in the technical aspects and skill in the diagnosis of mechanical problems. This will prevent inappropriate investigations and reduce patient suffering and anxiety.

● Guidelines for the Training of a General Surgeon with an Interest in Breast Disease[10]

The BASO Breast Specialty Group has also expanded the provision of guidelines to surgical training and has published recommendations laying down training requirements.

BASO are currently developing guidelines for the management of patients who are at increased risk of developing breast cancer owing to either a strong family history, the presence of a genetic mutation or a proliferative disorder acting as a marker for the future development of breast cancer.

Impact of evidence-based medicine

Evidence-based medicine is not new, and in 1990 the American Institute of Medicine stated that the attributes of good guidelines should be underpinned by the themes of credibility and accountability: '*the link between a set of guidelines and the scientific evidence must be explicit, and scientific and clinical evidence should take precedence over expert judgement.*'[11] Guidelines constructed by professional opinion or unsystematic literature reviews are subject to criticism and potential bias,[12,13] and therefore the most recent generation of guidelines[9,18] are based on systematic review of the evidence as defined as '*an efficient scientific technique to identify and summarise evidence on the effectiveness of interventions and to allow the generalisability and consistency of research findings to be assessed and data inconsistencies to be explored.*[14]

Earlier guidelines were developed to achieve changes in organisation and were consensus based, but currently they aim to achieve best practise and assure quality by evidence-based medicine as was recommended in the Guidelines for Purchasers—Improving Outcome in Breast Cancer.[8] However, the reliance on evidence was small and the majority of recommendations and statements were by professional consensus. There was no indication of where evidence-based recommendations were used and no attempt to indicate the quality of the evidence.

The two publications *Guidelines for the Management of Metastatic Bone Disease* from Breast Cancer in the United Kingdom and the Scottish Intercollegiate Guidelines Network (SIGN) *Breast Cancer in Women* have for the first time in the field of breast cancer addressed the need for evidence-based guidelines. The study design classification used by BASO and SIGN originates from the American Agency for Health Care Policy and Research (AHCPR).[15]

The criteria set out by the AHCPR guideline recommendations are graded to compartmentalise them into those based on strong evidence from those based on weak evidence. This grading is based on an objective analysis of study design and quality and a more subjective assessment of the clinical relevance and validity of the evidence.[16,17]

Classification of evidence levels

Ia   Evidence obtained from meta-analysis of randomised controlled trials

Ib   Evidence obtained from at least one randomised trial

IIa Evidence obtained from at least one well designed controlled study without randomisation

IIb Evidence obtained from at least one other type of well designed quasi-experimental study

III Evidence obtained from well designed non-experimental descriptive studies, such as comparative studies, correlation studies and case studies

IV   Evidence obtained from expert committee reports or opinions and/or clinical experiences of respected authorities.

Classification of grades of recommendations

A   Requires at least one randomised controlled trial as part of a body of literature of overall good quality and consistency addressing specific recommendation (evidence levels Ia, Ib)

B   Requires the availability of well conducted clinical studies but no randomised clinical trials on the topic of recommendation (evidence levels IIa, IIb, III)

C   Requires evidence obtained from expert committee reports or opinions and/or clinical experiences of respected authorities. Indicates an absence of directly applicable clinical studies of good quality (evidence level IV).

The grading does not relate to the importance of the recommendation but to the quality and strength of the supporting evidence.

Examples of evidence-based guidelines from SIGN and the BASO metastatic bone disease guidelines include:

- Radiotherapy after wide local excision
  Radiotherapy should normally be given to the breast after wide local excision
  Evidence level Ib, grade of recommendation A
- Radiotherapy after axillary clearance
  After axillary clearance the axilla should not normally be irradiated
  Evidence level III, grade of recommendation B
- Management of small well differentiated invasive carcinomas
  An axillary node sample is required to determine nodal status
  Evidence level IV, grade of recommendation C.

For endocrine therapy of bone metastases

- When considering second-line endocrine therapy, look for evidence of endocrine sensitivity of the disease
  Evidence level Ib, grade of recommendation A
- There is a wide range of oestrogen receptor (ER) status, and the absolute level of ER as well as other predictive factors should be obtained before deciding whether endocrine therapy is appropriate
  Evidence level IIA and III, grade of recommendation B
- On failure of second-line endocrine therapy consider third-line endocrine therapy (if tumour previously hormone sensitive) or chemotherapy
  Evidence level IV, grade of recommendation C.

Although the move toward a critical appraisal of evidence is welcomed within guidelines, further development is required. For example the guidelines on the *Management of Metastatic Bone Disease* is a 19-page document with a huge number of recommendations of which only 18 are obviously evidence based, and of these only seven recommendations are based on a level of evidence to merit grade A recommendation. Only 26 of the 100 SIGN guidelines are grade A (**Table 9.2**).

BASO guidelines		SIGN guidelines	
Grade of recommendation	No of recommendations	Grade of recommendation	No of recommendations
A	7/18	A	26/100
B	4/18	B	32/100
C	7/18	C	42/100

Table 9.2

These guidelines require regular updating and an increased number of recommendations based on randomised trials. This should encourage clinicians involved in breast cancer care to participate in clinical trials.

Place of guidelines in clinical practice

An emphasis on quality and accountability is becoming increasingly important for medical professionals. Instigated by problems over self-regulation that did not seem to be working effectively in some areas, the government has demanded to see more explicit standard setting and improvement in the quality of the service.

The General Medical Council, partly in response to public fears over standards of clinical practice and partly as its continuing drive to improve such standards, made firm commitments on behalf of the profession in two recent publications *Good Medical Practice* and *Maintaining Good Medical Practice*. These are the guiding principles that underpin all medical practice but more pointedly set out to drive the improvement in standards inherent in clinical governance.

The provision and implementation of guidelines in the management of breast cancer will play a key part in the local programmes of clinical governance.

Acknowledgement

We thank Mr Hugh Bishop for his help and advice with this chapter.

References

1. Quality Assurance Guidelines for Surgeons in Breast Cancer Screening. NHSBSP Publication No 20, 1992.

2. Guidelines for surgeons in the management of symptomatic breast disease in the United Kingdom. Eur J Surg Oncol 1996, 22 (suppl A).

3. Breast Cancer Minimum Standards of Care. Cancer Relief MacMillan Fund provision of breast services in the United Kingdom. The advantage of specialist breast units.

4. Provision of breast services in the United Kingdom. The advantage of specialist breast units. Reports of a working party of the British Breast Group. September, 1994.

5. A policy framework for commissioning cancer services. Prepared by an expert advisory group on cancer to the Chief Medical Officer of England and Wales, 1994.

6. Quality assurance guidelines for surgeons in breast cancer screening. NHSBSP Publication No 20 (Revised 1996).

7. Guidelines for surgeons in the management of symptomatic breast disease in the United Kingdom (1998 Revision). Eur J Surg Oncol 1998; 24: 464–76.

8. Guidance of purchasers: improving outcomes in breast cancer. The Manual and Research Evidence. NHS Executive (1996) Cat 539 1p7K.

9. BASO guidelines for the management of metastatic bone disease in breast cancer in the United Kingdom. Eur J Surg Oncol 1999; 25: 3–23.

10. The training of a general surgeon with an interest in breast disease. Eur J Surg Oncol 1995; 21 (suppl A).

11. Field MJ, Lohr KN (eds). Institute of Medicine Committee to advise the Public Health Service on Clinical Practise Guidelines. Clinical practise guidelines: directions for a new program. Washington DC: National Academy Press, 1990.

12. Antman EM, Lau J, Kupelnick B *et al.* A comparison of results of meta-analyses of randomised controlled trials and recommendations of clinical experts. Treatment for myocardial infarction. JAMA 1992; 268: 240–8.

13. Woolf SH. Practise guidelines, a new reality in medicine. II: methods of developing guidelines. Arch Intern Med 1992; 152: 946–52.

14. Mulrow CD. Rationale for systematic reviews. BMJ 1994; 309: 597–9.

15. US Department of Health and Human Services. Agency for Health Care Policy and Research. Acute pain management: operative or medical procedures and trauma. Rockville, MD: The Agency. Clinical Practice Guideline No 1. AHCPR Publication No 92-0023. p. 107.

16. Guyatt GH, Sackett DL, Sinclair JC *et al.* Users' guides to the medical literature. IX. A method for grading health care recommendations. Evidence-Based Medicine Working Group. JAMA 1995; 274: 1800–4.

17. Liddle J, Williamson M, Irwig L. Method for evaluating research and guideline evidence. Sydney: New South Wales Department of Health, 1996.

18. Breast cancer in women. A National Clinical Guideline. SIGN Publication No. 29.

19. Austoker J, Mansel RE, Baum M *et al.* Guidelines for referral of patients with breast problems. NHSBSP Publications 1995 1 SBN 187, 1997: 429.

10 Litigation in breast disease

T. Bates
R. Parkyn

Litigation in breast disease has accelerated at an alarming rate in many countries over the past few years, and in the USA legal action over delay in the diagnosis of breast cancer has reached such a proportion that the value of malpractice claims is second only to that for neurological damage to neonates.[1,2] Poor cosmetic outcome after cosmetic or reconstructive surgery is also a common cause for litigation, and the saga of Dow Corning and silicone breast implants has heightened public awareness and the expectation of recompense for real or perceived injury.[3]

The legal process does differ between countries and although the present account is based on civil law in England and Wales, the general principles used elsewhere are similar.

Doctors have been made increasingly aware of the need to warn patients of the risks involved with any procedure, be it diagnostic or therapeutic, and to seek informed consent having discussed the alternative options, which may include the likely outcome of taking no action. Patient information leaflets and more specific consent forms signed by the operating surgeon are now widely used but seem to have done little to stem the tide of litigation.

Basic principles

For a claimant (plaintiff) to succeed in law, he or she must satisfy the court (a judge, or, in some countries, a jury) that there was a failure or breach of duty of care (liability) and that as a foreseeable result the claimant incurred an injury (causation).

Liability

Duty of care

Any doctor—radiologist, surgeon or pathologist—owes each individual patient a duty of care. This is rarely an issue.

Breach of duty

If a patient is referred to a breast clinic and the standard of care falls below that which the patient could reasonably have expected from a breast specialist, there has been a breach of the duty of care.

The Bolam test

The Bolam test arises from the case of a patient who received electroconvulsive therapy and sustained fractures. Negligence was alleged because the patient was not given muscle relaxants and was inadequately restrained.[4] Some doctors would have used muscle relaxants or restraints, others not. The doctor was not found negligent because he acted in accordance with a practice accepted at the time (the publication date of guidelines must be taken into account) as proper by a responsible body of medical opinion even though other doctors adopt a different practice (the court may reject a body of opinion that is not formed on the basis of logic).[5] This case is cited in England; the 'Bolam test'.

The Bolam test requires a higher degree of skill from a specialist in his own specialty rather than from a general practitioner.

Consent

Great emphasis is now placed on warning patients of the risks of any proposed management, but the principle of informed consent remains largely untested in English law. The degree of disclosure 'must primarily be a matter of clinical judgement'.[6]

Causation

The second hurdle to be overcome by the claimant is to prove that the negligent act of the doctor, or more usually in the UK, the NHS Trust, which is vicariously liable for its employees (the defendant), actually caused an injury that was forseeable. Causation may be obvious where there is a poor cosmetic outcome from breast reduction, but it may be difficult to prove cause and effect where there has been a delay in the diagnosis of breast cancer. Such delay might, for example, occur due to failure to refer the patient from primary care, from false negative mammography results, from failure to do a triple assessment, from misinterpretation of fine needle aspiration cytology (FNAC) or from the misfiling of a positive test result.

Did the delay necessitate more severe treatment?

Where the patient has had a mastectomy it is often plausible to suggest, on the balance of probabilities, that an earlier diagnosis would have made conservative surgery with conservation of the breast a real option. When the patient received chemotherapy it is sometimes argued that this would not have been necessary if the diagnosis had been made sooner when, for example, the axillary lymph nodes would probably have been negative. This line of argument is, however, open to counterattack on the basis that failure to give chemotherapy would have omitted the only treatment likely to have made a real difference in prognosis.

Does delay in diagnosis reduce lifespan?

This is a controversial area because there is public expectation, which over the years has been promoted by doctors, that earlier diagnosis offers a better chance of a cure and a longer lifespan. Where expert opinion is divided, the court often prefers the evidence in favour of delay having caused a reduced survival time.

Does delay in diagnosis reduce the chance of a cure?

Loss of a chance of cure is not a concept endorsed by the English courts,[7] but it is a cause for action in the USA. Cure is a difficult concept in breast cancer and this is discussed further below.

The burden (level) of proof

In civil litigation the court determines the facts which means that the judge makes a decision on the balance of probabilities—more likely than not (51 v 49%). This level of proof is of course very different from criminal cases where proof is required beyond reasonable doubt.

Delay in the diagnosis of breast cancer

Phases of delay

Phase 1: patient delay

When a woman first becomes aware of a breast cancer she may delay seeking advice for fear of the diagnosis or the treatment, she may be over-optimistic about the likely diagnosis or may deny the probability that she has cancer. The causes of patient delay are not relevant to the present discussion. Delay is longer on average in ethnic or disadvantaged populations and at the extremes of age, but the absence of a palpable lump may also be an important factor in falsely reassuring a woman that her symptoms are not serious.

Phase 2: delay in primary care

The general practitioner (GP) or primary care physician who may see many patients with symptomatic breast disease each year but only one or two with breast cancer is in an increasingly difficult position. The patient's perception is that she needs to see a specialist but the GP is certain that the condition is benign especially in younger women. Breast cancer is very uncommon in women under 35 (3% of cancers), but when it does occur it is more difficult to diagnose.

It is usually inappropriate for a GP to use FNAC unless there is a history of recurrent cysts. To rely on a negative mammogram result without an expert clinical examination or FNAC to complete a triple assessment may increase the risk of false reassurance, although the evidence for this consensus opinion is not supported by the available data.[8] The GP is therefore faced with referring most women over 35 with breast symptoms for a specialist opinion without significant delay.

The specialist referral centre is also faced with the problem that women under age 35 lead to the majority of the diagnostic workload (66%) have the fewest number of breast cancers (3%)[9] and, paradoxically, produce the highest rate of medical malpractice claims.[2]

Administrative delay

Administrative delay between primary and secondary care may extend to an unacceptable interval of many weeks, and the UK government has recently acted to reduce this to a maximum of 2 weeks. However, the associated prioritisation of referral letters from GPs may be counterproductive if non-urgent cases have to wait longer, as several studies have shown that about 25% of breast cancers are found in patients who were non-urgent referrals.

Phase 3: after specialist referrals

This occurs in the setting of specialist diagnosis between the first visit to the breast clinic and the definitive diagnosis and treatment of breast cancer.

The North American experience

Two recent studies have been commissioned by the Physician Insurers Association of America (PIAA),[1,2] an association of 33 insurance companies representing over 90 000 physicians. Failure or delay in the diagnosis of breast cancer was the commonest cause of all medical litigation in the USA, and in terms of indemnity payout is second only to claims resulting from neurologically impaired newborn babies.[2] One of the most striking features of both studies was the relatively young age of the plaintiffs. In the earlier study women under 50 years of age accounted for 69% of the plaintiffs and received 84% of the indemnity paid.[1] These values are all the more surprising when it is considered that only 25% of breast cancers occur in women under 50 years.[10] In 487 cases where liability was admitted by the defendant, the mean delay was 14 months. The most common reasons cited for the delay were, in descending order, the physical findings failed to impress, failure to adequately follow-up the patient, a negative mammogram report, the mammogram misread and failure to do a biopsy. False negative and equivocal mammography results, whether used to diagnose a breast lump or as part of a screening programme was cited in 80% of the cases, and not surprisingly radiologists were the most common defendants. Radiologists are particularly at risk when the patient refers herself, since the triple assessment is incomplete without a clinical examination and a biopsy if appropriate. Mean damages of US$227 000 were awarded for delays of less than 5 months. The mean payout for all delays was US$301 000, with higher payouts being awarded for longer delays and to younger patients.[2] There are now statistical models for predicting the outcome and size of indemnity payout in malpractice lawsuits for breast cancer.[11]

That younger women, with the lowest incidence of breast cancer, have the highest incidence of malpractice claims is a paradox that may be explained by clinical lack of awareness or by unrealistic expectations of the ability to diagnose breast cancer in younger women. In any event, the diagnosis is more emotive especially when the patient has young children because the economic consequences of a reduced lifespan are more severe.

Diagnosis of breast cancer

Approximately two thirds of patients presenting at a symptomatic breast clinic are under 36 years of age and most will have benign disease, since only 3% of breast cancers occur in this age group.[12] Triple assessment, comprising an expert clinical examination, imaging by mammography and/or ultrasonography together with a needle biopsy, is the foundation upon which clinicians diagnose breast complaints. High degrees of accuracy have been quoted for these diagnostic modalities, but it is not well appreciated that the sensitivity and specificity of these tests are severely reduced in younger women. It has been suggested recently that perfection of diagnosis would require removal of every solid mass,[13] but this would represent a retrograde step.

If such a policy were adopted in the UK, the ratio of benign to malignant biopsies would increase considerably beyond the ratio of 1:1, recommended in the British Association of Surgical Oncology (BASO) guidelines for management of breast disease.[14,15] The practice of defensive medicine will certainly be encouraged by a private healthcare system, a litigious public and tests where sensitivity falls below 95%. Doctors were warned as medical students against the practice of defensive medicine, but the current medicolegal situation has reversed conventional wisdom.

To quantify the efficacy of diagnostic tests, the terms sensitivity, specificity, accuracy and positive predictive value are calculated. The sensitivity of a test in this setting is the ability to diagnose breast cancer and identifies the percentage of false negative cases. It is generally defined as $TP/(TP + FN) \times 100$, where TP is a true positive result and FN a false negative result. However, for sensitivity to be valid there must be accurate knowledge of the total number of false negative cases. Accuracy will be improved by establishing a link with the appropriate cancer registry, but the problem has been underlined by the difficulty in identifying all interval cancers in the NHS Breast Screening Programme.[16] The sensitivity of an investigation will also seem to be improved if inadequate samples are excluded from the calculations.

The specificity of a test identifies the percentage of false positive cases. Specificity is defined as $TN/(TN + FP) \times 100$ accuracy as $(TN + TP)/(TN + FN + TP + FP) \times 100$ and the positive predictive value usually as $TP/(TP + FP) \times 100$, where TP is a true positive result, TN a true negative result, FP a false positive result and FN a false negative result.

Physical examination

About 70% of all breast cancers are clinically palpable, but in tumours measuring 0.6–1 cm diameter this figure falls to 50%.[17] The larger the breast and the greater the density of breast tissue the more difficult physical examination becomes. Cyclical changes in breast parenchyma that occur during the menstrual cycle may necessitate repeated examination at different phases of the cycle, and it has been suggested that the optimal time to examine premenopausal women is 1 week after the onset of the menstrual period. However, a study of breast self-examination in six towns in the UK showed a nonsignificant negative effect.[18] This has not been satisfactorily explained, but if an operation in the early part of the menstrual cycle is deleterious[19] it might be speculated that physical examination would have the same effect. Coexisting benign lumps, scars and distortion produced by previous surgery, the ridge of tissue above the inframammary fold and the underlying ribs all add to the uncertainty of clinical examination. The small but real risk of breast cancer during pregnancy should also be appreciated. The changes in breast tissue in preparation for lactation increase the difficulties of clinical examination and may be a pitfall for the obstetrician who wishes to reassure an anxious patient at a prenatal assessment. Other difficulties include inflammatory cancers presenting as an infection, the presence of a silicone implant with an associated fibrous capsule and the effect of hormone replacement therapy (HRT) on the density of breast parenchyma, which increases both clinically and radiologically.

The sensitivity of clinical examination for the detection of breast cancer, carried out by a senior and a junior member of the surgical team in women aged 30–39 years was as low as 25%.[20] A sensitivity of 90% can only be expected in older women when the atrophic nature of the breast parenchyma and the low incidence of benign disease combine to make clinical diagnosis a relatively simple task.

The low sensitivity of clinical examination, the low incidence of breast cancer and the large numbers of young women attending breast clinics must largely explain why failure of physical findings to impress the physician was one of the most common reasons for delay in diagnosis of breast cancer in the PIAA study.[2]

Mammography

A false negative mammography result is one of the principal reasons for delay in diagnosis of breast cancer,[1,2,10,21,22,23] because a negative mammogram result gives the clinician and patient a false sense of reassurance that the condition is benign. How much reliance can be put on a negative mammogram result? Some authors suggest that the sensitivity of diagnostic mammography is greater than 90%, but these findings are not universal.[24] The age of the patient is an important factor in false negative reporting. The high radiographic density of the breasts in younger women and after exposure to HRT in older women make detection of a similarly dense tumour more difficult.

Further analysis of the data from the Health Insurance Plan Project study has estimated that the mean time that the diagnosis of breast cancer can be advanced by screening (lead time) is 1.7 years,[25] and other estimates vary from 0.4 to 3.0 years.[26,27] It is therefore probable that some cancers detected after the initial (prevalent) screening mammogram (interval cancers) were in fact present at the time of the prevalent mammogram but not detected. It has been shown that 25% of the cancers detected at the second screening mammogram (the incident screen) which is carried out 3 years after the initial (prevalent) screen in the NHS Breast Screening Programme (BSP), represent a false negative finding on the first X-ray film.[28] Data from the Breast Cancer Detection Demonstration Project (BCDDP) revealed that both clinical examination and mammography were less sensitive in women under 50 years.[10] Interval cancers are more often node positive, but this may be due to length bias, where those cancers detected in the interval between screens are more aggressive than prevalent cancers detected at the initial screen. By expressing the number of interval cancers as a percentage of the total number of cancers detected, it is evident that the number of cancers not detected by the initial screen is inversely proportional to the age of the patient. Thirty six per cent of cancers in women aged 40 attending for screening were not detected by the prevalent screen compared with just 9% in those aged 75.[10] Screening issues are well discussed by Wright and Mueller.[29]

Ultrasonography

The use of ultrasonography to augment mammography has expanded since the mid-1990s. The expertise of breast radiologists in the use of this technique has improved considerably owing to specialisation in breast imaging and from improvements in the performance of equipment. It is now considered good practice to carry out ultrasonography in a patient of any age complaining of a lump, especially when this is not detectable on clinical or mammographic examination. There is a trend for ultrasound-guided core biopsy to replace FNAC, but either or both techniques are currently acceptable.

Fine needle aspiration

FNAC of breast lumps has become the principal method for obtaining a tissue diagnosis of a palpable lump, since it is both cost effective and obviates the need for open biopsy and associated complications. How much reliance can be placed in the result obtained from a fine needle aspirate? Dixon reports that the sensitivity of FNAC can be increased from 66 to 99% by restricting the biopsy to one aspirator.[20] By comparison, the sensitivity of fine needle aspiration in women under 36 years was found to be reduced to 78% in two small series.[12,30] Dixon found that the accuracy of this investigation is not related to the age of the patient, and the sensitivity of FNAC in women under 36 years was 100% if inadequate samples were excluded from the calculations.[20]

When comparing studies of FNAC it should be known whether inadequate samples were included in the calculations of sensitivity and the length of follow-up for interval cancers. Reviews on the effectiveness indicate that a satisfactory sample is obtained in 89–98% of specimens. In a review of 112 reports of FNAC of breast masses by Layfield,[31] the overall accuracy was over 95%, but concern was raised over the range of false negative and false positive reporting (from 1–35% and up to 18%, respectively) and of unsatisfactory specimens (1–68%). Despite the introduction of FNAC, delay in diagnosis of greater than 50 days still occurred and 85% of such delays were in women under 55 years. It is possible that aspiration cytology in isolation could fail to detect breast cancer in 25% of women under 36 attending a breast clinic. A sampling error, where the clinician fails to sample the actual tumour, is probably more common than failure to achieve an adequate sample with a minimum of five clumps of epithelial cells or from misinterpretation of the cytology.[33] Where a lump is very small or indefinite but is apparent ultrasonographically, current practice is moving towards an ultrasound-guided core biopsy.

Efficacy of triple assessment

If it is assumed that breast cancer detection by clinical examination, mammography and FNAC are independent of each other, it is possible to calculate the rate at which all three tests will give a false negative result for a particular patient. The false negative rates of the three investigations[9,12,30] have been multiplied and expressed as a percentage (**Table 10.1**). It is very probable that the sensitivities of these tests are not totally independent of each other and therefore the predicted rate that all three tests will be false negative for an individual is a conservative estimate. The sensitivity of the three tests means that for a woman under 36 years with breast cancer there is at least a 12.3% chance that all three tests will give a false negative result. If the generally accepted overall sensitivities are taken, the chance that all three tests will produce a false negative result decreases to approximately 1 in 1000 patients. However, the data from which these sensitivities are calculated will be skewed towards the older age groups and the rate of false negative triple assessment may be as high as 4%.[33]

Curability of breast cancer

Since survival measurements are made from the date of histological diagnosis, earlier detection of the tumour by mammographic screening will improve survival data without necessarily having any real impact on cure. This phenomenon is known as lead-time bias.

	False negative rate	
	Women <35 years	Overall
Clinical examination	0.75	0.12
Mammography	0.75	0.12
Fine needle aspiration cytology	0.22	0.05
All three false negatives (%)	12.3	0.072

Table 10.1 False negative rate of triple assessment in women under 35 compared with generally quoted results.[9,12,30]

Is breast cancer a curable disease? Five and 10-year survival rates are useful in the comparison of different treatment regimens but are not synonymous with cure.

Crude cure rates seldom take account of the histological nature of the breast cancer. In a study of 133 long-term survivors of breast cancer,[34] 10% were, on histological review, considered to have benign disease. Of the remaining 119 survivors with a definite diagnosis of breast cancer more than two thirds had a special type of invasive cancer (e.g. cribriform, tubular), tumours that are generally considered to be less aggressive than invasive ductal or lobular cancer.

Haybittle has discussed three concepts of cure: statistical cure, clinical cure and personal cure.[35]

Three concepts of cure

Statistical cure: death from all causes

Statistical cure can be applied to a group of patients rather than to individuals by comparing the survival of a group of patients treated for breast cancer with the survival of an age-matched normal population. If, after a long period of follow-up, a fraction of the original group of patients shows an annual death rate from all causes similar to the age-matched normal population that fraction can then be said to be statistically cured.

By expressing the observed number of deaths in the treated group as a ratio of the expected number of deaths in the age-matched normal population (O/E ratio), statistical cure would be shown by a ratio of unity. In four long-term studies of patients treated for breast cancer, statistical cure has not been convincingly shown. In a French study from Villejuif, the 95% confidence intervals included unity between 15 and 25 years but over the next 5 years the ratio was significantly greater than one.[36] In the Cambridge study, which followed 704 patients for 31 years, the O/E ratio and 95% confidance intervals were always greater than unity. In the Edinburgh study, the O/E ratio reached 1.47 at 17–20 years (95% confidence limits 1.00 to 2.07) and in the Birmingham study the O/E ratio was 1.34 (0.95 to 1.84) at 35 or more years. Even after 40 years an excess mortality in young patients treated for breast cancer has been shown by Rutqvist.[37] The evidence is *against* a statistically cured group and it seems that a population of patients who have had breast cancer will *always* have a higher death rate from all causes than a matched control population, even after 20 or 30 years.

Clinical cure: free of breast cancer at post mortem examination

Clinical cure is shown if a group of patients treated for breast cancer is at no greater risk of dying from breast cancer than an age- and sex-matched normal population.[35] This definition of cure as applied to a disease considered fatal is used by actuaries for life insurance policies. To establish a clinical cure for breast cancer would be the most satisfactory outcome of any study, but accurate reporting of the cause of death for all participants in such a study is essential, which perhaps explains the paucity of data relating to clinical cure. Long-term studies have failed to show a clinical cure for breast cancer. The Edinburgh study showed that 15–20 years after initial treatment patients were 20 times more likely to die of breast cancer than the normal population. In the Cambridge study[35] deaths from breast cancer were 19 times the expected rate between 20 and 25 years and 15 times between 25 and 35 years. An excess mortality in patients with breast cancer has also been reported after 18 years in Stockholm and Connecticut.[38]

Personal cure

Personal cure relates to the individual. Personal cure can be claimed if the patient has no further symptoms from breast cancer at the time of death and the patient dies from another cause. Accurate death certification is essential and in the Cambridge study 26% of deaths were assessed as being from another cause, without overt signs of breast cancer being present. Mueller investigated the cause of death in 3558 patients with breast cancer, reported to the Upstate Medical Center Cancer Registry, Syracuse New York, and found that 20 years after diagnosis 80% of women diagnosed as having breast cancer were dead; 88% of these deaths were due to breast cancer.[39] Cancer of the breast was the ultimate cause of death in 96.5% of patients aged 21–50 years at the time of diagnosis, 90.0% in the group aged 51–70 and 77.5% in the group aged 71–100. It is only in the oldest group of patients that death from other causes competes significantly with breast cancer, so that a personal cure rate of 22.5% can be claimed. If adjuvant therapy postpones death rather than eliminating the disease completely, the lifespan of patients will be increased. Such an increase in lifespan would result in more deaths being due to other causes and the number of personal cures would increase.

Cancer control window

The theory that early detection of a tumour leads to cure depends on the concept that at the time of earlier detection and treatment the tumour will not have metastasised. There is therefore a theoretical window of opportunity to cure patients with cancer by surgery. The period of time between the earliest possible detection of the cancer and the time at which the tumour metastasises has been described as the cancer control window (**Fig. 10.1**).[40] If the tumour

Figure 10.1
A theoretical window of opportunity (the cancer control window) in the surgical treatment of breast cancer exists if the tumour can be diagnosed and excised prior to dissemination. Angiogenesis and the potential for lymphovascular spread occurs at an early stage of tumour growth. After Spratt and Spratt, reference 40.

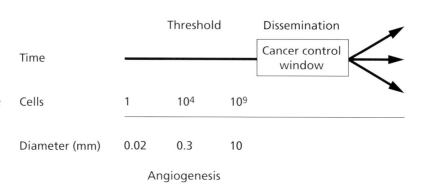

Figure 10.2
Possible effect of chemotherapy on survival of an individual patient with node-positive breast cancer. Chemotherapy may extend the life of a patient with lymph node metastases by 18 months. After Early Breast Cancer Trialists' Collaborative Group, reference 41.

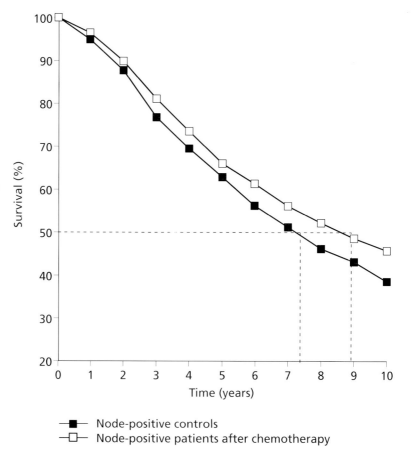

has already metastasised by the time it reaches the threshold size for detection, there is no window and only effective systemic therapy could cure the patient. Adjuvant chemotherapy has been shown to increase survival in women with node-positive disease, although by less than 10% of the treated population.[41] If, however, the life table graph is read horizontally it can be estimated that adjuvant chemotherapy will prolong survival in an individual patient by about 18 months (**Fig. 10.2**).

Tumour doubling time

Patients presenting to a symptomatic breast clinic typically have a tumour diameter of 3 cm. Assuming the cancer cell has a 10 μm diameter and exhibits exponential growth, this equates to 10^{10} cells and 33 tumour doublings. The threshold diameter for detection of a breast cancer by physical examination is 1 cm; such a tumour consists of 10^9 cells and is the result of 30 doublings. It is possible for mammography to detect tumours as small as 2 mm diameter, which equates to a tumour of 10^7 cells and about 23 tumour doublings. Assuming a constant doubling time, early detection of breast cancer is a misnomer, since at least two thirds of the biological life of the tumour will have been completed at the time of detection.[42] In medicolegal terms, if the mean delay in diagnosis was 10 months, for a cancer with a doubling time of 90 days such a delay would equate to the number of cells increasing by one order of magnitude (i.e. from 10^9 to 10^{10} cells); (**Fig. 10.3**). This does represent a major increase in tumour load but it is a very short period of the lifespan of the tumour and it is difficult to be sure that this period of delay would have a significant effect. In civil law, however, the court wants to know whether such an effect is more likely than not to have had any effect on a patient's prognosis.

Figure 10.3
Tumour doubling time: the effect of a 10-month delay. Graphic representation of tumour growth for a breast cancer with a doubling time of 90 days, assuming an exponential growth pattern. Growth rates (measured by the number of cells, the number of tumour doublings and the size of the tumour) of tumours that begin as a single cell and as a group of 1000 cells are plotted. By the time of diagnosis, typically two thirds of the tumour's life will have passed. The effect that a 10-month delay in diagnosis would have on the size of the tumour is shown (shaded). After Plotkin and Blankenberg, reference 42.

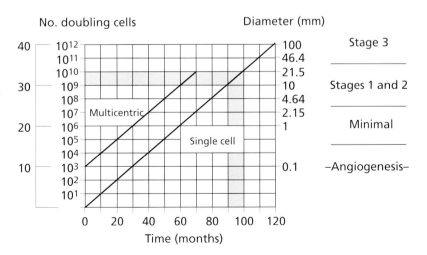

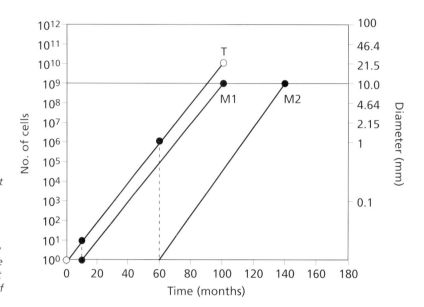

Being unable to sustain growth by diffusion, a growing spheroid of cells induces angiogenesis when it has a diameter of 0.3 mm, equivalent to 10^4 cells (12 doublings).[40] It is after this point that vascular dissemination of tumour cells becomes a possibility. Lymph node metastases are often encountered at the time of surgical excision, and Rutqvist found that 61% of women under 51 had axillary disease at the time of surgery.[37] The volume of a metastatic tumour is slightly less than the original tumour volume (1–2 logarithms difference in the number of cells). Assuming the growth rate of the metastasis approximates to that of the primary tumour, it is possible to estimate the time at which the tumour must have metastasised (**Fig. 10.4**). Not infrequently this would have occurred long before the threshold size for detection of the primary tumour.[42]

Tubiana has shown that the probability of dissemination for breast cancer is log normally distributed, demonstrating considerable variation between individual cancers.[43] The time interval between treatment of the primary tumour and detection of distant metastasis depends on four variables: the size of the tumour at time of metastatic dissemination, the size of the tumour at treatment, the doubling time of the tumour and the doubling time of the metastases. Breast cancer represents a continuum from slow-growing tumours with late axillary involvement and distant dissemination to the most aggressive rapidly growing and early metastasising subtype. In medicolegal terms only one of the four variables is considered, namely the delay in treatment that is likely to be related to the size of the tumour at detection. It is generally assumed by the patient and the legal profession that delay in diagnosis and treatment is the cause of the metastasis rather than the inherent biology of the tumour itself.

As with other cancers it is generally accepted that breast cancer begins as a single cell or a small group of cells, which exhibit an exponential growth pattern. The length of time taken for a tumour to double in size is known as the doubling time and is usually expressed in days. The percentage of cells in S phase (as measured by the thymidine labelling index (LI)) is closely related to the percentage of tumour cells engaged in proliferation. The duration of the S phase as a proportion of the cell cycle is relatively constant for human tumour cells.[43] A potential doubling time calculated from the labelling index *in vitro* is always much shorter than the actual doubling time observed *in vivo* because the potential doubling time takes no account of cell loss. In some tumours up to 90% of cells produced may be lost.

Actual doubling times for breast cancers have been estimated by measuring the size of mastectomy scar recurrences and also by serial mammographic evaluation, both estimations assume exponential growth of the tumour.[44,45] There is great variation in the magnitude of doubling times between different breast cancers, from less than 25 days to more than 1000, and tumour doubling times seem to exhibit a log normal distribution.[44] Survival after treatment for breast cancer also approximates to a log normal distribution, but it cannot be assumed that differences in patient survival are due entirely to differences in tumour growth rate.

Pearlman[44] categorised patients as having fast (<25 days), intermediate (26–75 days) and slow (>76 days) growing tumours based on a measurement of tumour doubling time; 5-year survival rates were 5%, 62% and 100%, respectively (**Fig. 10.5a**). If, however, patient survival is plotted against the lifespan of a patient, expressed as the number of tumour doublings that a patient survived (e.g. a patient who survived 6 years and had a tumour doubling time of 25 days would have survived 88 tumour doublings), the differences in survival between the fast-growing and intermediate/slow-growing tumours disappears (**Fig. 10.5b**). This implies that there was little therapeutic response for any of the patients, despite there being differences in the actual periods of survival; i.e. patients tended to survive a similar number of tumour doublings.

Although lymph node metastases are more commonly found in fast-growing tumours,[45] it would be wrong to assume that the survival of patients was entirely a consequence of tumour doubling time. Galante emphasises the importance of the metastatic potential of the tumour, suggesting that within fast-, intermediate- and slow-growing tumours there may be subsets with high and low metastasising potential.[45]

Liability for a breach of duty of care

The following vignettes have been constructed to illustrate the kind of issues that arise in medicolegal breast cancer cases, most of which concern either a

Figure 10.5
(a) Survival after mastectomy scar recurrences correlated with tumour growth. The cumulative percentage of survivors of 68 patients with mastectomy scar recurrences, correlated with tumour growth rate (fast, intermediate, slow). All patients with slow growing tumours survived 5 years, few patients with fast growing tumours survived 5 years.
(b) Survival correlated with number of tumour doublings.[44] Cumulative percentage survival of patients expressed in terms of the number of tumour doublings, correlated with tumour growth rate (fast, intermediate and slow). Difference in survival for the three categories are largely eliminated. This implies that there was little difference in the therapeutic response for any of the patients, despite differences in the actual time of survival. Patients in this series tended to live the same number of tumour doublings.
From Pearlman, reference 44.

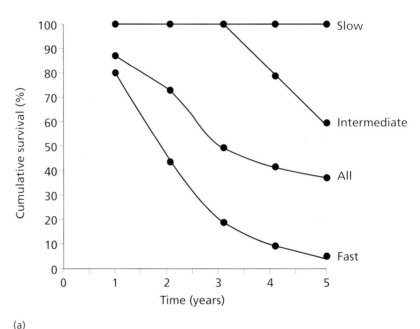

(a)

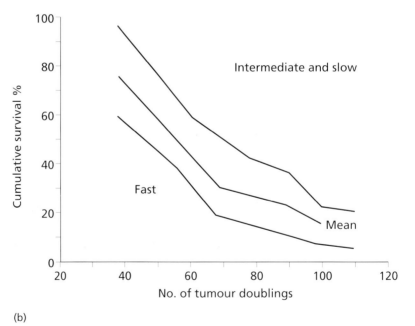

(b)

delay in diagnosis or a poor cosmetic outcome after cosmetic or reconstructive surgery. There are, however, other issues that arise, which include a pneumo-thorax caused by FNAC and a false positive cytology result leading to unnecess-ary surgery.

None of the vignettes is an accurate description of any one case, all of which have individual variations. The comments after each vignette should not be taken as a definitive opinion but do raise issues that are discussed in conference with counsel. The level of care must be taken in the context of the time at which the incident took place because the practice of breast surgery and investigation is changing rapidly. If any authority or guideline is quoted it must have been in the public domain at the time the advice was given or the treatment took place. Some allowance of time taken for dissemination of information must also be made.

Vignette 1

Pneumothorax at FNAC

A 32-year-old dental nurse presented with a lump in the tail of the left breast. Ultrasonography gave a negative result, and an experienced clinical assistant in the breast clinic carried out a FNAC. He unfortunately pierced the pleura and caused a pneumothorax, which required admission to hospital and pleural drainage. The patient was not warned of the risk and complained of persistent chest pain over a period of many months.

Comments:

- Did the clinician fail in a duty of care by advancing the needle too far or by failing to warn the patient? The literature suggests a risk of 1:10 000,[46] and it has been suggested that at this level of risk a warning may do more harm than good in heightening the anxiety of an already nervous patient who might well decline a necessary test in consequence. However, a show of hands at a recent medicolegal conference indicated that this injury is more common than the literature suggests. It is not rare to strike a rib during FNAC and it is only a matter of chance whether the rib or the space is entered. Perhaps the injury is more common than is recognised and that the consequent pain of a pneumothorax is perceived to be in the breast.
- The literature indicates that the needle pass during FNAC should always be tangential to the chest wall, but there is now considerable debate as to whether this is alway practical. A deep-seated lump may be pulled away from the chest wall with the non-aspirating hand to avoid a pleural puncture.
- A recent case in the English courts ruled this injury to be negligent, which was an unexpected judgement. It is an unfortunate fact of current medicolegal practice in the UK that if the patient receives legal aid the defendant does not recover their costs even when the case is successfully

defended. There is therefore a reluctance on the part of health authorities to defend cases in court and an even greater reluctance to appeal a judgement that seems open to doubt.

- In resisting a claim of negligence it is important to be able to show that the clinician was experienced in the technique. Were this to be a trainee it would be important to show that he or she was properly supervised. It is important that clinicians are aware of the risk of pneumothorax, which is most common in the tail of the breast of a thin patient.

- Pneumothorax can rarely be caused by the radiologist at needle localisation or by aspiration of a postoperative seroma of the axilla or the post-mastectomy space.

Vignette 2

False positive cytology result/lymphoedema/alteration of records

A 60-year-old woman was referred to a breast clinic with a clinically suspicious lump in the breast. Mammography was also suspicious of malignancy (R4), and the cytology result was malignant (C5). The patient had a wide local excision and an axillary lymph node clearance for what subsequently proved to be a histologically benign condition. She complained of a poor cosmetic outcome and a painful swollen arm, which she had not been warned about. The nursing records state that 'patient was warned of the risk of lymphoedema.'

Comments:

- A false positive cytology result is a rare but potentially devastating event. From a medicolegal standpoint an external expert review of the cytology should be the first step. If one or more experts are agreed that the cytologist acted reasonably in reporting the slides as unequivocally malignant, attention should then focus on the surgeon.

- The surgeon has to be aware that a false positive cytology result may occur in the best hands (1:1000), and for this reason many surgeons will not carry out a mastectomy without histological confirmation from a core biopsy. A full axillary clearance for a benign condition is a potentially major injury, and it is unfortunate that this patient developed lymphoedema.

- The risk of lymphoedema is not well quantified as it may occur a long time after the treatment, vary considerably in extent and may occur after a variety of treatments—or even without intervention. It is well recognised that radical radiotherapy to the axilla after an axillary node clearance carries an unacceptable risk, but radiotherapy after a positive-node sample may carry a higher risk than radiotherapy or clearance alone.[47] Communicating the potential risk of lymphoedema to the patient of about 1:10 is a difficult task because whatever treatment option she may choose or be guided towards carries some risk.

● The tense of the warning about lymphoedema indicates that this was a retrospective note made after the event.

Judges place most credence on handwritten contemporaneous records, which are often brief and poorly legible. Any addition, alteration or amendment to the record must be clearly identified as such by signing and dating the record. Any temptation to alter the record after the event must be firmly resisted even if it is a computer-generated entry. Lawyers are constantly on the alert for alterations to the records, which are often quite obvious.

Senior counsel: 'nurses are always doing it—doctors do it too, but they are usually a little more subtle'.

Vignette 3

Cosmetic defect after benign biopsy / benefit of preoperative diagnosis

A 50-year-old woman who was free of symptoms was invited to attend the NHSBSP. Mammography showed a suspicious lesion in one breast, and a diagnostic excision biopsy was carried out after stereotactic wire localisation. The pathology proved benign, but the specimen weight was not recorded. The cosmetic outcome was unsatisfactory, with loss of volume and distortion of the nipple.

Comments:

● The current quality guidelines for the NHSBSP indicate that 80% of benign excisional biopsies should weigh less than 20 g.[48] The target in the original guidelines was 90%, but the current UK national average indicates that over 50% of such biopsies weigh in excess of this target.[49] Failure to record the weight immediately places the surgeon in a difficult position, but it is also important to document that an explanation of risk has been given to the patient. The surgeon who is experienced in the use of this technique is more likely to achieve an appropriate biopsy with the minimum of tissue loss.

● Surgeons are sometimes tempted to carry out a larger biopsy in the hope that the operation will be both diagnostic and therapeutic. This is a hazardous strategy because if the biopsy proves benign there may be an unnecessary cosmetic defect and if malignant an inadequate resection may require further surgery.

● Preoperative diagnosis by core biopsy is clearly preferable to excisional biopsy. The national average for preoperative diagnosis of cancers in the NHSBSP is 71%, but a rate of 90% is now being achieved in several centres.[49]

Vignette 4

Failure of preoperative assessment and postoperative management

A 65-year-old woman presented with a small but obvious carcinoma in the tail of the left breast. The surgeon carried out fine needle aspiration, which showed malignant cells (C5), and he carried out a wide local excision of the tumour without preliminary breast imaging and without carrying out an axillary node sample. The tumour was grade 2, but the resection margins and the presence of vascular invasion were not reported. The patient started taking tamoxifen, but was not referred to an oncologist for consideration of radiotherapy.

Comments:

- The management of this patient falls short of an acceptable standard in several respects but until such time as she develops evidence of recurrence, which may never occur, any harm remains potential.
- A preoperative mammogram may have shown widespread malignant microcalcification or multifocal tumours, and in this situation conservative surgery would not have been appropriate. There may also have been an undetected cancer in the contralateral breast.
- Reliance on C5 cytology for conservative surgery may be acceptable where the surgeon is absolutely confident of the cytologist and the imaging is unequivocally malignant (R5). That was not the situation in this case.
- To manage a patient with conservative surgery without knowledge of the resection margins and not to refer her for consideration of radiotherapy is unacceptable. An unacceptably high rate of local recurrence of the order of 35% is to be expected.
- It is clear that this case was not discussed at a multidisciplinary meeting. The case history would certainly have alerted a member of the team to the inappropriate management.
- Knowledge of the axillary node status is considered to be important and is recommended in all current guidelines.

Vignette 5

Failure to carry out a triple assessment

A 32-year-old woman who mentioned a lump in the breast was seen in the general surgery clinic of a surgeon with a breast interest. On examination the surgeon found some indefinite thickening but no discrete lump. He did not therefore carry out a FNAC but arranged for ultrasonographic examination and asked to review her in 2 months.

When she came back for review she was seen by a junior trainee who noted the same findings. She had not yet had ultrasonography which he therefore expedited. This was carried out by a general radiologist and showed an indeterminate opacity corresponding with the lump of which the patient complained.

Eventually an excisional biopsy was carried out which showed an invasive ductal carcinoma, grade 3. At subsequent definite surgery 5 months after the initial consultation one of six axillary nodes was positive.

Comments:

There are several issues here.

- When a breast specialist sees a patient in a general clinic there is an increased risk of delay in diagnosis because there is:
  1. No preliminary imaging
  2. No immediate reporting of FNAC
  3. No breast care nurse
  4. No multidisciplinary meeting.

- An interval of 2 months between consultations is rather long and there is significant value in seeing the patient in a different phase of the menstrual cycle, usually at 6 weeks.
- It is accepted that there is no value in carrying out FNAC where there is no physical sign, but when the patient mentions a lump and the clinician finds some thickening at the same site, further investigation is indicated. One of the commonest causes of delay in diagnosis of breast cancer in the American PIAA study was that the physical signs failed to impress the clinician.[1,2]
- Ideally ultrasonography (or mammography in patients >35) should be carried out before FNAC, and if there is an abnormality an ultrasound-guided core biopsy of a solid lesion may be carried out.
- Where the clinician is aware of a long delay in carrying out diagnostic tests he or she should consider whether the expected delay is acceptable.
- Breast imaging requires a specialist in breast radiology. A breast radiologist would have carried out, or at least suggested, ultrasound-guided core biopsy and would be in close liaison with the breast clinic on a day-to-day basis, as part of the team.
- A pre-operative diagnosis would have prevented a diagnostic operation and would have facilitated a single therapeutic intervention.

Vignette 6

Radiological delay in diagnosis

A 54-year-old woman attended for the second round of breast screening (the incident screen) and was found to have an opacity on mammography that proved malignant. Having been shown the films she asked to see the previous films taken 3 years ago. When these were reluctantly produced it was obvious to her that the cancer was present 3 years previously.

Comments:

- A quarter of screen-detected cancers are apparent with hindsight 3 years and, very occasionally, 6 years earlier. Most often the tumour is only seen as one of several similar opacities on the original mammograms.
- Such a 'missed diagnosis' may be obvious to a radiologist in the knowledge of the outcome, but if the mammograms are interspersed with normal films, as in the screening situation, more often than not they will be passed as normal. In perhaps one third of such cases expert opinion will state that any competent breast radiologist working to an acceptable standard should have reported the abnormality, and in this situation liability has to be admitted.
- It is important in any screening programme that the number of women who have benign mammographic abnormalities who are recalled for further tests and even excision biopsy is kept to a minimum. The radiological quality standard for recall rate is 7%.
- Breast radiologists in the BSP who have a high detection rate (sensitivity) for breast cancer also have a high recall or false positive rate (low specificity). Conversely, radiologists with a lower detection rate recall fewer patients unnecessarily.
- A recent Appeal Court judgement in a controversial cervical screening case has ruled that relatively minor abnormalities that eventually proved malignant should have been referred for more expert opinion. If this level of sensitivity were to be required of breast screening, it might put the whole programme at risk.
- The net result of the increasing medicolegal threat to breast radiologists has been an increase in the recall rate and the core biopsy rate of any doubtful lesion. The recruitment of radiologists into breast imaging is also proving difficult.
- The increasing use of ultrasonography, the use of ultrasound-guided core biopsies and the specification (and cost) of the equipment have placed breast imaging outside the field of activity for the general radiologist. The breast surgeon may be similarly compromised unless fully trained in the technique which he or she uses on a day-to-day basis.
- The practice of repeating mammography after an interval for an appearance that is very probably benign may be difficult to defend if it eventually proves malignant. This particularly applies to microcalcification where core biopsy with specimen radiography to confirm a representative sample is the safest course.

- To be certain that an abnormality is benign on the strength of an apparently representative core biopsy is difficult. If microcalcification is present it is essential to radiograph the cores for confirmation. Benign radial scars are often seen in juxtaposition to a cancer, and it is agreed that an excisional biopsy is appropriate.

Vignette 7

False negative FNAC results—trainees in the diagnostic setting / lobular carcinoma/young women, delay in diagnosis

A 38-year-old woman was referred to a breast clinic with a breast lump. Preliminary mammography was negative and a specialist registrar (senior trainee) found an indefinite lump of which he was not suspicious. He carried out FNAC but failed to achieve an adequate specimen (C1). The result was not available at the time of the clinic visit. At follow-up appointment 6 weeks later she was seen by another specialist registrar who repeated the FNAC. On this occasion cytology showed an adequate sample of benign ductal cells (C2). She was discharged from the clinic but re-presented 6 months later with a lobular carcinoma at the same site.

Comments:

- Trainees must be adequately supervised and only permitted to see patients by themselves when their trainer is satisfied that they are entirely competent and understand local management protocols. The 1995 guidelines (BASO Breast Surgeons Group)[14] required that a trainee should also have been attending the breast clinic for at least 2 months. This latter requirement has been omitted from the current revision of the guidelines.[15]
- There is a learning curve in achieving adequate samples on FNAC, and it is likely that this will be achieved more quickly with immediate reporting of cytology as the trainee has immediate feedback and is then faced with repeating the procedure immediately. The rate of inadequate breast FNAC samples (C1) should be monitored for each clinician. This should be less than 20%, but an adequate sample of benign ductal cells (C2) does not ensure a representative sample of the palpable lump.
- A false negative cytology result may be due to cytological misinterpretation, but more commonly it is due to sampling error.
- Clinicians should be aware that lobular cancers are prone to false negative mammogram results. There is also an increased rate of inadequate cytology (C1) and of difficulty with false negative interpretation (C2).
- The diagnosis of breast cancer in young women is difficult and delay is more common. The cause of this delay is multifactorial but includes the

large number of women with benign breast disease who have firm nodular breasts, which are more difficult to examine clinically and on imaging. The sensitivity of a triple assessment, which is 99% in post-menopausal patients, may fall below 90% in young women and will lead to some false negative assessments, with consequent delay in diagnosis.

- In the situation where a patient complains of a lump but on clinical examination or mammography nothing is obvious, ultrasonography is particularly useful. If a lesion is seen, a guided core biopsy is probably superior to ultrasound-guided FNAC.

- Risk management of delay in the diagnosis of breast cancer should be an important item for any employing authority in the same way that neurological damage to babies carries a high risk profile. Trainees must be carefully supervised and should not be brought in to fill an unforeseen hiatus of out-patient care in the breast clinic. Strict adherence to local protocol is essential.

Vignette 8

Poor cosmetic outcome after reconstruction by a breast surgeon

A 52-year-old woman with multifocal cancer was advised to have a mastectomy by a breast surgeon, but after discussion with the breast care nurse she requested an immediate reconstruction. He offered her a tissue expander, which was inserted at the time of mastectomy. It was not possible to achieve symmetry with the large contralateral breast and breast reduction was carried out with a poor cosmetic outcome. She was subsequently referred to a plastic surgeon.

Comments:

- Patient expectation of a good cosmetic outcome is less demanding after reconstruction than for cosmetic surgery of the breast. Nevertheless there is a growing demand for more sophisticated reconstruction and a better outcome.

- The first question that must be addressed is the adequacy of training in reconstructive surgery that the surgeon has received. If that training was entirely appropriate the second question is whether the standard of advice and operative skill was such that the patient could reasonably have expected. Very often a poor outcome is owing to bad luck rather than poor judgement, and provided the patient has been warned of the risk she does not have a case against the surgeon. However, unless the answer to both questions is in the affirmative, the surgeon is liable, and in the sphere of cosmetic and reconstructive surgery the damage is self evident, i.e.

causation is less of an issue than liability. With delay in diagnosis the converse is the case.

- It is not infrequently the case that a general surgeon who has become a breast surgeon will also have become competent in the use of implants and tissue expanders. A surgeon will have often attended a training course on the use of the latissimus dorsi (LD) flap, and as this is a robust and safe flap its use by surgeons without a formal training in reconstructive surgery has on the whole proved satisfactory. However, an LD flap usually requires the addition of an implant.

- The best long-term result for reconstruction after a mastectomy is from the use of solely autologous tissue, and a transverse abdominis myocutaneous (TRAM) flap is the most successful in this respect. Some breast surgeons have mastered the art of a pedicled TRAM flap, but the most versatile version is a free flap where a microvascular anastomosis of the blood supply is made in the axilla or to the internal mammary artery. This reconstruction is usually beyond the capability of a breast surgeon, but when it is a matter of a delayed reconstruction this option is open to the patient by referral to a plastic surgeon.

The move towards immediate reconstruction at the time of mastectomy has made it more difficult to offer the patient what may be the most appropriate reconstruction for her. This tension may not yet have surfaced as a medicolegal issue, but patients who have been offered less than the best may feel that their advice was below that which they could reasonably have expected.

Impact of the NHSBSP in the UK

The NHSBSP has had an impact in several ways in the UK:

- Many breast surgeons were trained as general surgeons but with the passage of time and the call for subspecialisation now provide a breast service at the local district general hospital, usually with the help of a colleague who may have another specialist interest. Both surgeons are on call for general surgical emergencies, and neither have a formal training in reconstructive or cosmetic surgery.

- Surgeons used to manage most patients with breast cancer by mastectomy and may or may not have referred patients who are node positive to the radiotherapist. Latterly patients have been given adjuvant tamoxifen, but there has been an increasing call for conservation of the breast. This pressure to avoid mastectomy whenever possible, heightened with the start of the NHSBSP in 1988/89. Sooner, or sometimes later, it was learnt that failure to give radiotherapy after conservative surgery led to an unacceptably high local recurrence rate. Yet the proportion of patients receiving radiotherapy post-conservative surgery after 10 years of the screening programme is still only 75%. Some patients have particularly good prognosis tumours such as would be eligible for the BASO 2 trial (grade 1, node negative, <2 cm diameter with clear resection margins and no vascular invasion). Some patients decline radiotherapy, but together with those patients with a tumour with a good prognosis these cases do not amount to 25%.

- The NHSBSP has for the first time enabled a close and rather public audit of radiologists, pathologists and surgeons. Radiologists will know their own detection and recall rates. Standard Detection Ratios, which allow for differences in case-mix, are compared between screening units and are published. An interval cancer is one that presents within 3 years of the most recent mammogram or whatever the duration of screening interval. In most screening units the previous mammograms of all interval cancers that are notified are reviewed so that the radiologist will be acutely aware of his or her false negative results.

- Radiologists in the breast screening programme are expected to review 10 000 films per annum to maintain their expertise, but it is unlikely that any radiologist doing purely symptomatic (not screening) work would achieve this level of exposure. It is axiomatic that patients with screen-detected cancer should receive the same quality of care as symptomatic patients, and vice versa. This is not always easy to achieve.

- The borderline between atypical ductal hyperplasia and low-grade ductal carcinoma in situ (DCIS) may be very difficult to determine. Pathologists in the screening programme are periodically sent a set of specimen slides, which they are required to score as benign or malignant.

- Inevitably in this closely audited situation some professionals are shown to be outliers, which has led to medicolegal action in both radiology and surgery. Retraining and revalidation or opting out of the specialty may be a difficult choice.

- Audit of the surgical and oncological treatment of breast cancer eventually followed the earlier example of radiology and pathology, and inevitably there have been variations in the level of care, which have often amounted to no more than the limitation of current knowledge. The mastectomy rate for small screen-detected invasive breast cancers (15–20 mm) varies by surgeon, but it also varies by region so that the highest rate in 1997/98 was in Trent (43%) and the lowest in south west Thames (17%).[49] That is not to suggest that some women in Trent are necessarily having an inappropriate mastectomy as it is also possible that some women in the South West Thames region are having inadequate surgery.

- Variations in radiotherapy techniques have also been highlighted by the screening programme, and suboptimal treatment schedules have led to changes.
- The management of symptomatic breast cancer has not been audited in the same way as screen-detected cancer, but this will eventually be the case.
- There has been considerable pressure on the occasional operator to stop work in a given subspecialty. In breast surgery it may take many years for any difference in outcome due to suboptimal surgery to become apparent. An increased local recurrence rate would be the first difference to emerge but that would be entirely dependent on the availability of good data. It is quite possible that a unit providing suboptimal management of *in situ* and invasive breast cancer will also have poor data, and if patients are lost to follow-up, local recurrence rates may seem to be lower than expected.
- Breast cancer carries a high profile and once a perceived problem with a screening unit or hospital enters the public domain, considerable anxiety is generated in the local population. The breast screening programme has now set up a rapid-reaction force to assist the local audit team. It has become clear that openness is the best policy, and any attempt to withold potentially embarrassing information is counterproductive.

Causation

In a case of delay in diagnosis it is relatively straightforward to establish whether or not there has been a breach of duty of care, and if, on the advice of expert opinion, the defendant has failed the Bolam[4] test the interval between that breach and the diagnosis of breast cancer can be readily calculated. There have usually been several clinic visits, and it is often a point at issue as to which consultation amounted to a breach of duty of care. On this decision will depend the actual length of time for which causation will be calculated.

The next hurdle to be overcome by the plaintiff (the patient) is to satisfy the court on the balance of probability that this period of delay actually caused her predictable harm. The public and the judiciary have the expectation that has been encouraged by the medical profession that an early diagnosis carries a better outlook for the treatment of cancer and a better chance of a cure. It is not surprising therefore that protestations of lead-time bias and predeterminism tend to fall on deaf ears.

Having established liability for a delay in diagnosis and the length of the delay, a case will be made that less severe treatment would have been required with earlier diagnosis, e.g. a mastectomy would not have been necessary. It will also be argued that psychological damage has ensued.

The main difficulty, however, centres around the question as to whether the plaintiff has incurred a reduced expectation of life or if, as is so often the case by the time the matter comes to court, she has already died; would she have lived longer?

Expert opinion is often divided, and the court will make a judgement on the position that sounds most convincing on the day. As already explained, the level of proof is more likely than not as opposed to scientific level of proof required by scientists to prove or disprove the null hypothesis, i.e. that the delay in diagnosis made no difference to the length of survival.

Richards has recently carried out a systematic review of the literature on the effect of delay in diagnosis of breast cancer. After allowing for lead-time bias Richards found that a reduction in 5-year survival with a delay of 3–6 months survival is reduced by 7% and for a delay of more than 3 months by 12%.[50]

Dische has extrapolated a 1.8% decrease in survival from Richards data for each 1 month delay up to 6 months.[51] Published in the same issue of the *Lancet* Sainsbury *et al.* report no such effect but with the apparently contradictory finding that the patients with the shortest delay had the worst prognosis. This latter finding has been previously reported by Afzelius, who found that the rapidly growing breast cancer with the worst prognosis is immediately apparent to the first clinician the patient consults.[52] The very slowly growing tumour with a good prognosis may be more difficult to diagnose.

The survival curves for patients with the best prognosis tumour, which would be grade 1, node negative, have a prognosis that is not very different from the normal population, and clearly a formula based on the findings in Richards' study to assess reduction in survival from each month of delay would be inappropriate. If it is accepted, however, that this is a real effect, it would have to be argued that some tumours with a worse prognosis would have a greater loss of survival.[51]

Whether delay in the diagnosis of breast cancer causes a worsened outcome is a controversial issue because there is a possibility that the outcome may in some cases be predetermined and that earlier diagnosis may result in a longer time with knowledge of breast cancer but no change in the natural history of the disease.

The following vignettes have been constructed to illustrate some of the issues that arise once liability has been accepted and the question of causation arises. The comments should not be taken as definitive because in an area of considerable uncertainty they reflect the authors' opinion.

Vignette A

A 32-year-old woman was referred to a breast clinic with a lump in the breast. Ultrasonography showed an indeterminate opacity 1.0 cm in diameter consistent with a fibroadenoma, but no sample was taken by FNAC or core biopsy.

She was discharged from the clinic but returned a year later with a clinical carcinoma at the same site. This measured 2.1 cm ultrasonographically and on pathological examination was grade 3 and one of four nodes were positive.

Liability for a delay in diagnosis and treatment was admitted for failure to carry out a biopsy at the first visit.

Comments:

- The Nottingham Prognostic Index (NPI)[53] is often used to calculate the difference in outcome from the change of the value of the index over the period of delay.
- The NPI is calculated as follows:
  NPI = 0.2 × tumour size (cm) + node status (1–3) + grade (1–3).
- This index has proved to be a robust indicator of prognosis, but from a medicolegal standpoint it has the following drawbacks:
  1. The tumour grade remains constant.
  2. The node status at the time of the breach of duty is usually unknown. The axillary lymph nodes are always presumed negative by the plaintiff but this is supported by tables for grade and tumour size, which show the probability of positive nodes. Only in grades 2 and 3 tumours, which are greater than 2.5 cm in diameter, does the probability of positive nodes rise above 50%. Therefore on the balance of probabilities, which is the legal test, the nodes would have been negative.
  3. The tumour size is a weak determinant of prognosis in the NPI:
     Size 1.0 cm = 0.2
     Size 2.1 cm = 0.42

- The NPI score at the first visit was 4.2: Size = 0.2, node = 1 (presumed negative), grade = 3.
- The NPI a year later was 5.42: Size = 0.4, nodes = 2, grade = 3.
- The prognosis groups on NPI scores are as follows[53]:

Group	NPI	15-year survival (%)
Good	<3.4	80
Medium	3.41–5.4	42
Poor	>5.41	13

- The patient has therefore moved from the medium prognosis group with a 42% survival at 5 years to the poor prognosis group with a very low long-term survival. If, however, the tumour had only increased to 2.0 cm, the patient would have remained within the medium prognosis group (**Fig. 10.6**).

Figure 10.6
*Comparison of
survival between
medium and poor
prognosis groups.
Nottingham
Prognostic Index.
After Galea et al.,
reference 53.*

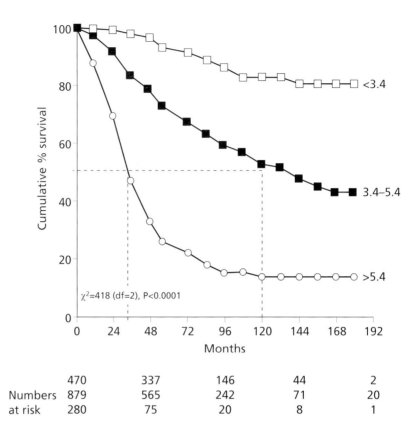

	470	337	146	44	2
Numbers	879	565	242	71	20
at risk	280	75	20	8	1

- It is possible to further subdivide the NPI subgroups to reduce the number of anomalies or to extrapolate individualised survival plots. The NPI is often used by expert opinion, but it has not been validated as a method for calculating differences in survival in this way.
- If this method is used, allowance should be made for lead-time bias, which in this case should be 1 year.

Vignette B

A 40-year-old woman presented with a lump in the breast, and a triple assessment was carried out. The tumour measured 1.5 cm on imaging and the cytology of the FNAC was reported as benign (C2). She was discharged from the clinic but 2 years later returned with a carcinoma 3.0 cm in diameter on histology. The tumour was grade 1 and the four axillary nodes sampled were clear.

Review of the original cytology indicated that this had been underreported, and an expert opinion graded the slides unequivocally malignant (C5).

Liability was admitted. The patient was treated by wide local excision and radiotherapy to the breast.

Comments:

- It is important that the standard of care provided in the triple assessment —in this case by the cytologist—is judged by the standard to be reasonably expected of a cytologist working at the same level. It is therefore inappropriate to ask a world expert in the specialty to judge the opinion of a doctor from a district general hospital. This principle is sometimes overlooked.
- The NPI has only changed from 2.3 to 2.6, and although the tumour has doubled in size over the 2-year period of delay, it remains within the good prognosis group. The treatment would have been the same with an earlier diagnosis and therefore there is no causation on this test.
- A grade 2 tumour could also double in size and if node negative would remain within the medium prognosis group. Again there would be no proof of causation when tested on the NPI. However, the Richards[50]/ Dische[51] formula would indicate a reduction of 12% at 6 months. If 2% per month was extrapolated to 2 years (for which there is no evidence), survival time would be reduced by 50%.

Vignette C

A 50-year-old woman responded to an invitation for mammographic screening and was recalled for magnification views of a localised area of microcalcification in one breast. There was soft tissue opacity, and the appearance was judged benign. She was returned to routine screening but 3 years later the second round of screening films showed an obvious carcinoma at the same site. This was an infiltrating carcinoma (2.0 cm in diameter, grade 2) with an extensive *in situ* component. Four of 10 nodes were positive: NPI = 5.4.

An external opinion from a breast screening radiologist rated the original films as suspicious of DCIS (R4) and stated that the focus of microcalcification should have been biopsied by any competent breast radiologist.

Comments:

- Practice has changed owing to fear of medicolegal action, and a radiologist is more likely to advise biopsy of microcalcification now than 3 years previously. It is important that the radiologist is judged on what was considered reasonable at the time the original decision was made.
- Whether clinical delay in the diagnosis of breast cancer affects the outcome is controversial and is discussed elsewhere. Delay which is due to radiological misinterpretation tends to be a matter of years rather than months. If 3-yearly breast screening by mammography does reduce the

number of deaths from breast cancer by about 25% it is more likely than not that a delay in diagnosis of 3 years between two screens will affect survival in a proportion of cases.

- The potential loss of survival in this particular case would be considerable as the original lesion would, on the balance of probabilities, be an area of high-grade DCIS without evidence of invasion. This lesion would carry a near-normal expectation of life if it had been adequately treated at age 50. At age 53 the patient now has a poor prognosis tumour and more likely than not will fail to reach retirement age.

Vignette D

A 30-year-old woman was referred to a general surgeon with a lump in the breast in January 1989 but was seen by a succession of three registrars (surgeons in training). Initial ultrasonography showed a 1 cm opacity consistent with a fibroadenoma, but the FNAC was reported as mildly atypical (C3) and the pathologist noted 'consider biopsy to confirm.' The registrar took no action because the pathologist always seemed to make equivocal reports and a 6-month follow-up appointment was given, which was subsequently repeated by two other registrars. The GP did not wait for the third appointment but referred the patient again to the surgeon who saw her for the first time in March 1990. The surgeon immediately diagnosed breast cancer. In the event the slides were underreported and liability for the delay was admitted. This was a grade 3, 4 cm diameter and heavily node-positive tumour: NPI = 6.8. The patient was initially treated by wide local excision and radiotherapy alone. She was not given chemotherapy or hormone treatment until she developed bone secondaries 16 months later. The oestrogen receptor status was not determined (1990).

Liability was admitted for the delay in diagnosis and the failure to give chemotherapy at the time of diagnosis of the primary tumour. This case is similar to Taylor *v* W. Kent (1997),[54] where causation was disputed, and although a catalogue of diagnostic and therapeutic errors were admitted the amount of damages awarded did not relate to the severity of the negligence (see later).

- To ignore an invitation to consider a biopsy because the pathologist 'always says that' suggests a failure of communication between clinician and cytologist. It is clear that there was no multidisciplinary meeting.
- To arrange a 6-month follow-up for a breast lump that is presumed benign is illogical. A follow-up at 6 weeks would have been appropriate, at which time an excisional biopsy or repeat FNAC would have been optimal in a woman aged 30. An ultrasound-guided core biopsy would not have been standard practice in 1990.

- The place of a trainee giving an independent opinion in a breast clinic is discussed elsewhere. It is unlikely that all three registrars measured up to the stated criteria—but these were not published until 1995.
- The judge was faced with five expert witnesses. It was agreed that when the patient was first seen she would have had a grade 3, 1 cm, node-negative tumour and that chemotherapy would not have been given in 1989. The tumour had increased in size to 4.0 cm in the 14 months of delay, and opinion was divided as to whether this was potentially curable. Inevitably the experts for the plaintiff were far more optimistic than those for the defence, but in the event the judge preferred the latter. The trial proceedings make good reading.[54] The Woolf recommendation that there might be only one expert responsible to the court is controversial, but the concept that experts should not be in the pocket of one party is more widely welcomed.
- The effect of the delay of 15 months in giving chemotherapy was also a matter of considerable variation between the experts. The estimated reduction in life years ranged between a few months and 5 years. 'Doing the best that I can on the basis of all the evidence, I consider that on the balance of probabilities, the negligent failure to provide Mrs T. with adjuvant chemotherapy in 1990 caused her to die 18 months before, sadly she would have died anyway.'

    One can only have sympathy with the judge in taking an average of the opinions on offer (**Fig. 10.2**).

- There was considerable sympathy for the family of the deceased patient who were awarded damages. Unfortunately the damages amounted to less than the defence had already paid into court. The plaintiff could have taken the damages but chose to contest the case for a larger sum on the advice of their experts. Civil litigation rules resulted in the family winning the case but receiving no damages.

The medicolegal implications of silicone implants

Any discussion regarding the medicolegal aspects of breast disease must inevitably focus at some point on the saga of the silicone breast implant. Notwithstanding the rising trend towards litigation in breast cancer, these cases pale into insignificance when compared with the half a million women who joined in class action suits for damages from silicone implants.

On reflection, the events that transpired in the USA courtrooms were perhaps one of many skirmishes between science and the law, with abuse of expert witnesses, anecdote and fear. Whatever the philosophy, the outcome was that in 1995 the principal manufacturer of silicone implants, Dow-Corning, filed for Chapter 11 bankruptcy.[3] Although litigation has predominantly been aimed at the manufacturers of breast implants it is perhaps only a matter of time before individual surgeons who inserted the implants will be sued if the manufacturer is already bankrupt.

The saga is fascinating and is well covered by Renwick.[55] From the mid-1950s silicone had been injected into the breasts of some Asian women for breast augmentation. Unfortunately these injections produced granuloma with hard nodular areas within the breast, which led to subsequent concern over possible systemic effects which were first raised in Japan in the early 1960s. Silicone-gel-filled prostheses were first used in 1964, and there have been varying estimates of between one and two million for the number of women having prosthetic augmentation.[56] Several types of prostheses have been used in the past, but regardless of the type there has been ongoing concern about mechanical problems and the potential for autoimmune disease.

Mechanical problems included (a) fibrous encapsulation, (b) 'bleeding' of silicone-gel between the implant envelope and the fibrous capsule and (c) the possibility of implant rupture causing migration of silicone into the breast and other body tissues. Moderate numbers of women have had local pain and discomfort related to infection around the prothesis.[57]

From 1980 there were sporadic anecdotal references in the literature, where an association between silicone-gel implants and autoimmune disease was proposed. This subsequently led to a hypothesis that connective tissue disease was induced by the silicone implant. Scleroderma was the most commonly reported connective tissue disease, although the symptomatology of the various connective disorders described was often non-specific,[58] it coincided with the common pattern of complaint from the general community in patients who had never been exposed to silicone.

In 1977, several litigants reporting ruptured prostheses were awarded above US$ 170 000. In 1982, lawyers in San Francisco gained access to 800 pages of internal documents from Dow-Corning, which suggested that basic investigations on the safety and efficacy of long-term silicone implantation had not been performed. In addition there were complaints that reports of 'bleeding' and fibrous contraction around the prosthesis had not been further investigated, and subsequently one litigant was awarded US$ 1.7 million. This was followed in 1988 by a further two cases with awards above US$ 7 million, but on this occasion there was considerable media coverage. Subsequently numerous silicone implant support groups were formed as a result of media publicity on the speculation that connective tissue disease was caused by the implants.

In 1991 the commissioner for the Food and Drug Administration in the USA placed a moratorium on the use of silicone-gel implants on the grounds that they had not been proven safe. By 1992 the number of cases was rapidly becoming exponential, with the development of class actions. One notable Texan case, however, involved a single litigant who was subsequently awarded US\$ 25 million for a ruptured prosthesis and influenza-like symptoms.[59] This judgement associated with extensive media coverage resulted in a huge expansion in the number of litigants despite the fact that no scientific evidence had been produced to support a definite link between silicone implants and systemic disease of any kind.

In 1994, 200 000 litigants joined in a class action, but by May 1995 this number had increased to 480 000. Under siege, Dow-Corning filed for Chapter 11 bankruptcy and thereafter legal action was subsequently instituted against its parent company Dow-Chemical.

In 1997, alleging they had been misled as to the safety of breast implants, 200 plastic surgeons from Pennsylvania joined in a class action against Dow-Corning leading from their own defence of law suits by their patients alleging lack of informed consent.[60]

From 1994 various cohort and epidemiological studies have been reported, with a consensus that supports the Medical Devices Agency of the Department of Health in the UK, which published an extensive review and concluded that 'there is no evidence of an increased risk of connective tissue disease in patients who have had silicone gel breast implants.'[61]

One study was reported in February 1996 suggesting a possible increased relative risk in connective tissue disease of 1.24 in women with implants.[62] However, the authors also alluded to a potential significant bias within their study, and most likely the relative risk was lower. Statistically, at most approximately 2000 of the 2 million women exposed to breast prostheses would have connective tissue disease based on the normal incidence in the community, and should the relative risk be doubled or trebled then the number of women reporting these disorders should increase only to between 4000 and 6000. One can only surmise that perhaps 400 000 of the litigants had symptoms unrelated to their breast prostheses. In addition, although some women have undoubtedly been 'injured' by their prostheses through mechanical problems such as infection or rupture, a 1994 study reported that effectively only 1.5% of all prostheses had either bled silicone or had leaked.[57]

How could it be that with a lack of scientific epidemiological evidence supporting a link between systemic disease and breast implants that such penalties be imposed upon the manufacturers? The answer lies firstly in the concept of 'proof beyond reasonable doubt' versus 'probability' of liability, with the desired aim not to determine the ultimate 'truth' but more to resolve a dispute between the plaintiff and the defendant. In a criminal court the standard of proof would be 'beyond reasonable doubt,' and this would equate to a scientific acceptance of a 'causation hypothesis' demonstrating 95% confidence intervals, which is usually that required by journal editors for publication. Secondly, in criminal law it would be preferred by the community that some criminals be acquitted rather than an innocent party be jailed. By analogy, a 'safe decision' was preferred above 'a scientific decision.' In the context of a public health issue such as breast implants in a civil court, a standard of proof of 'more likely than not' and a 'safe decision,' a jury was perhaps always more likely to find in favour of the plaintiff.

There was, however, another major feature of the litigation in that adequate safety and efficacy testing before marketing had not been performed by Dow-Corning, and there was therefore little evidence that breast implants were safe because the manufacturers had not fulfilled their responsibility to look for dangers. Although there have been numerous claims for damage against the tobacco industry, until recently none had been successful on the grounds that the risks of smoking had been known to and accepted by the plaintiff. In the case of breast implants, the plaintiffs had allegedly not been properly warned by the manufacturer or subsequently through their surgeons of potential dangers.

Legal argument also brought focus on the issue of scientific evidence in the courtroom. Until 1993 the 'Frye rule'[63] or 'general acceptance rule' determined the admissibility of scientific evidence within the courtroom. Essentially, for evidence to be accepted, the basic scientific principle should have already gained general acceptance within the scientific community. This rule was, however, overturned in 1993 when in the Daubert case[64] the Supreme Court of the USA determined that the Frye rule had been surpassed by the federal rules of evidence, which essentially said that all relevant evidence was admissible. In particular no single test of the validity of any evidence, such as the publication of evidence in a peer review journal, could be used to exclude that particular evidence. To this end it could seem that speculation and anecdote rather than peer reviewed scientific evidence may well have played a part in the courtroom decisions regarding silicone breast implants.

Although ultimately it may well be generally accepted that there is no association between breast implants and connective tissue disease, certainly some women were appropriately compensated for mechanical harm. There is also little doubt that Dow-Corning had considerable time to conduct appropriate safety investigations, to investigate complaints regarding failure of prostheses and to warn potential users of their implants of potential complications. This did not occur and rather than using the court room to defend its position Dow-Corning decided to seek bankruptcy.

Poor cosmetic outcome

Where surgery is undertaken in the management of breast cancer, clinical experience suggests that litigation arising from a poor cosmetic result is very uncommon. Perhaps this relates to patients' greater concerns regarding the diagnosis of malignancy and their ultimate survival rather than cosmesis. However, this situation could change with the increasing practice of breast conservative surgery rather than mastectomy in the management of early breast cancer, or when the latter procedure has been carried out there is now considerable demand for reconstruction. The patient may claim that a mastectomy is a much poorer cosmetic outcome than breast conservative surgery leading to a claim for damages. This may have some basis in fact should there have been reasonable indications to support the use of breast conservative surgery and had not that option been discussed with the patient. Furthermore, when mastectomy is advised there should be evidence of discussions regarding either immediate or later breast reconstruction.

With the greater use of clinical practice guidelines and with more literature available for patient information prior to surgery it is increasingly unlikely that such situations will arise. Informed consent is paramount in this situation, and it will undoubtedly be to the clinician's benefit to appropriately record that such alternative issues, options and potential complications of surgery have been discussed. The use of a properly trained breast care nurse to augment and reinforce the surgeon's advice is an additional protection that is now seen as an essential requirement in the practice of breast surgery.

On the other hand, cosmetic breast surgery poses greater expectations from the patient and potentially more risks for the surgeon. Beauty is in the eye of the beholder, and at times it can be difficult to convey a picture of the ultimate appearance preoperatively and more importantly to interpret the acceptance and understanding of the outcome by the patient.

Misplacement of the nipple after breast reduction is a potent source of litigation, which is only avoided by meticulous preoperative measurement and marking.

Evidence that appropriate discussions about potential risks and complications and poor cosmetic outcome in the realm of cosmetic surgery needs to be adequately recorded with perhaps the use of appropriate information brochures, photographs and video material to adequately explain the proposed procedure. In addition the surgeon should consider obtaining both standard evidence of consent as well as evidence that the literature has been both received and understood.

Auditing of operative results may also be required in the future to demonstrate that a particular complication was simply bad luck and within the expected percentage risk of this occurrence. Audit evidence may well confirm that a particular surgeon's complication rate was at or below the accepted rate for that particular procedure. Alternatively audit evidence that a particular surgeon had a complication rate far exceeding the accepted norm may well lead to litigation should that information become available to the patient. This fact has undoubtedly been responsible for the reluctance of some practitioners to undergo peer review or self-auditing processes. In addition the storage and availability of such data have undoubtedly caused some anxiety to hospital-based peer review and audit committees, raising the question of what is privileged material. However, in a specialty of surgery where success or failure are not a matter of mortality but of a value judgement and where complications will inevitably be underreported, any audit would lack the finality of the cardiac surgeon's results. The general principle of informed consent seems again to be at the forefront of defensive medical practice.

Clinical practice guidelines

Clinical practice guidelines have been promoted as systems that will assist both the practitioner and patient to reach appropriate decisions about healthcare management, although there has been considerable scepticism that their main purpose is cost containment. There has, however, been a significant variability in treatment patterns offered for early breast cancer both nationally and regionally, dependent on local resources, practitioner experience and patient acceptance of various treatment patterns. Because of this, and the fact that the general public may regard the spectrum of breast cancer as a single entity, there exists a perception that various treatments offered by some individual practitioners may not have resulted in the optimal result expected by the patient. This in itself may lead to a significant increase in the number of medicolegal claims.

To overcome this difficulty, hospitals and institutions have often adopted clinical practice guidelines to restrict variation in clinical practice in the hope that this will reduce the number of medicolegal incidents. If the practitioner followed established guidelines a poor outcome could be more likely attributed to misadventure rather than mismanagement.

Garnick *et al.* quite correctly point out that for practice guidelines to have any influence on the number of medicolegal events they should be developed for those specific conditions that commonly result in medical negligence claims.[65] They should be widely accepted by practitioners, completely integrated into clinical practice and be simple and readily interpreted in the courts. It would seem that breast cancer could offer such an opportunity for a successful set of practice guidelines.

There is, however, still considerable concern regarding the medicolegal implications of clinical practice guidelines. Carrick *et al.* reported that whereas 41% of surgeons surveyed believed that guidelines would protect them against medicolegal claims, 37% believed that they would increase their exposure to claims.[66] Of interest, significantly more breast surgeons compared with general surgeons believed that their exposure to claims would increase. This may reflect a wish to fine tune and individualise treatment for individual patients.

Carrick reported that 80% of surgeons thought that guidelines would be helpful, suggesting that they had been generally accepted, but only 37% of surgeons routinely gave relevant associated literature (*A Consumers Guide to the Clinical Guidelines*) to all or more than half of their patients. Nattinger *et al.* reported on the effect of legislative requirements on the use of breast conservation surgery.[67] The rates of breast conservation surgery versus mastectomy were examined, comparing centres where there were no state laws specifically requiring a disclosure of treatment options with other sites that had such legislation. They concluded that such legislation had only a slight and transient effect on the rate of use of breast conservation surgery. Is it difficult for clinical practice guidelines to be fully integrated into clinical practice?

Woolf compared various methods employed for the development of clinical practice guidelines.[68] Firstly, there was informal consensus development, where various organisations or societies simply gathered expert panels and eventually arrived at a general consensus decision. Secondly, there was formal consensus development, consisting of a similar process except that the discussion and investigation by survey was more structured and developed—perhaps more accurately reflecting the predominant opinion. However, with any consensus statement the final result is likely to reflect the thoughts of the dominant group and could also be influenced significantly by political, personal and regional dynamics. The third method consisted of evidence-based guidelines where the association between recommendations and supporting research was more transparent. The value of guidelines relates to the strength of the scientific support but evidence-based guidelines are limited by the small numbers of clinically validated studies.

Finally, explicit guideline development uses components of both the evidence-based approach and expert opinion to establish an accepted consensus. Further methods have been developed to assist with simplicity and interpretation, which include the use of a four-point rating system to identify the evidence base for any key decision. This last approach has been adopted by the National Health and Medical Research Council (NHMRC) of Australia through its Standing Committee on Quality of Care and Health Outcomes

(QCHOC). The system recommended assigns level 1 to 4 ratings to the various key points. The NHMRC guidelines are not designed to be rigid procedural paths nor were they designed to be prescriptive.[69] Whether or not they can influence the explosion of medical litigation related to breast disease within Australia remains to be seen.

That clinical practice guidelines are gaining greater notoriety relates to the management of early breast cancer and are surgeon oriented. Numerous studies have shown that the greatest cause for litigation, however, relates to a delay in diagnosis, which is often lodged at the GP level rather than the specialist. In addition, radiologists rate highly among those practitioners being sued. In Australia clinical practice guidelines directed towards GPs have been released, aimed at categorising women into low, middle and high risk groups. The general thrust of the guidelines relates to the triple diagnostic test of clinical examination, mammography and FNAC. The use of clinical practice guidelines for the investigation of symptomatic breast disease may well improve the outcome for the population in general but a small percentage of patients will continue to experience a delay in diagnosis.

The fact that a GP followed guidelines and arranged for a triple assessment may not protect from litigation. The practitioner should quantitate the individual perceived risk for that patient in terms of a negative triple assessment, and thereafter it should be the patient's choice as to whether or not that level of risk is acceptable or the patient would warrant an open biopsy.

Hurwitz reports that written guidelines cannot be cross examined in British courts as they are regarded as here-say evidence.[70] It is likely that in time the courts will take greater notice of protocols and guidelines after reform of the legal system following the Woolf report[71] and these documents will play an important part in 'expert evidence.'

Within Australia a new professional list was established in the common law division of the Supreme Court of New South Wales.[72] This list is designed to deal with professional negligence and in particular medicolegal cases. The Chief Justice, in announcing the establishment of the list, implied that the major objective of the list 'was to reduce delay and costs, increase the number of settlements and improve communication between parties.' The list in particular examines the role of the expert witness. The expert witness is now to be provided with a schedule to the practice note, which in turn sets out expectations under the list of the part to be played by an expert in the proceedings. The schedule also requires the expert to record or annex in the report their qualifications and their basic assumptions underlying their opinions and to specify examinations, tests or investigations used and literature relied on in support of their opinions. But *de facto* in Australia it is likely that such experts would have had considerable exposure to (if not been party to) the development of the clinical practice guidelines, and as a result it is likely that these guidelines will in time be accepted as reasonable management.

Clinical practice guidelines do not necessarily need to be directed at the larger population of practitioners but may have a role in individual practice situations. On a smaller scale, individual practitioners should have documented their own guidelines for secretarial staff such as office reminder systems and guidelines for recall, probably computerised, to facilitate the recall of patients for further follow-up and to ensure that appropriate test results have been received and acted on.

The identification of patients requiring scheduled examinations, screening procedures and follow-up arrangements will be essential to avoid potential litigation.

Within Australia these particular points have been highlighted by the recent Malycha *v* Kite case, where considerable damages were awarded to a patient undergoing a delay in diagnosis.[73] Although the medical care by the practitioner was deemed to be above reproach, a breakdown in either office or laboratory procedure resulted in a delayed follow-up of a positive cytology result. Although the patient failed to return for further follow-up or to ring for the results, the judge ruled that the patient was absolved of the responsibility and that there was a breach of duty by the practitioner. These findings have had significant implications in current office management procedures within Australia, and although in general terms clinical practice guidelines refer to the management of medical conditions they may, in turn, be directly related to office and secretarial management.

The award of damages

The sole remedy available to the successful claimant in medical negligence litigation is an award of damages—a sum intended to restore the plaintiff, so far as money is able, to the position she would have been in but for the negligent act. Explanation and apology, desirable though they may be, are not within the power of the law.

The award is made up of two components: general and special damages. General damages are intended to compensate for pain, suffering and loss of amenity and are based on judicial guidelines, which are upgraded to allow for inflation. Special damages are specific to the individual plaintiff and include past losses, which can be identified with some accuracy, and future losses, which can only be estimated. It is the future loss of earnings and the costs of providing care for the plaintiff and/or dependents that generate claims of very high value. Awards well in excess of £1 million are common for infants brain damaged at birth who may have a normal life expectancy and require complex care throughout. A young woman with dependent children earning a high income will also attract a high value award if she (or her surviving spouse) can demonstrate that her premature death resulted from lack of care. The all-or-none principle adopted in English law means that the successful plaintiff will normally recover damages in full, although in one recent case where the claimant was held to have lost an 80% chance of cure, a deputy high court judge directed that damages should be calculated accordingly.[74] It is important to note that in English law the magnitude or perceived culpability of the negligent act has no bearing whatsoever on the sum awarded and that the principles of calculating the value of a claim are followed whether the matter is settled by direct negotiation or is heard in court where damages, if not agreed, are determined by a judge sitting without a jury. This contrasts with the position in the USA where cases that proceed to trial (the minority) rely on jury decisions which can, and often do, incorporate an element of 'aggravated or exemplary (punitive) damages', a sum the jury considers warranted by the wrongfulness of the defendant's act. The extent to which this affects the magnitude of the award can be seen by comparing the average value of claims concluded by settlement (US$ 282 244) with the US$ 869 766 secured by jury verdict in the 1995 USA PIAA survey.[2]

Costs of litigation

Legal services are expensive, and in the PIAA survey[2] the costs incurred when cases concluded by settlement versus jury verdict were US$ 26 166 and US$ 100 926, respectively. Costs accrue merely because a claim has been investigated thoroughly and must be met even if the claim is of low value or is not pursued.

The Woolf report

In a review of the UK civil justice system, Lord Woolf singled out medical negligence cases as being worthy of special attention.[71] The difficulty of proving both causation and negligence, which arises more particularly in medical negligence than in other personal injury cases, accounts for much of the excessive cost. The root of the problem, however, lies less in the complexity of the law or procedure than in the climate of mutual suspicion and defensiveness, which is still all too prevalent in this area of litigation. Patients feel let down when treatment goes wrong, sometimes because of unrealistic expectations as to what could be achieved. Doctors feel they are under attack from aggrieved patients and react defensively. The patients' disappointment is then heightened by what they perceive to be a refusal to acknowledge fault and an attempt to cover up.

Lord Woolf identified medical negligence as the area generating most expense, delay and confrontation and the highest proportion of claims that failed. In cases valued at less than £12 500, the median figure for the costs of litigation was 137% of the value of the claim. This financial background has a profound effect on the conduct of litigation. The general rule is that 'costs follow the event'—the unsuccessful party is responsible for the costs of both sides. Privately financed claimants are therefore reluctant to pursue actions where the chances of success are equivocal. In the UK if the plaintiff (the patient) is supported by legal aid and loses the case, the costs are not recoverable by the defendant (the provider). The health authority/defence society or practitioner cannot recover their own costs, even if successful; whereas if unsuccessful, they will be responsible not only for all their own but for all the claimant's costs as well. It is small wonder there is a pressure to settle low value claims, even if defensible. Perhaps more importantly there is reluctance to appeal when an important point of principle has been left uncontested.

It has been estimated that over 90% of medical negligence claims that reach litigation are legally aided because of the high costs of medical litigation. Most often the defendant is the health authority or Trust and expenses incurred by plaintiff and defendant are, therefore, funded from the public purse. Medical negligence cases more commonly involve unacceptable delays in resolution and have lower success rates than other personal injury claims.

It is anticipated that two recent changes in the UK will improve the position of the plaintiff and reduce the need for litigation. Firstly, the NHS Litigation Authority administers a voluntary scheme, which acts as a mutual insurer for those Trusts that participate (Clinical Negligence Scheme for Trusts). Secondly, jurisdiction of the NHS ombudsman is to be extended to include complaints against all NHS staff, once the internal complaints system has been exhausted. The latter is a free service, which provides an inquisitorial investigation but has no jurisdiction over financial compensation.

The recommendations of the Woolf report are intended to improve the resolution of disputes between patients and physicians and to reduce delays and costs while treating both parties fairly. The recommendations include:

1. Training health professionals in the rudiments of medical negligence law.
2. The General Medical Council should consider whether a rule of professional conduct is needed to clarify the responsibility of healthcare professionals to their patients when they discover an act or omission in which they may have been negligent.

3. The NHS should improve methods of tracing former hospital staff.
4. A prelitigation protocol for medical negligence cases. Claimants should notify defendants with a written intention to sue 3 months before action. If liability is disputed, defendants should provide a reasoned answer.
5. Alternatives to litigation, such as the health service ombudsman, should be proffered to patients by solicitors.
6. The special lists on the Queen's Bench should include a medical negligence list of judges familiar with medical negligence cases.
7. Training trial judges in medical issues.
8. Standard tables to quantify medical negligence claims.
9. Courts should facilitate a pilot study of the various 'fast track' options for dealing with claims under £10 000, so that these claims can be litigated on a modest budget.

Shortcomings of the present system for the plaintiff include (a) the delay in resolving claims, (b) the low success rate of medical litigation compared with other personal injury litigation owing to the difficulty in proving both causation and negligence and (c) the fact that unmeritorious cases are often pursued whereas clearcut claims are often defended for too long. Physicians are concerned that, for financial reasons, Trusts may wish to reach an out of court settlement rather than pursue an expensive defence in court. However, the new Civil Procedure Rules, 1998 have introduced a fundamental change to medical negligence litigation in England and Wales. There are now tight timetables in order to reduce delays to a minimum, and medical experts will be required to address their report to the court and not to the party from whom the expert has received instructions (part 35).[75] 'The expert witness has a duty … to provide objective unbiased opinion to the court on matters within his expertise, never assuming the role of an advocate.'

Risk management

Failure of communication and poor physician–patient relationships often prompt patients into taking legal action. A woman who feels that her complaints have been taken seriously and investigated thoroughly is less likely to sue her clinician. In cases where the patient–physician relationship breaks down, referral to another specialist may be the best course of action.

That 'early diagnosis' of breast cancer is a misnomer and the probability that delay in diagnosis may not adversely affect survival will not be intuitively obvious to the plaintiff, her family or the legal profession. The best defence against allegations of injury is to make a timely diagnosis of breast cancer, and this must remain the goal of those responsible for treating patients with breast disease. However, when allegations of delay are made, it is easier to construct a defence showing that no breach of duty occurred rather than to debate whether the delay, or the inherent malignancy of the tumour, was the proximate cause of injury. Extensive risk management strategies have been proposed for radiologists and clinicians in an attempt to improve the quality of patient care and to reduce the likelihood of defending costly legal cases.[2,76,77] The recommendations of the PIAA study, covering the most common problems, are tabulated.[2] Many of these recommendations will be best realised by the establishment of a multidisciplinary approach to the care of breast patients. Other recommendations, such as the physical examination by radiologists, of all women attending screening mammography would require considerable additional resources.

Risk management recommendations: PIAA, 1995[2] (text in brackets are authors' additions)

All practitioners involved in the diagnosis of breast cancer should:

- Document all patient complaints relative to the breast (a gynaecological history: menarche, age of first pregnancy, termination of pregnancy, breast feeding, menopause/hysterectomy, oral contraceptive use, HRT).
- Document any family history of breast cancer (including the age of the first-degree relative at diagnosis and bilaterality).
- Document the results of previous mammographic studies.
- Document the recommendations for subsequent diagnostic studies and follow-up.
- Follow up with other consultants the results of investigations.
- Achieve a tissiue or cytological diagnosis in those with a palpable mass and a negative mammogram.
- Use appropriate diagnostic tests even in the case of pregnancy.

Primary care physicians including obstetricians/gynaecologists should:

- Not abandon diagnostic pursuit because the clinical findings are unimpressive.
- Perform a thorough breast examination on every woman as part of the physical examination regardless of age or complaints.★
- Undertake appropriate studies to rule out malignancy if a mass is detected.
- Be sure that the patient understands the need for further studies and document the fact.

- Perform regular follow-up examinations on patients who present with breast complaints.†

    ★ This recommendation must be contentious.

    † This recommendation runs counter to BASO guidelines[15] that less than 10% of new patients should be seen more than twice.

Radiologists should:

- Repeat a study if a mammogram results in a film of poor technical quality.
- Recommend a repeat study, additional views, follow-up studies and other imaging modalities (ultrasound examination) etc., as appropriate if the mammogram results are equivocal.
- Be sure an adequate physical examination was performed and documented.‡
- Compare the results of the present study with previous studies.
- Promptly report findings to the referring physician; if the patient was self-referred, the result should be sent directly to her. If there is any suspicion of an abnormality, the patient should be advised and told to consult her physician or surgeon promptly.
- If performing a screening mammogram on a self-referred patient, be sure to do a thorough breast examination or advise the patient of the importance of a physical examination to complement the mammographic study. In cases where the patient is self-referred, the radiologist should ensure that the patient receives proper follow-up visits. Double reading (two radiologists) increases the sensitivity of screening mammography.

    ‡ This would cause difficulty for screened patients.

Surgeons should:

- Always perform an adequate examination and document findings, especially when the referring physician's findings were unimpressive.
- Ensure the correct lesion was removed, in both open and needle procedures when performing a biopsy. An X-ray film of the open biopsy (specimen) should always be taken.
- Promptly report consultation and biopsy results to the referring physician.
- (Obtain a tissue or cytological diagnosis of all palpable abnormalities, even if the imaging is negative.)

Acknowledgement

Much of this chapter is based on the definitive article by BT Andrews and T Bates. Delay in the diagnosis of breast cancer: medico-legal implications. Breast 2000; 9: 223–7.

References

1. Physician Insurers Association of America. Breast Cancer Study, 1990.

2. Physician Insurers Association of America. Breast Cancer Study, 1995: 1–27.

3. Price JM, Rosenberg ES. The silicone gel breast implant controversy: the rise of expert panels and the fall of junk science. J R Soc Med 2000; 93: 31–4.

4. Bolam *v* Friern Hospital Management Committee [1957] 2A11 ER 118, 1957 1WLR 582.

5. Bolitho *v* City and Hackney Health Authority [1997] 4 All ER 771; 1997 3 WLR 1151.

6. Sidaway *v* Bethlem R. Hospitals [1985] AC 871.

7. Brahams D. Loss of chance of survival. Lancet 1996; 348: 1604.

8. Salih A, Webb WM, Bates T. Does open-access mammography and ultrasound delay the diagnosis of breast cancer? Breast 1999; 8: 129–32.

9. Dixon M, Sainsbury R. Assessment and investigation of common symptoms. In: Handbook of diseases of the breast. Edinburgh: Churchill Livingstone, 1993: 8–35.

10. Lannin DR, Harris RP, Swanson FH *et al.* Difficulties in diagnosis of carcinoma of the breast in patients less than fifty years of age. Surg Gynec Obstet 1993; 177: 457–62.

 11. Zylstra S, Bors-Koefoed R, Mondor M *et al.* A statistical model for predicting the outcome in breast cancer malpractice lawsuits. Obstet Gynaecol 1994; 84: 392–8.

12. Yelland A, Graham MD, Trott PA *et al.* Diagnosing breast carcinoma in young women. BMJ 1991; 302: 618–20.

13. Donegan WL. Evaluation of a palpable breast mass. N Engl J Med 1992; 327: 937–42.

14. The Breast Surgeons Group of the British Association of Surgical Oncology. Guidelines for surgeons in the management of symptomatic breast disease in the United Kingdom. Eur J Surg Oncol 1995; 21(suppl A): 1–13.

15. The Breast Surgeons Group of the British Association of Surgical Oncology. Guidelines for surgeons in the management of symptomatic breast disease in the United Kingdom (1998 Revision). Eur J Surg Oncol 1998; 24: 464–76.

16. Woodman CBJ, Threlfall AG, Boggis CRM *et al.* Is the three year breast screening interval too long? Occurrence of interval cancers in NHS breast screening programme's north western region. BMJ 1995; 310: 224–6.

17. Wolfe JN. Analysis of 462 breast carcinomas. Am J Radiol 1974; 121: 846–53.

18. Ellman R, Moss SM, Coleman D *et al.* Breast self-examination programmes in the trial of early detection of breast cancer: ten year findings. Br J Cancer 1993; 68: 208–12.

19. Badwe RA, Gregory WM, Chaudray MA *et al.* Timing of surgery during menstrual cycle and survival of premenopausal women with operable breast cancer. Lancet 1991; 337: 1261–4.

20. Dixon JM, Anderson TJ, Lamb J *et al.* Fine needle aspiration cytology, in relationships to clinical examination and mammography in the diagnosis of a solid breast mass. Br J Surg 1984; 71: 593–96.

21. Mitnick JS, Vazquez MF, Plesser KP *et al.* Breast cancer malpractice litigation in New York State. Radiology 1993; 189: 673–6.

22. Joensuu H, Asola R, Holli K *et al.* Delayed diagnosis and large size of breast cancer after a false negative mammogram. Eur J Cancer 1994; 30A: 1299–302.

23. Tennvall J, Moller T, Attwell R. Delaying factors in primary treatment of breast cancer. Acta Chir Scand 1990; 156: 591–6.

24. Walker QJ, Langlands AO. The misuse of mammography in the management of breast cancer. Med J Australia 1986; 145: 185–7.

25. Walter SD, Day NE. Estimation of the duration of a pre-clinical disease state using screening data. Am J Epidemiol 1983; 118: 865–6.

26. Dubin N. Benefits of screening for breast cancer: application of a probabilistic model to a breast cancer detection project. J Chron Dis 1979; 32: 145–51.

27. Fox H, Moskowitz M, Saenger L *et al.* Benefit/risk analysis of aggressive mammographic screening. Radiology 1978; 128: 359–65.

28. Daly CA, Apthorp L, Field S. Second round cancers: how many were visible on the first round of the UK National Breast Screening Programme, three years earlier? Clin Radiol 1998; 53: 25–8.

29. Wright CJ, Mueller CB. Screening mammography and public health policy: the need for perspective. Lancet 1995; 346: 29–32.

30. Ashley S, Royle GT, Corder A *et al.* Clinical, radiological and cytological diagnosis of breast cancer in young women. Br J Surg 1989; 76: 835–7.

31. Layfield LJ, Glasgow BJ, Cramer H. Fine needle aspiration in the management of breast masses. Pathol Ann 1989; 24: 23–62.

32. Bates AT, Bates T, Hastrich DJ *et al.* Delay in the diagnosis of breast cancer: the effect of the introduction of fine needle aspiration cytology to a breast clinic. Eur J Surg Oncol 1992; 18: 433–7.

33. Jenner DC, Middleton A, Webb WM *et al.* In-hospital delay in the diagnosis of breast cancer. Br J Surg 2000; 87; 914–9.

34. Dixon JM, Page DL, Anderson TJ *et al.* Long-term survivors after breast cancer. Br J Surg 1985; 72: 445–8.

35. Haybittle JL. Is breast cancer ever cured? Rev Endocrine-Related Cancer 1983; 13: 13–18.

36. Le MG, Hill C, Rezvani A *et al.* Long-term survival of women with breast cancer. Lancet 1984; ii: 922.

37. Rutqvist LR, Wallgren A. Long-term survival of 458 young breast cancer patients. Cancer 1985; 55: 658–65.

38. Ederer F, Cutler SJ, Goldenberg IS *et al.* Causes of death among long-term survivors from breast cancer in Connecticut. J Natl Cancer Inst 1963; 30: 933–47.

39. Mueller CB, Ames F, Anderson GD. Breast cancer in 3,558 women: age as a significant determinant in the rate of dying and causes of death. Surgery 1978; 83: 123–32.

40. Spratt JS, Spratt SW. Medical and legal implications of screening and follow-up procedures for breast cancer. Cancer 1990; 66: 1351–62.

41. The Early Breast Cancer Trialists Group. Systemic treatment of early breast cancer by hormonal, cytotoxic or immune therapy: 133 randomised trials involving 31000 recurrences and 24000 deaths among 75000 women. Lancet 1992; 339: 1–15, 71–85.

42. Plotkin D, Blankenberg F. Breast cancer—biology and malpractice. Am J Clin Oncol 1991; 14: 254–66.

43. Tubiana M, Koscielny S. Cell kinetics, growth rate and the natural history of breast cancer. The Heuson Memorial Lecture. Eur J Clin Oncol 1988; 24: 9–14.

44. Pearlman AW. Breast cancer—influence of growth rate on prognosis and treatment evaluation. A study based on mastectomy scar recurrences. Cancer 1976; 38: 1826–33.

45. Galante E, Gallus G, Guzzon A *et al.* Growth rate of primary breast cancer and prognosis: observations on a 3- to 7-year follow up in 180 breast cancers. Br J Cancer 1986; 54: 833–6.

46. Christie R, Bates T. The risk of pneumothorax as a complication of diagnostic fine needle aspiration or therapeutic needling of the breast. Should the patient be warned? Breast 1999; 8: 98–9.

47. Forrest APM, Everington D, McDonald CC *et al.* The Edinburgh randomised trial of axillary sampling or clearance after mastectomy. Br J Surg 1995; 82: 1504–8.

48. National Coordination Group for Surgeons Working in Breast Cancer Screening. Quality assurance guidelines for surgeons in breast cancer screening, NHS Breast Screening Programme Publication No. 20, 1996.

49. NHS Breast Screening Programme and British Association of Surgical Oncology. An audit of screen detected breast cancers for the year of screening April 1997 to March 1998. NHS Breast Screening Programme, 1999.

50. Richards MA, Westcombe AM, Love SB *et al.* Influence of delay on survival in patients with breast cancer: a systematic review. Lancet 1999; 353: 1119–26.

51. Dische S, Bentzen G, Bond S. The influence of delay in diagnosis of breast cancer upon outlook. Clin Risk 2000; 6: 4–6.

52. Afzelius P, Zedeler K, Sommer H *et al.* Patients' and doctors' delay in primary breast cancer. Acta Oncol 1994; 33: 345–51.

53. Galea MH, Blamey RW, Elston CW *et al.* The Nottingham Prognostic Index in primary breast cancer. Br Cancer Res Treat 1992; 22: 207–19.

54. Taylor *v* West Kent Health Authority [1997] 8 Med LR 251–7.

55. Renwick SB. Silicon breast implants: implications for society and surgeons. Med J Aust 1996; 165: 338–41.

56. Terry MB, Skovron ML, Garber S *et al.* The estimated frequency of cosmetic breast augmentation among US women, 1963 through 1988. Am J Public Health 1995; 85: 1122–4.

57. Duffy MJ, Woods JE. Health risks of failed silicone gel breast implants: a 30 year clinical experience. Plast Recontr Surg 1994; 94: 295–9.

58. Reilly PA. Fibromyalgia in the workplace—a management problem. Ann Rheum Dis 1993; 52: 249–51.

59. Angell M. Science on trial: the clash of medical evidence and the law in the breast implant case. New York: WW Norton, 1996.

60. Medical and legal aspects of breast implants, Mar 1997. [Posted by Janet Van Winkle, American Silicone Inplant Survivors (AS-IS), member of board of editors.]

61. Medical Devices Agency. Silicone implants and connective tissue disease. London: Department of Health, 1995.

62. Hennekens CH, Lee Im, Cook NR *et al*. Self reported breast implants and connective tissue diseases in female health professionals. A retrospective cohort study. JAMA 1996; 275: 616–21.

63. United States *v* Frye, 293 F1013 (DC Cir 1923).

64. Daubert *v* Merrel Dow Pharmaceuticals Inc, 509 US 579 (1993).

65. Garnick DW, Hendricks AM, Brennan TA. Can practice guidelines reduce the number and costs of malpractice claims? JAMA 1991; 266: 2856–60.

66. Carrick SE, Bonevski B, Redman S *et al*. Surgeons' opinions about the NMRC clinical practice guidelines for the management of early breast cancer. Med J Aust 1998; 169: 300–5.

67. Nattinger AB, Hoffman RG, Shapiro R *et al*. The effect of legislative requirements on the use of breast conserving surgery. N Engl J Med 1996; 335: 1035–40.

68. Woolf SH. Practice guidelines: a new reality in medicine. Methods of developing guidelines. Arch Intern Med 1992; 152: 946–52.

69. Clinical practice guidelines for the management of early breast cancer. NHMRC, Australian Government Publishing Service.

70. Hurwitz B. Clinical guidelines and the law. BMJ 1995; 311: 1517–18.

71. Woolf HK. Medical negligence. In: Access to justice: final report to the Lord Chancellor on the civil justice system in England and Wales. London: Stationery Office, 1996: 169–96.

72. Professional List Australia. Common law division of the supreme court of New South Wales, 1999.

73. Kite *v* Malycha, South Australia. (Judgement No. S6702).

74. Judge *v* Huntington Health Authority [1995] 6 Med LR 223.

75. Civil Procedure Rules, 1998.

76. Brenner RJ. Medico-legal aspects of breast imaging: variable standards of care relating to different types of practice. Am J Roentgenol 1991; 156: 719–23.

77. Osuch JR, Bonham VL. The timely diagnosis of breast cancer: principles of risk management for primary care providers and surgeons. Cancer 1994; 74: 271–8.

Index

Pages numbers in italics refer to tables and figure